Scripture and Science
A Physician's Reflections on Judaic Doctrine

Scripture and Science
A Physician's Reflections on Judaic Doctrine

Harold Speert, M.D.

Lately, Special Lecturer in Obstetrics and Gynecology
College of Physicians and Surgeons,
Columbia University
and
Consultant in Obstetrics and Gynecology
The Presbyterian Hospital
New York, New York

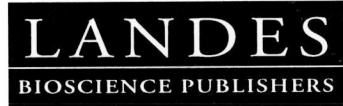

SCRIPTURE AND SCIENCE

R.G. LANDES COMPANY
Austin, Texas, U.S.A.

U.S. and Canada Copyright © 1995 R.G. Landes Company
All rights reserved. Printed in the U.S.A.

Please address all inquiries to the Publisher:
R.G. Landes Company, 909 Pine Street, Georgetown, Texas, U.S.A. 78626
or
P.O. Box 4858, Austin, Texas, U.S.A. 78765
Phone: 512/ 863 7762; FAX: 512/ 863 0081

U.S. and Canada ISBN 1-57059-256-X

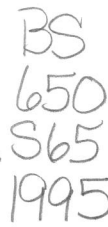

Library of Congress Cataloging-in-Publication Data

Speert, Harold, 1915-
    Scripture and science : a physician's reflections on Judaic doctrine / Harold Speert.
    p. cm.
Includes bibliographical references and index.
ISBN 1-57059-256-X
1. Bible and science. 2. Medicine in the Bible. 3. Bible. O.T.—Criticism, interpretation, etc.
I. Title.
BS650.S65 1995   95-18835
296.3'875—dc20   CIP

Cover Painting by John Huston for the label of Château Mouton Rothschild 1982

DEDICATION

To the memory of my parents:

Samuel Speert (1878-1962)

Ella Frances Becker Speert (?1878-1950)

CONTENTS

Preface viii
1. The Doctrinal Sources 1
2. Creation and Other Cosmic Events 7
    Creation 7
    Some Other Cosmic Events 11
    Earth's Variable Rotation 13
    Meteorites, Craters, and Extinctions 14
    Summary 20
3. The Plagues of Egypt and the Exodus 23
    Blood 24
    Hail 25
    Fire 26
    Darkness 27
    Insects 28
    Locusts 29
    Death 31
    The Exodus 32
    Water 37
    Manna 38
    Quails 38
    The Theophany at Mt. Sinai 39
    Jericho 40
    Summary 42
4. Medicine in the Bible 45
    Sanitary Code of the Israelites 45
    Sexually Transmitted Disease 47
    Water for Jerusalem 48
    Skin Ailments 50
    Leprosy 50
    Hemorrhoids 52
    Plague 52
    Job's Disease 53
    Smallpox 54
    Colitis 54
    Heat Stress 55
    Hypoglycemia 55
    Alcohol: Its Use and Abuse 56
    Neuro-Psychiatric Disorders 58
    Dreams 62
    Gigantism 65
    Resuscitation 66
    Senility 68
    Summary 69

CONTENTS

5. **Biblical Obstetrics** 73
   - Fertility and Infertility 73
   - Conception 76
   - Midwives 76
   - Antenatal Care 78
   - Abortion and Miscarriage 80
   - Duration of Pregnancy 80
   - Labor 81
   - Position for Delivery 82
   - Cesarean Section 83
   - Monsters 84
   - Multiple Births 84
   - Maternal Death 85
   - Puerperium 86
   - Care of Infant at Birth 86
   - Sudden Infant Death Syndrome 87
   - Weaning 87
   - Summary 88

6. **The Disease of Theories** 91
   - Summary 93

7. **The Conjugal Relationship** 95
   - Polyandry 95
   - Polygamy 96
   - Concubinage 96
   - Homosexual Marriage 97
   - Menstruation and Cohabitation 98
   - Menstrual Mythology 99
   - Saliva 103
   - Blood 103
   - Other Secretions 103
   - Cut Flowers 104
   - Other Effects of Menotoxin 104
   - Conception and the Laws of Niddah 105
   - Artificial Insemination 107
   - Niddah and the Sex Ratio 108
   - Summary 109

CONTENTS

8. Fertility and Its Control **113**
    Contraception 113
    Sterilization 118
    Applied Genetics 120
    Tay-Sachs Disease 122
    Abortion 123
    Execution in Pregnancy 125
    Intervention During Pregnancy 125
    Sex Selection 126
    Artificial Insemination 127
    In Vitro Fertilization 128
    Ovum Transplantation 129
    Surrogate Motherhood 130
    Frozen Embryos 131
    Summary 132

9. Circumcision **139**
    Biblical Background 140
    The Operation 142
    Circumcision in the United States 143
    Timing of Circumcision 144
    Physiologic Sidelights 145
    Pros and Cons of Routine Circumcision 146
    Summary 151

10. Kashruth: The Dietary Laws **155**
    Forbidden Foods 155
    Laws of Slaughter 164
    The Hind Quarter 166
    Meat and Milk 166
    Modern Interpretation 168
    Summary 168

11. Conservation: of Earth and Person **171**
    The Sabbath 171
    Retirement 174
    The Land 175
    The Gaia Hypothesis 179
    Summary 180

CONTENTS

12. **Separatism** 183
    Shaatnez 184
    Demographics 186
    World Jewish Populations 187
    Who is a Jew? 205
    The Chosen People 206
    Summary 209
13. **Medical-Ethical Issues** 213
    The Role of the Physician 213
    Doctor-Patient Relationship 215
    AIDS 216
    Alzheimer's Disease 217
    Organ Transplantation 218
    End-of-Life Decisions 220
    Active Euthanasia 222
    Autopsy 224
    Summary 226
14. **Scriptural Miscellany** 229
    Physical Exercise 229
    Gourd Poisoning 233
    Pi 235

Index 239

PREFACE

The Bible is a rich source of subjects for scientific commentary and research. I have examined some scientific facets of the theories of creation and other cosmic events; the plagues of Egypt; the Exodus of the Israelites; the Biblical dietary laws and those of the Sabbath and conservation; the concept of "the chosen people" and separatism; medicine in the Bible; some issues of current interest in medical ethics, including the role of the physician, the doctor-patient relationship, AIDS, Alzheimer's disease, organ transplantation, end-of-life decisions, euthanasia, and autopsy; a few miscellaneous subjects including mathematical pi, physical exercise, and gourd poisoning; and because of my special interest in obstetrics, have devoted separate chapters to Biblical obstetrics, eclampsia, a dreaded complication of pregnancy, the conjugal relationship, fertility and its control, and circumcision. In this study I have restricted myself to the Hebrew Scriptures: the Bible, or *Tanach* (Torah, Prophets, and Writings), the Talmud, and subsequent commentaries including some *responsa*; using, except where otherwise noted, the English translation in the Authorized King James Version.

To those who have already tilled this field I am much indebted: particularly Julius Preuss, for his encyclopedic *Biblisch-Talmudische Medizin* (Karger, 1911), which has been ably translated into English by Fred Rosner (*Biblical and Talmudic Medicine*, Sanhedrin Press, 1978); Charles Brim, for his *Medicine in the Bible* (Froben Press, 1936); Rev. P.M. Shepherd, for his "The Bible as a Source Book for Physicians," (*Glasgow Medical Journal*, 36, 1955, 348-395); and my late colleague Robert Greenblatt, for his stimulating essays in *Search the Scriptures* (Lippincott, 1963).

The philosophers of the Renaissance attempted to shield themselves against the persecution of the Church with the scholastic dictum that "what is true in religion may be false in science." Sarna, a current commentator,[1] has likewise insisted that attempts to reconcile Biblical accounts of creation with the findings of modern science are naive and that any apparent correspondence ingeniously demonstrated between them is mere coincidence. Similarly, few believe that the Biblical proscription of pork is based on its causal association with trichinosis; or that the authors of the Bible knew of the medical benefits of circumcision, or of the relation of the consumption of animal fat to arterial disease. An increasing number of modern commentators, on the other hand, denying that religion and science contradict, have found what Joseph Soloveitchik[2] and C.A. Coulson[3] have called complementary approaches to reality. William James[4] had concluded, earlier, that science and religion "are both of them genuine keys for unlocking the world's treasure-house," that the world is "so complex as to consist of many interpenetrating spheres of reality, which we can...approach in alternation by using different conceptions and assuming different attitudes." Without science, Einstein once remarked, religion is lame.

The conflicts that some have seen between religion and science cease to exist when one accepts the premise that they are based, as are various other disciplines, on differing methodology, propositions, and theories. To question whether a poem, a painting, or a symphony is "true" is clearly meaningless. Euclidean geometry and Newtonian physics have not been invalidated by the theory of relativity, nor the wave theory of light by the quantum theory. Light acts with the properties of waves under certain conditions, as corpuscles under others. Science never leads to absolute certainty; its conclusions are always subject to revision. The issue was well stated by Kasher:[5] "There can be no contradiction between the affirmation of a particular proposition within the context of one discipline and the negation of the same proposition within the context of another discipline, since what we are really confronted with...are two totally different concepts of the truth - the one defined by the methodology of the one discipline, the other defined by the methodology of the other." The oft-told parable, attributed to the astrophysicist Arthur Eddington,[6] tells of the student of deep-sea life who, using a net with 3-inch mesh, concluded after bringing up repeated samples, that the waters contained no fish less than 3 inches wide.

The philosophy of Maimonides, dedicated to the compatibility of the presuppositions of science and the tenets of Judaism, continues to be explored in the light of modern advances in cosmology, atomic physics, and molecular biology. At a conference at the Carter Center of Emory University, Atlanta, Georgia, in late 1989 leaders from 32 Christian denominations and representatives of Islamic, Judaic, and Native American groups concluded that medical science and religion should not be considered incompatible or in opposition to each other.

The Torah, in the view of most scholars and in agreement with early-14th century Jewish philosopher Gersonides, has many layers of meaning, not limited to that obvious in a casual reading. Ben Bag Bag, the Hebrew sage who was drawn from heathenism to the study of the Torah by Hillel in the first century C.E., urged his students: "Delve in it and delve in it again, for everything is in it; contemplate it continually, and wax grey and old over it, but do not depart from it, for everything you want to know is found within it."[7] Scholars still explore the Torah's text for new insight. Modern research continues to find new interfaces between Scripture and Science. If we adopt the approach of some commentators, that much of Biblical wording is purely figurative, not to be taken literally, and that its true meaning requires further study, we find a common ground for the Genesis account of creation and the Big Bang theory of modern physics. Fred

Hoyle, author of the name, found it "curious that, while most scientists eschew religion, it actually dominates their thoughts more than it does those of the clergy."[8]

Many of the miracles or wonders of the Bible have been explained by modern scientists as the working of nature. Natural phenomena have been adduced, for example, in explanation of the plagues of Egypt, the parting of the waters of the Red Sea, and the manna that fed the Israelites in the desert. I have sought, in the pages that follow, to present a survey of views and a commentary; interpretation is for the reader. The problem of evidence in matters of religion is not amenable to solution. As noted by Soloveitchik,[9] "the believer does not miss philosophic legitimation; the skeptic will never be satisfied with any cognitive demonstration."

I record with gratitude my indebtedness to Rabbi Carla Freedman for her critical reading of my manuscript.

H.S.
Keene, New York 12942

References

1. Sarna NM. Understanding Genesis. New York, Jewish Theological Seminary of America McGraw-Hill 1966:2-3.
2. Soloveitchik JB. The Halakhic Mind. Seth Press, Macmillan 1986.
3. Coulson CA. Science and Christian Belief. University of North Carolina Press 1955:chapter 3.
4. James W. The Varieties of Religious Experience, (1902). New Hyde Park, NY University Books 1963:122-123.
5. Kasher A. Fundamental assumptions for discussion on religion and science. Tradition, 10. 1968:87-89; quoted by Fred Rosner in Modern Medicine and Jewish Ethics. Ktav and Yeshiva University Press 1986.
6. Eddington A. The Nature of the Physical World. Cambridge University Press 1928:16.
7. Ethics of the Fathers. 5:25.
8. Quoted by Paul Davies in The Mind of God. New York, Simon and Schuster 1992:223.
9. Soloveitchik JB. loc. cit., p. 118.

BIOGRAPHY

A native of Baltimore, Md., Harold Speert, M.D., is the world's foremost historian of obstetrics and gynecology. He received his B.A. and M.D. from the Johns Hopkins University and his training in obstetrics and gynecology at the Johns Hopkins Hospital, Barnes and St. Louis Maternity Hospitals, and New York's Roosevelt Hospital. During World War II he did aeromedical research for the Army Air Forces, and after the cessation of hostilities served as chief of obstetrics and gynecology at Wright-Patterson Field Regional Hospital in Ohio. From 1947 to 1986 he taught and practiced at the Columbia-Presbyterian Medical Center in New York, and for shorter periods at the Mt. Sinai Hospital in New York and as Consultant Gynecologist at the Elizabethtown Community Hospital in Elizabethtown, New York. He is the author of more than 100 papers dealing with the physiology of reproduction, the pathology of pregnancy, gynecologic cancer, and the history of obstetrics and gynecology; as well as the following books: Obstetric Practice (with A.F. Guttmacher), Iconographia Gyniatrica, Obstetric and Gynecologic Milestones, The Sloane Hospital Chronicle, Obstetrics and Gynecology in America: A History (published by the American College of Obstetricians and Gynecologists), and the autobiographical As I Remember It.

He is a Diplomate of the American Board of Obstetrics and Gynecology and a Life Fellow of the American College of Obstetricians and Gynecologists, the American College of Surgeons, and the New York Academy of Medicine. Retired from practice, he lives with his wife in the Adirondack village of Keene, New York.

CHAPTER 1

THE DOCTRINAL SOURCES

Judaic doctrine is founded on the Torah, the Talmud, the Teachings (Midrashim), and a never-ending flow of Responsa from rabbinic authorities.

The Torah, for over two and one-half millennia "the keystone of Jewish life, the starting point of Christendom, and the background of Islam,[1] known also as the Pentateuch or Five Books of Moses (Genesis, Exodus, Leviticus, Numbers, and Deuteronomy), has been characterized as "a book of dubious authorship, implausible time shifts, linguistic eccentricities, bewildering narrative leaps... the definitive text of our civilization, the basic source of its myth and history.[2] Modern scholars believe it to be a collection of works written over eight to ten centuries before being fixed in its official Hebrew text and declared sacred, about 400 C.E. The oldest known surviving scroll of the Torah dates from about the ninth century. The recently discovered (1947) Dead Sea Scrolls contain older texts.

Few serious students of biblical history, with the exception of some Orthodox Jews and Christian fundamentalists, still believe that the Torah was received by Moses, i.e. dictated to him by God—or indeed, written by any one person. Modern scholarship recognizes several strands in the fabric of its authorship. Thomas Hobbes, Isaac La Peyrère, and Baruch Spinoza had already denied the role of Moses in the Torah's composition when my obstetrical forebear, Jean Astruc[3] (1684-1766), proposed what came to be known as the documentary Hypothesis.[4] Astruc attributed the contradictions and lack of order in Genesis to its multiple authorship, manifested in two primary documents and several fragmentary secondary ones, woven together by an editor. Astruc's contemporary, J.G. Eichhorn, called attention to different forms of the divine name, as had Astruc, and noted further diversities in vocabulary and literary style throughout the Pentateuch. Julius Wellhausen (1844-1918), in his classical studies in the last quarter of the 19th century, found traces of four prior sources, persons or schools, subsequently labeled J, E, D, and P, which have served as the basis of later Biblical scholarship.

The J source is distinguished by its use of YHWH (Yaweh or Jehovah) for the name of God; its text comprises most of Genesis and is embedded throughout Exodus and Numbers. It is attributed to an author or authors living in the Southern Kingdom, or Judah, after the death of King Solomon, in the ninth century B.C.E. The E source, so called because of its reference to God as Elohim, was imputed to authorship in the Northern Kingdom, or Israel, some think contemporaneously with J. Others ascribe E's contribution to a somewhat later date, in the eighth century B.C.E. Together these two sources make up most of the Pentateuchal narrative.

The D source contributed most of Deuteronomy, the book containing the law code and religious reforms believed to have been instituted by King Josiah about 621 B.C.E. The P (for Priestly) source, from the sixth century B.C.E., presented an alternative to the versions of J and E, with special interest in rituals and sacrificial laws, and genealogical details. The joining together of these versions and their editing, or redaction (R), was carried out, it has been suggested,[5] by Ezra the Scribe, an advocate of the Aaronid priests, who rose to a position of leadership as the Jews were returning from exile in the late sixth century B.C.E. and seeking to rebuild their homeland and their place and mode of worship.

Thus the Torah, as we now know it, represents centuries of disparate traditions melded into one book, the eternal text of Israel. A Greek version, in the third century B.C.E., the earliest translation from the Hebrew, was termed the Septuagint because of the legend that it was written by 70 (or 72) Palestinian Jews in 70 days, a belief based upon a letter, long since known to be spurious, from Aristeas to Philocrates, Greek functionaries. The Greek translation is now attributed to Egyptian Jews, working independently of one another and at different times.

Those who looked to the Torah for guidance in the conduct of their lives found need for further explication or more exact definition of many of its terse provisions. This need was met in part by an "oral Torah," a body of law, some believed, imparted to Moses, as was the written law, during his 40 days and 40 nights on Mount Sinai, but not written down. The concept of a two-fold Torah became increasingly important in rabbinic teaching after 70 C.E.,[6] the year of destruction of Jerusalem and the Second Temple by the Romans.

Then as now, theological differences existed among the Jews. And then as now, they aligned themselves into three principal groups. During the first century before and the first century of the Common Era, according to Josephus Flavius, the Judean historian, the major philosophic movements were those of the Sadducees, the Pharisees, and the Essenes. The Essenes were a small, highly disciplined group of men, mostly celibate, who lived a monastic life of study and prayer, separated from the rest of the community. Reminiscent of the current schism among authorities on American Constitutional law was the disagreement between the Sadducees and the Pharisees on the nature and source of Jewish law. The Pharisees, mostly laymen, embraced the unwritten regulations and "traditions of the fathers," which were passed on from generation to generation; while the more conservative Sadducees, many of them priests, insisted that only the written doctrine could be considered valid.

For many years the oral law remained literally and exclusively oral, for it was viewed as improper to put in writing that which God had not commanded Moses to record. Some scholars, notably Rabbi Akiba, feeling the need to preserve the oral law and ensure its perpetuation, began its compilation during the early years of the second century C.E., and by about the year 200 it had become codified in Hebrew and made public in the Galilee. The principal redactor of this, the Mishnah, was Judah ha-Nasi, the foremost rabbinic scholar of his time. The Mishnah was his major legacy.

The Mishnah is divided into the following six orders (*sedarim*); each, into tractates, 63 in all; each of which is divided, in turn, into chapters:

    1. *Zeraim* (Seeds): dealing with time and place for benedictions and prayers; agricultural matters, including tithes of harvests to priests, Levites, and the poor; and Sabbatical years, when the land was to lie fallow.

    2. *Moed* (Feasts): tractates on the holy days and Temple dues.

    3. *Nashim* (Women): dealing with matters affecting women and the family, including betrothal, marriage, divorce, and adultery.

    4. *Nezikim* (Damages): ten tractates on property rights, legal procedures, ethical maxims, and idolatry.

    5. *Kodashim* (Holy things): dealing with sacrificial offerings and other Temple matters.

    6. *Teharot* (Purifications): twelve tractates on ritual uncleanliness.

An English translation of the Mishnah by Herbert Danby[7] ran to 789 pages of small print.

Elaboration of the Mishnah during the third, fourth, and fifth centuries, by exposition, amplification, and commentary on each paragraph by rabbinic scholars known as *amoraim* (teachers), resulted in a large, multivolume work, written in the Aramaic vernacular, the Gemara. Joined with the Mishnah, the combined text formed the Talmud.

Two versions of the Gemara, and hence of the Talmud, came into being. The Jerusalem or Palestinian Talmud, the earlier and smaller, dating from the first half of the fifth century, was edited hastily and incompletely, because of the pressures of Christianization by the Romans. The Babylonian Talmud, on the other hand, compiled during the next century or two under conditions of greater stability and peace in the religious academies of Babylon, whose Jewish community had superseded that of Palestine in culture and influence, showed the result of more leisurely preparation and more thorough editing, and became the preferred and authoritative version.

Supplementing the Torah and concerned primarily with law, the Talmud served also as an encyclopedia of Jewish culture, a summation of a thousand years of intellectual, religious, and social achievement.[8]

Companions to the Torah and commonly bound together with it in one volume, the *Tanach* (an acronym from its three components), are the book of Prophets, *Nev'im*, (Joshua, Judges, 1 Samuel, 2 Samuel, 1 Kings, 2 Kings, Isaiah, Jeremiah, Ezekiel, Hosea, Joel, Amos, Obadiah, Jonah, Micah, Nahum, Habbakuk, Zephaniah, Haggai, Zechariah, and Malachi) and the Sacred Writings, *Ketuvim*, (Psalms, Proverbs, Job, Song of Songs, Ruth, Lamentations, Ecclesiastes, Esther, Daniel, Ezra, Nehemiah, 1 Chronicles, and 2 Chronicles). The *Tanach*, known also as the Old Testament, is perhaps more properly called the Hebrew Bible, because of the implication in the name that the Old Testament is completed only in the New Testament and that together they comprise a continuous work.[9]

Although the Talmud supplemented the Torah it did little to probe the meanings beyond the Torah's cryptic verses. This the sages attempted through their *midrashim*. Some were expositional, others homiletic. Together they resulted in a vast literature of ethics and legend in the form of a commentary on the Torah, compiled between the fourth and thirteenth centuries. Lawmaking thus became an ongoing process, producing the categorical religious imperatives of *halakhah*. Digests of the *halakhah*, major codifications of the laws of practice and conduct accepted as authoritative, were produced by the *Mishneh Torah* of Moses Maimonides, about 1178, the *Arba'ah Turim* of Jacob ben Asher (c. 1270-1340), and the *Shulchan Arukh* of Joseph Caro, in 1564.

By the thirteenth century the systemized disciplines of history and theology had begun to supersede the *Midrash*.[10] Haphazard *midrashim* were now being replaced by formal *responsa*, binding opinions by designated rabbinic authorities, some brief, others in the form of lengthy treatises, on questions of *halakha*. When a rabbi was faced with a difficult legal question that he could not answer with confidence, he raised his question with the regional *gaon*, usually the head of a religious academy, or *yeshivah*. The published answer, or *responsum*, established a legal precedent for the consideration of other rabbis in their subsequent deliberations.

Initially most questions of Jewish law were referred to the academies in Babylonia, the recognized centers of Talmudic authority. As these began to decline, in the tenth and eleventh centuries, and centers of religious study spread to North Africa, Spain, Italy, and the Rhineland, local rabbis submitted their questions to Talmudic luminaries of their generation, wherever located. Almost every great rabbi of the Middle Ages is credited with authorship of many *responsa*. Huge quantities survive and have been collected, classified, indexed, and computerized in Israel.[11] Bar Ilan University houses some 253 volumes of responsa.

Fresh *responsa* continue to be added by every generation. In America each of the three major branches of Judaism (Orthodox, Conservative, and Reform) maintains its own committee of designated rabbinic scholars for *responsa* research and authorship, helping maintain Jewish law as a living tradition.

The foregoing outline provides a background for the evolution of Judaic doctrine. In the pages to follow I shall point out not the *basis* or *reason* for some of the commandments and ordinances but rather their *interface* with science and the synergism between science and religion.

NOTES AND REFERENCES

1. Plaut WG. In: *The Torah*, Union of American Hebrew Congregations 1981; xix.
2. Atlas J. In: *Congregation*. Rosenberg D, ed. Harcourt Brace, Jovanovich 1987;189.
3. Astruc is best known in medical circles for his inauguration of regular academic instruction for midwives in France in 1745 and for his six-volume *Traité des Maladies des Femmes*. Paris 1761-1765.
4. *Conjectures sur les Memoires Originaux Dont il paroit que Moyse s'est servir pour composer le livre de la Genese*. Brussels 1753.
5. Friedman RE. *Who Wrote the Bible?* Summit Books 1987.
6. Seltzer RM. *Jewish People, Jewish Thought*. Macmillan 1980; 216.
7. Danby H. *Mishnah*. Oxford Univ Press 1933.
8. Bokser BZ. *The Wisdom of the Talmud*. Philosophical Library 1951.
9. Alter R. *The Art of Biblical Narrative*. Basic Books 1981; ix.
10. Strack HL. *Introduction to the Talmud and Midrash*. 5th ed. Jewish Publication Soc of America 1931.
11. Goldenberg R. In: *Back to the Sources*. Holtz BW, ed. Summit Books 1984:160.

CHAPTER 2

CREATION AND OTHER COSMIC EVENTS

CREATION

HOW DID OUR UNIVERSE COME INTO BEING?

According to the Torah, "In the beginning God created the heaven and the earth. And the earth was without form, and void; and darkness was upon the face of the deep. And the Spirit of God moved upon the face of the waters. And God said, Let there be light: and there was light. And God saw the light, that it was good: and God divided the light from the darkness... And God said, Let there be a firmament in the midst of the waters, and let it divide the waters from the waters. And God made the firmament, and divided the waters which were under the firmament from the waters which were above the firmament... And God said, Let the waters under the heaven be gathered together unto one place, and let the dry land appear: and it was so... And God said, Let there be lights in the firmament of the heaven to divide the day from the night; and let them be for signs, and for seasons, and for days, and years: And let them be for lights in the firmament of the heaven to give light upon the earth; and it was so. And God made two great lights; the greater light to rule the day, and the lesser light to rule the night; he made the stars also. And God set them in the firmament of the heaven to give light upon the earth, And to rule over the day and over the night, and to divide the light from the darkness... And God saw every thing that he had made, and, behold, it was very good... Thus the heaven and the earth were finished..." (*Genesis* 1:1-7, 9, 14-18, 31; 2:1)

Had God been experimenting? And had He made, and destroyed, other universes before finding one to His liking—one that was *very good*? A *midrash* states that our world resulted from God's seventh effort at creation.[1]

The early philosophers took different positions on our origins. Plato (427?-347? B.C.E.) held that the world had been created *from* an undefined "something," and the ordering of pre-existent random, disorderly motion. His pupil Aristotle (384-322 B.C.E.), who rivaled and at times outshone his mentor, held a variant view, insisting, that the heaven is "ungenerated and indestructible"[2] and hence must always have existed, "actually and perfectly," permanent and without beginning. No thing, he argued, can be produced from nothing. Since matter and form, existing now, are in constant motion, he added, they must have been ever moving. Time also can never have begun, and "there could not be a before or an after if time did not exist."[3]

Jewish philosophers, of later date, embraced the traditional interpretation of the Torah, Maimonides (Moses ben Maimon, 1135-1204) asserting that it was indeed possible for God to have willed the creation of the world out of absolutely nothing,[4] that causation by the divine will supersedes and is unlimited by natural law. Although an admirer of Aristotle, Maimonides insisted that the universe is not eternal, that it was created by God. Gersonides (Levi ben Gerson, 1288-1344) agreed that the world was created by an act of God's will, but rejected Maimonides' assertion that the world could have been brought into being out of absolutely nothing; and proposed the alternative view that the world was created from a shapeless, amorphous mass.[5]

The development of natural science and the increasing freedom permitted to literary and historical criticism resulted in open expressions of doubt that all truth is contained in the Scriptures or that all contained in the Scriptures is true. Even before the new astronomy of the Polish physician Nicholaus Copernicus (1475-1543), the English clergyman John Colet (1467?-1519) attributed the apparent discrepancies between the story of creation and natural science to knowledge limitations in writing of the Bible. In 1616 the theologians of the Church's Holy Office condemned Galileo Galilei's proposition that the sun is immobile in the center of the universe and that the Earth undergoes a diurnal rotation. Admonished by Pope Paul V, Galileo made the promise, which he later broke, not to "hold, teach, or defend" this heretical doctrine.

More than $3^1/_2$ centuries later, astronomers are returning to the Biblical view of creation. In 1978 the astrophysicist Robert Jastrow wrote: "At this moment it seems as though science will never be able to raise the curtain on the mystery of creation. For the scientist who has lived by his faith in the power of reason, the story ends like a bad dream. He has scaled the mountains of ignorance; he is about to conquer the highest peak; as he pulls himself over the final rock, he is greeted by a band of theologians who have been sitting there for centuries."[6]

The so-called "steady state" model, essentially that of Aristotle, in which the universe has no beginning and no end, was popular among scientists until the early 1960s. Its adherents had no need to confront the birth of the universe, with all its attendant uncertainties, for according to the steady state model the universe always was and always will be as we see it now. The steady state concept has since been rejected by virtually all cosmologists. Neither evidence nor explanation has been provided for the continuous creation of mass from nothing; and the discovery of cosmic radiation and quasi-stellar radio sources (quasars) has provided strong evidence that the universe was different in the past.[7] Most modern cosmologists have embraced the "Big-Bang" theory of the origin of the universe.

According to Einstein's theory of general relativity the universe began in a singularity (a place in space or time at which some quantity becomes infinite) of density. A cosmological adaptation of this concept was proposed in 1922 by Alexander Friedmann, Russian mathematician and meteorologist, whose model was rediscovered a few years later by Georges Lemaitre, a Belgian priest and physicist.[8] The term "Big-Bang" was coined during a series of radio talks by Fred Hoyle in England during the late 1940s.

The Big-Bang model of creation rests on four groups of observations: (1) the outward motion of the galaxies from us, in all directions, discovered by Hubble in 1929, evidence of expansion of the universe and of its explosive beginning; (2) good agreement between the age of the universe, as estimated from the rate of motion of the galaxies, and the age of the Earth, as measured by the radioactive decay of its uranium ore; (3) radio waves from outer space, which had been predicted as an essential remnant of a hot, younger universe, and which were actually discovered in 1965; and (4) the chemical composition of the universe, approximately 25% helium and 75% hydrogen, explicable in terms of atomic processes in the infant universe.[9] The other elements in the universe, such as those responsible for the form and function of the Earth, and the heavier chemical elements, are quantitatively insignificant. Oxygen and carbon make up only a trace of the total mass of the universe. The Cosmic Background Explorer, a satellite launched in November, 1989, provided precise measurements of the cosmic background radiation, extraordinarily close to the spectrum predicted by the Big-Bang model.

If the galaxies are moving away from one another now, they must have been closer together in the past. Assuming that this backward extrapolation can be continued, there was a moment in past time when all matter in the universe was compressed into a state of almost infinite density. Calculating from the rate of expansion, astronomers estimate this point, when the Big Bang occurred, at 10 to 15 billion years ago. They predict that, at the current rate of expansion, the universe will double its size in another 10 to 15 billion years.

The mass about to become the universe, compressed to infinite smallness, was therefore infinitely hot. As it expanded, its temperature decreased. One second after the Big Bang the temperature would have fallen to about 10,000 million degrees; 100 seconds later, to 1,000 million degrees.[10] The universe was still too hot and dense to permit the combination of nuclei and electrons into atoms, as they eventually did, when the temperature fell to about 3,000°K. (2727°C.) Until it cooled to this point, before the stars and galaxies were formed, the early universe consisted only of an "ionized and undifferentiated soup of matter and radiation."[11]

According to the inflationary hypothesis, to which many but not all cosmologists subscribe, the early compressed universe, released by a reversal of its gravitational force underwent an exponential inflation, increasing in about 1/000,000,000,000,000,000,000,000,000,000,000 second from the size of a tennis ball to its present girth, 10 billion or more light years in radius. Stephen Hawking and Roger Penrose provided mathematical proof in 1969 of Einstein's cosmological singularity, concluding that the universe must have had a beginning and may possibly have an end. "The present evidence," Hawking wrote, ". . . suggests that the universe will probably expand forever, but all we can really be sure of is that even if the universe is going to recollapse, it won't do so for at least another ten thousand million years..."

The rate of expansion, he explained, is the result of several factors, including the initial explosive force, the mass of the universe, and the power of gravitational forces. If the expansion rate after the Big Bang had been smaller by even one part in a hundred thousand million million, the universe would have recollapsed before attaining its present size. If, on the other hand, it had been greater by as little as one ten-thousandth of one percent, the stars and planets could not have formed. "The odds against a universe like ours emerging out of something like the Big Bang" by chance, Hawking mused, "are enormous." "The cosmos," Ian Barbour added, "seems to be balanced on a knife edge."[12]

When first formed, the Earth was very hot and without atmosphere. As the universe expanded and cooled, emissions from the Earth's rocks formed an environment containing hydrogen sulfide and other gases, capable of supporting some primitive forms of life, but no oxygen. The release of oxygen by these early organisms brought a gradual change in the atmosphere to its present composition, allowing the evolution of fishes, birds, and a myriad of complex land creatures, including humankind.

Rarely does unanimity prevail among scientists. Hannes Alfvén, winner of the Nobel Prize in Physics in 1970 and proponent of his alternative theory of "cosmic plasma,"[13] dismissed the Big Bang as a myth.

Physicists remind us of the incredibly delicate balance within our chemical elements. If the strong nuclear force (the attractive force between proton and neutron) were even slightly weaker, the universe would contain only hydrogen; if only slightly stronger, the hydrogen would all have been converted to helium. In either case stable stars could not have formed and familiar, basic compounds such as water would not exist. The nuclear force is barely sufficient for the formation of carbon, an essential element of organic life; if slightly stronger, all carbon would have been converted to oxygen.[14]

One-half millennium ago Isaac Abrabanel (1437-1508), Jewish philosopher, theologian, and commentator, who served as minister of state under Ferdinand and Isabella before the expulsion of the Jews from Spain in 1492, had already theorized that if the sun had been larger or nearer the Earth, its heat would have destroyed our planet; and had it been placed farther away, the Earth would have been locked forever in a frozen winter.[15]

According to modern cosmologists many possible universes would be consistent with Einstein's equations, but ours is one of only a few in which the physical parameters even approach compatibility with organic life. A small change in any would render our universe uninhabitable. Through the maze of their mathematical equations and their mass of physical data some see evidence of design. Hawking speaks of "clear religious implications." Barbour concludes "that both biological forms and the physical conditions favorable for life must be the product of an intelligent designer because it is inconceivably improbable that they could have occurred by chance....The doctrine of creation...is an affirmation of dependence on God and the essential goodness and orderliness of the world."

In the twilight of his life Nobelist Isaac Bashevis Singer wrote: "No matter how the human brain might grow, it will always come back to the idea that God created heaven and earth, man and animals, with a will and a plan, and that, despite all the evil life undergoes, there is a purpose in Creation and eternal wisdom."[16]

SOME OTHER COSMIC EVENTS

In 1950 Immanuel Velikovsky dropped a bomb on the scientific community, in the form of a book.

A cluster, in cosmology, is an agglomeration of galaxies, grouped together more closely than would be predicted if scattered at random through space, typically about 15 million light years in diameter. Larger bunching of galaxies, to a diameter of about 150 million light years, is known as a supercluster. Among the early students of superclusters was Gérard de Vaucouleurs, then of the Australian National University and from 1964 Professor of Astronomy in the University of Texas at Austin. His work on the subject, reported in 1953, was rejected initially by scientific authorities. First there was complete silence, then denials. One authority stated, in 1956: "We have no evidence for the existence of galaxy superclusters." In 1959 another added: "Superclustering is nonexistent." Another told his students: "It's complete nonsense.

You shouldn't pay any attention." Decades later, asked why he thought his work on superclusters was resisted, De Vaucouleurs replied: "Because it did not come from a member of the establishment. As one of them told me years later, 'If it doesn't come from us, I don't believe it.' There is only one true church."[17]

Early in my professional career I had a somewhat similar experience. The editors of The American Journal of Obstetrics and Gynecology had accepted for publication my historical essay based on the first meeting of the American Gynecological Society (1876), the self-designated elite of the specialty, and suggested that I prepare similar essays on the Society's subsequent annual meetings, for publication in book form. Informed of this project, the Society's Council expressed its strong disapproval—that anyone not a Fellow of the Society should presume to write its history—and "suggested" that the editors (read "coerced the editors to") request my voluntary withdrawal of the initial essay.[18]

The reception accorded Velikovsky's *Worlds in Collision*[19] therefore came as no surprise to me. Immanuel Velikovsky had studied natural sciences at the University of Edinburgh; history, law, and medicine in Moscow; biology in Berlin; neurophysiology in Zurich; and psychoanalysis in Vienna. In 1939 he came to New York and practiced psychiatry until moving to Princeton in 1952, where he pursued independent research until his death in 1979.

Prominent among Velikovsky's theses, initially rejected by the scientific establishment but subsequently confirmed, were the claims: (1) that global catastrophes, collisions, and near-collisions, of extraterrestrial origin, had occurred in the past, resulting in mass faunal extinctions; (2) that electromagnetism, in addition to gravity and inertia, is a major force in cosmic processes; and that a magnetosphere exists above the terrestrial ionosphere (confirmed by Van Allen in 1958 and known as the Van Allen Belts); (3) that the solar system has a recent history, that youthful features are detectable on Venus and Mars, and that the former is a newcomer to the planetary system (perhaps only 3500 years old); and (4) that a steep thermal gradient exists a few feet under the lunar surface, remnant magnetism in lunar rocks; that their thermoluminescence dating would provide evidence of the recentness of the last heating, and melting, of the lunar surface; and that traces of hydrocarbons or their derivative carbides would be found on the moon—all of which predictions were confirmed by the Apollo moon landings (1969-1972).

The Macmillan Company, Velikovsky's publisher, had already made a large printing of *Worlds in Collision* when a few politically prominent members of the American scientific establishment learned of the book; and some, without having read it, organized an effective protest against its publication. Under the threat of a boycott of its highly profitable textbook division, the Macmillan Company was forced to abandon its planned publication, which was taken over by Doubleday, a company not subject to the same coercion.

Velikovsky later reminisced, in the preface to his *The Test of Time*: "I was compelled by logic and by evidence to penetrate into so many premises of the house of science. I freely admit to having repeatedly caused fires, though the candle in my hand was carried only for illumination." "Never, before Velikovsky," commented William Mullen, "have so many disciplines been united to illuminate those major events which myths were first to describe."[20]

In the fifteenth century before the Common Era, Velikovsky concluded, the planet Earth was scorched by fire and swept by hurricanes and huge tides; and seven centuries later (776-687 B.C.E.) the Earth was approached repeatedly, its axis and orbit disturbed, by Mars, which had already been displaced from its path by contact with Venus, all three planets assuming new positions in the solar system. As a result of these cosmic catastrophes, planetary atmospheres were exchanged, with the transfer of the carbon clouds of Venus and some of the Martian atmosphere to the Earth.

These disasters and the fires, hurricanes, and tides they produced, Velikovsky believed, are recorded in the Scriptures and permit natural explanation of the plagues at the time of the Exodus, the passage through the sea, the theophany at Mount Sinai, the messages of the Prophets, and other wonders of Biblical time.

EARTH'S VARIABLE ROTATION

Joshua, in pursuit of the Amorites, implored the sun and moon to stop in their courses: "And he said in the sight of Israel, Sun, stand thou still upon Gibeon; and thou, Moon, in the valley of Ajalon. And the sun stood still, and the moon stayed, until the people had avenged themselves upon their enemies....So the sun stood still in the midst of heaven, and hasted not to go down about a whole day." (*Joshua* 10:12-13)

A large comet, passing close to the Earth, could have disrupted its normal movement; or, as Velikovsky suggested, even if the Earth's rotation remained undisturbed, its axis might have tilted in a strong magnetic field, with the sun's apparent loss of several hours of its diurnal movement and with the increase in the length of one day.

Disparate sources provide independent supportive evidence of the event. The Mexican *Annals of Cuauhtitlan* (known also as the *Codex Chimalpopoca*), which contains records of incidents dating beyond a millennium before the Common Era, tells of a cosmic catastrophe in the remote past in which the night persisted for a long time. With no communication between the eastern world and the Americas, the authors of these annals could not have known of the Hebrew Scriptures; nor the authors of the latter, of the Mexican annals. Additionally, Velikovsky relates, a Spanish scholar named Sahagun, who followed

Columbus to America in the early 16th century and recorded the traditions of the American natives, wrote of their belief in a meteorologic aberration of ancient time, when the sun rose only slightly above the horizon, where it appeared to remain stationary, and when the moon too seemed to stand still, with the increase in the length of one night.

Modern geodesists and cosmologists, from precise determinations of the Earth's angular velocity, have been able to demonstrate variations in our planet's rotation over time scales ranging to centuries and longer. These variations they have imputed (1) to stresses applied from outer sources, and (2) to changes in the Earth's moment of inertia from the redistribution of matter within it, as resulting from the gravitational action of the sun, moon, and other extraterrestrial bodies, from deformations resulting from surface stresses caused by fluctuations in the fluid flow in the Earth's liquid metallic core, and especially by the torques generated by atmospheric motions, and from mass redistributions caused by earthquakes, melting snow, and, on geologic time scales, by mantle convection and the movements of tectonic plates.[21]

In addition to changing the Earth's course, extraterrestrial confrontations probably caused reversals in the Earth's polarity. A flash of lightning, striking a magnet, can produce a reversal of the magnet's poles. Electrical contact between the Earth and another cosmic body, Velikovsky reasoned, could similarly have resulted in the exchange of the former's north and south magnetic poles. Lava, when it solidifies after a volcanic eruption, assumes a magnetization dependent upon the orientation of the Earth's magnetic field at that time. But, as geologists had already pointed out, some igneous rocks are polarized oppositely from the present direction of the local magnetic field. Assuming that the magnetization of the rocks occurred as the magma cooled and that their positions have remained unchanged, earth scientists concluded that the Earth's polarity has been completely reversed within recent geologic time.[22]

Egyptian annals record the reversal of east and west in various epochs, with the sun rising in the west and setting in the east. Plato likewise wrote of "disruptions of every possible kind" in the Earth's course. Changes in the Earth's magnetic field, with reversal of north and south magnetic poles, are now believed to have occurred at intervals of hundreds of thousands of years. Records exist of 48 such reversals during the past 3 million years.[23] "Was the cosmic catastrophe that terminated a world age in the days of the fall of the Middle Kingdom and of the Exodus," Velikovsky asks, "one of these occasions...?"

METEORITES, CRATERS, AND EXTINCTIONS

The globular clusters that illumine our skies, each an aggregate of about a million stars, are the oldest star assemblages in the universe. Observations of one, known as 47 Tucanae, in the southern sky, of about 150 clusters in our galaxy, published in 1991 by astronomers at the Space Telescope Science Institute in Baltimore, the Australia Telescope National Facility in New South Wales, and the University of Manchester, have shown it to be rife with violence. The ancient stars that populate the cluster's core, each about two or three times the mass of our sun and apparently at least 10 billion years old, are still (or again) burning hydrogen, shown by their blue color, evidence of having regained their youth from collisions and near-collisions with their neighbors. Some of them sustain the cluster from collapse into a black hole under their own gravitational force, the scientists suspect, by acting as slingshots, ejecting other stars from the cluster's center.[24]

For nearly two centuries scholarly suspicion has existed, now replaced by scientific certainty, that stones fall from the sky. Astronomers have identified 184 asteroids whose orbits have crossed that of the Earth, some discharging showers of rock in their errant flights, others actually plunging into the Earth. Corroborative evidence of asteroidal merger with the Earth is provided by abnormally high concentrations of iridium at the suspected sites of impact, a metal rare in the Earth's mantle but common in asteroids; and by distinctive markings on quartz crystals which have been reproduced in the laboratory but only under the force of extremely high pressures, as would result from collision with an extraterrestrial body or an atomic blast.

A hole in the Earth's crust one-half mile in diameter, created 50,000 years ago in northern Arizona and discovered in 1891 by G.K. Gilbert, was regarded as evidence of headlong collision with a small comet or asteroid. No serious research was devoted to this find by the U.S. Geologic Survey, however, for nearly 60 years. On June 30, 1908 a ferrous mass with a calculated weight of 40,000 tons fell in the Central Siberian Uplands, with an estimated force of 12 megatons of TNT.

Additional evidence of impact craters resulted from a flurry of discoveries in the late 1920s. Another crater was found in Odessa, Texas in 1928. A few years later 13 craters and hundreds of iron meteorites were discovered at Henbury, Australia. Iron masses and two craters walled with silica glass impregnated with millions of metallic nickel-iron spherules (identifying their asteroidal origin), found among the shifting sands of the Arabian peninsula in 1933, were taken as proof of meteorite impact.

But uniformitarianism, a concept enunciated by James Hutton (1726-1797) and by Charles Lyell (1797-1875), was slow to die. Hutton, whose gravestone in Edinburgh memorializes him as "The Founder of Modern Geology," rejecting the Biblical version of creation, had stated in 1788 that "we find no vestige of a beginning—no prospect of an end." Lyell, born in the year of Hutton's death, embraced and extended the latter's teachings. He viewed the Earth as an efficient machine, operating independently of external forces, which, having been set in motion by God, would never be interfered with by Him. Only a minority of geologists, designated as "catastrophists," rejected the Hutton-Lyell concept. Uniformitarianism remained the fundamental principle of mainstream geology for nearly two centuries. It was clearly incompatible with the concept of impact craters. Until World War II most geologists regarded them as rare curiosities, unimportant to the established principles of their profession.

Interest in meteorites soared throughout the English-speaking world after the orbiting of Sputnik I, in October 1957. American astronauts, on their final Apollo 17 mission, in 1972, brought back from the lunar highlands rock aggregates, analysis of which showed their origin from impact rather than volcanic activity. Space vehicles, dispatched into the reaches of the solar system, were soon sending back images that showed impact craters to be the most common topographic feature on all planets and satellites with surfaces of rock or ice.

In 1979 Luis Alvarez and his colleagues at the University of California in Berkeley discovered large amounts of iridium at several sites around the world, in sediments of 65 million years ago, about the time the dinosaurs disappeared; and when they proposed bolide impact as a likely cause of the extinctions at the Cretaceous/Tertiary boundary they finally captured the attention of geologists: meteoritic impact was recognized as a major global phenomenon.[25]

The Alvarez team concluded that a large extraterrestrial object, perhaps 10 kilometers in diameter, had collided with the Earth, producing a thick cloud of dust that dispersed and blocked light from the sun, thereby halting photosynthesis and causing wholesale loss of life. Most of the calcareous plankton, marine reptiles, and dinosaurs became extinct; but some biologic groups including land plants, crocodiles, and many small invertebrates were spared. Others, as early as 1956, had related extinctions to extraterrestrial impacts, but it was the Alvarez report, followed almost immediately by similar observations by Ganapathy,[26] that provided the first hard evidence of such a link. Evidence accumulating in the early 1980s pointed to a periodicity in these biological crises, with extinctions linked with catastrophes as intervals variously estimated at 26-32 million years to 100-500 million years.[27]

Still to be sorted out was impact importance in relation to other possible causes of mass extinctions. Ursula Marvin, of the Harvard-Smithsonian Center for Astrophysics, pondered: "This process brings with it visions of random violence to the Earth on a scale never before contemplated: meteorite or comet impacts scar the lithosphere and generate towering tsunamis; exceptional impacts trigger magnetism, or shroud the globe in darkness and cold, poisoning life on land and in the sea or igniting wildfires that incinerate the world's flora to ashes...Could late-falling planetesimals have plunged through [the Earth's] crust and caused the inhomogeneity [and plate tectonics] of the mantle?...The Earth's own thermally unstable interior may have generated many of the phenomena we read in the geologic record but impacts certainly have played a major role in altering the Earth throughout its 4.6-billion-year history."[28]

In 1972 an asteroid with an estimated diameter of 260 feet sped through the upper atmosphere over northern United States and Canada. A smaller mass did likewise in 1989; and in January 1991 another passed the Earth within less than half its distance from the moon. New asteroids are being added to our skies, cosmologists believe, at the rate of about two a month.

In 1990 geologists obtained crucial evidence that a 180-kilometer-wide ring-shaped crater at a site named Chicxulub, on the north coast of Mexico's Yucatan peninsula, had been caused by the impact of an asteroid at the end of the dinosaurs' long reign on Earth. Samples of rock from drillings for oil exploration two decades earlier contained quartz crystals bearing the distinctive markings resulting from extreme impact; and some, in mineralogical tests, were similar to rocks that had been formed by melting in other craters, known to have been produced by impacts. Scattered debris in nearby Caribbean areas and around the Gulf of Mexico contained heavy concentrations of iridium. Dating by means of radiogenic isotopes showed the various deposits to be 64.5 to 65 million years old. In addition to these signs of an extraterrestrial impact, the catastrophe left evidence of a huge seismic sea wave, or tsunami, presumably having formed beneath at least 500 meters of water, producing a wave a kilometer or more in height and leaving a deposit containing ripple marks and bits of wood, which must have been washed off from the land.[29]

If, as Velikovsky alleged, the distortion of the Earth's path in Joshua's time was caused by the approach of a comet, the encounter was probably accompanied by a torrent of meteorites. The book of Joshua indeed tells of stones rained upon the Amorites:

"And it came to pass, as they fled from before Israel, and were going down to Beth-horon, that the Lord cast great stones from heaven upon them unto Azekah, and they died: they were more which died with hailstones [*barad*] than they whom the children of Israel slew with the sword." (*Joshua* 10:11)

Extraterrestrial planetary proximity may likewise have caused the destruction of Sennacherib's army. Sennacherib, son of Sargon, after mounting the Assyrian throne in 705 B.C.E., soon launched a great military campaign to the west. In 701 he invaded Judah and imprisoned its King Hezekiah, but was bought off with heavy tribute from destroying Jerusalem; whereupon he captured Babylon, in 689 B.C.E., and razed it to the ground. Sennacherib was murdered by his two sons in 681. The Scriptures tell of the forecast of his doom and of his army's decimation:

"Behold, I will send a blast upon him, and he shall hear a rumour, and shall return to his own land; and I will cause him to fall by the sword in his own land...And it came to pass that night, that the angel of the Lord went out, and smote in the camp of the Assyrians an hundred fourscore and five thousand: and when they arose early in the morning, behold, they were all dead corpses. So Sennacherib king of Assyria departed, and went and returned, and dwelt at Nineveh." (*II Kings* 19:7, 35-36; and *Isaiah* 37:7, 36-37)

According to the Talmud and Midrash, Velikovsky noted, the blast and scourge that destroyed the army of Sennacherib, the night after the return of the sun's shadow, in the spring of the year 687 B.C.E., were accompanied by a deafening din and a column of fire, inflicted by the archangel Gabriel. The archangel Gabriel was synonymous with the planet Mars, which, together with the archangel Michael, or the planet Venus, had also saved the people Israel at the time of the Exodus, centuries earlier. Michael and Gabriel came to be looked upon as Israel's guardian angels.

The great cosmic catastrophe of the middle of the second millennium B.C.E., which had been witnessed, described, and recorded independently among the traditions of various nations of the ancient world, was designated by Velikovsky as a "battle in the sky." Some regarded it as a fight between an evil monster, in the form of a serpent, and the light-god, who ultimately prevailed and saved the world.

A huge cometary mass, destined to become the planet Venus, had torn loose from Jupiter. The resultant spectacle was viewed from almost all parts of the world as a gigantic battle. As the comet and Earth approached, the latter's seas rose in massive tides. The gases, dust, and meteorites of the comet's tail disturbed the Earth's rotation and distorted its path; and the comet itself, attracted by the Earth, followed for a time its orbit. As the comet and Earth alternately approached and separated, violent electrical discharges occurred, a pillar of smoke resembling a great serpent arose from the comet's gases, and the Earth seemed to change its direction of rotation.

Amid the violent electrical exchange between the comet's head and tail, with their alternate attraction and repulsion, meteorites were rained upon the Earth. Divested of much of its atmosphere and of its electrical potential, the comet parted from the Earth and settled into its own orbit. Venus was born. The Earth resumed its normal course. Commented Isaiah: "The people that walked in darkness have seen a great light: they that dwell in the land of the shadow of death, upon them hath the light [of Noga, a Hebrew name for Venus] shined. (*Isaiah* 9:2)

Like other peoples, Velikovsky reasoned, the Hebrews saw in this great cosmic struggle a conflict between good and evil, a concept preserved in the Scriptures. A psalmist wrote: "O Lord God of hosts, who is a strong Lord like unto thee?...Thou rulest the raging sea...Thou hast broken Rahab [Hebrew name for the contestant with the Almighty] in pieces, as one that is slain...thou hast scattered thine enemies with thy strong arm. The heavens are thine, the earth also is thine: as for the world and the fulness thereof, thou hast founded them. The north and south thou hast created them." (*Psalm* 89:8-12)

The Prophets remembered the menace of Rahab in their prayers: "Awake, awake, put on strength, O arm of the Lord; awake, as in the ancient days, in the generations of old. Art thou not it that hath cut Rahab, and wounded the dragon?" (*Isaiah* 51:9)

A large comet or meteorite approaching but not making physical contact with the Earth would surely have disrupted the latter's movement. Velikovsky's scenario: "Points on the outer layer of the rotating globe (especially near the equator) move at a higher linear velocity than points on the inner layers, but at the same angular velocity. Consequently if the earth were suddenly stopped (or slowed down) in its rotation, the inner layers might come to rest (or their rotational velocity might be slowed) while their outer layers would still go on rotating. This would cause friction between the various liquid or semi-liquid layers, creating heat; on the outermost periphery the solid layers would be torn apart, causing mountains and even continents to fall or rise."

In the summer of 1991 an international conference on Near Earth Asteroids was held in San Juan Capistrano, California, attended by some 200 scientists, to consider means for saving our planet from future devastation. A committee of NASA scientists concluded in 1993 that nuclear technology offers the only hope of directing an asteroid from a collision course.

Mass extinctions of the Earth's species have occurred repeatedly. It is estimated that of the billions of species that have inhabited the Earth during the last $3^1/_2$ billion years 99.9% no longer exist.[30] Five great mass extinctions are revealed in fossil records, the best studied and most famous of the extinctions, because of its inclusion of the demise of the dinosaurs, 65 million years ago, being designated as the K/T (K for *kreta*, Greek for chalk, common among fossils of the Cretaceous period; and T for the Tertiary period of geologic time).

Among the possible causes of the extinctions scholars have considered climatic cooling, changes in sea level, and loss of habitat; but most attribute the extinctions to collisions of the Earth with bodies from outer space. David Raup and Jack Sepkoski, at the University of Chicago, reported finding fossil records of periodicity in the extinctions from meteorite impacts, huge chunks of debris from the solar system slamming into our planet, on average, once every 26 million years.

Earth scientists convened at Snowbird, Utah in 1981 and again October 20-23, 1988, when 60 talks were given on global catastrophes in world history and the relation of impacts and volcanoes to mass mortality.[31] Comet storms, it was widely agreed, have been responsible for many otherwise unrelated geophysical and astrophysical observations, including features of the fossil record, impact craters, and geomagnetic reversals. Mass extinctions of the past 600 million years, it was concluded, resulted primarily from impacts of extraterrestrial objects. Analysis of Cretaceous/Tertiary boundary sections from various sites throughout the world provided evidence that marine organisms had died out suddenly, their extinction consistently associated with the telltale elevation of iridium concentration and other bolide by-products in the boundary layer. Abrupt floral extinctions of 45% of the existing genera or species, estimated from the plant microfossil records across western North America, were likewise reported.[32,33] A 3-year field study (1987-1990) of bones of the dinosaurs from diverse taxonomic families in the Hell Creek Formation in the Great Plains of Montana and North Dakota, which records the last 2 to 3 million years of the Cretaceous period, provided additional evidence that the extinction of the dinosaurs was brought about by a catastrophic event, such as the crash of an asteroid or comet into the Earth; and offered no support for the alternative scenario of their demise, in which the decline in numbers was gradual, resulting from climatic change or other environmental factors.[34]

Let it not be thought, however, that all has been quiet within the bosom of Mother Earth herself. Some extinctions may have been caused by internally generated events. The cold waters off the coast of Canada were once warm, perhaps 100 million years ago, as evidenced by the fossil remains of alligators and crocodiles at the latitude of present-day Labrador. Marine geologists have produced evidence, in the form of oceanic plateaus, some as much as 2 kilometers beneath the sea and covering $1^1/_2$ million square kilometers, of submarine volcanic eruptions in the Pacific basin about 120 million years ago. The massive upheaval of gas-laden magma that produced these laval plateaus, they believe, released enough carbon dioxide to cause a major greenhouse effect with resultant global warming. A mere doubling of current atmospheric carbon dioxide concentration could have accounted for the presumed warmth; estimates based on sediments corroded by sea water carbonic acid suggest concentrations of carbon dioxide up to 12 times higher than today's. With the subsidence of the surge of volcanism in this mid-Cretaceous period, climatic cooling slowly occurred. The ice ages that followed made life impossible for the alligators and crocodiles in northern climates.[35]

Similarly, deep-sea borings off the coast of Antarctica and measurements of the oxygen and carbon isotopes in remains of the foraminifers, bottom-dwelling unicellular organisms, have related their decrease from a diverse community of 60 species to one of 17 survivors, to the oceanic warming from an outpouring of volcanic carbon dioxide-laden lava, the temperature of the bottom waters rising from about 10°C to 18°C, 57 million years ago.[36]

SUMMARY

The Biblical account of creation finds its counterpart in the Big Bang model, widely accepted by modern cosmologists, with explosion of a singularity, or infinitely compact mass, some 10 to 15 billion years ago, to form myriads of galaxies in the ever-expanding universe. Other Biblical events have been associated with global catastrophes, collisions, and near-collisions, of extraterrestrial origin.

NOTES AND REFERENCES

1. The first world was called *Heled*; the second, *Tevel*; the third, *Yabbashah*; the fourth, *Harabah*; the fifth, *Arka*; the sixth, *Adamah*; the seventh, *Eretz*. Ancient tradition, recalled the rabbinical authority Rashi (Rabbi Solomon ben Isaac, 1040-1105) in his Commentary to Genesis (11:1), told of periodic collapses of the firmament at intervals of 1,656 years, one of which occurred at the time of the Deluge; others were accompanied by conflagration.
2. Aristotle: "De Caelo" [On the Heavens]. Translated by JL Stocks. In: The Basic Works of Aristotle R. McKeon, ed. Random House 1941: 398-466.
3. Aristotle: On Man in the Universe. LR Loomis, ed. Walter J. Black 1943:xxiv.
4. Maimonides. The Guide for the Perplexed...Translated from original Arabic text by M. Friedländer, 2nd ed. Dover Pub 1956 (from 1881 and 1904 editions).
5. Taub JJ. The Creation of the World According to Gersonides. Scholars Press 1982:75.
6. Jastrow R. God and the Astronomers. WW Norton 1978:116.
7. Lightman A, Brawer R, eds. Origins: The Lives and Worlds of Modern Cosmologists. Harvard U. Press 1990:20.
8. Lemaitre G. A homogeneous universe of constant mass and increasing radius accounting for the radial velocity of extra-galactic nebulae. Annals of the Scientific Society of Brussels. 47A, 1927:49. English trans: Monthly Notices of the Royal Astronomical Soc, 1931; 91:483.
9. Lightman and Brawer (7), 1-2.
10. Hawking SW. A Brief History of Time. Bantam Books 1988.
11. Weinberg S. The First Three Minutes. Basic Books 1977; 54,75.
12. Barber I. Religion in an Age of Science. Harper and Row 1990; 135-136, 179-180.
13. Alfvén H. Cosmic Plasma. D Reidel Pub Co 1981.
14. Carr BJ, Rees MJ. The Anthropic Principle and the Structure of the Physical World. Nature 1979; 278:605-612.
15. Fields HJ. A Torah Commentary for Our Times. 1, Genesis. UAHC Press 1990;24.
16. Singer IB. Genesis. In: Congregation. Rosenberg D, ed. Harcourt, Brace, Jovanovich 1987:8.
17. Lightman and Brawer (7); 92-93.

18. Two decades later this essay, together with material from the Society's next 24 annual meetings, made a major chapter for my Obstetrics and Gynecology in America: A History. Amer Col Obstetr Gynecol 1980.
19. Velikovsky I. Worlds in Collision. Doubleday 1950.
20. Velikovsky Reconsidered. by the editors of Pensee, Sidgwick and Jackson 1976; 246.
21. Hide R, Dickey JO. Earth's variable rotation. Science 1991; 253:629-637.
22. Fleming JA. Ed Terrestrial Magnetism and Electricity. McGraw-Hill 1939; 32:326.
23. Research News: A core-mantle link? Science 1991; 252:1617.
24. Flam F. The private lives of globular clusters. Science 1991; 253:739.
25. Alvarez LW et al. Extraterrestrial cause for the cretaceous-tertiary extinction. Science 1980; 208:1095-1108.
26. Ganapathy R. A major meteorite impact on the earth 65 million years ago; evidence from the Cretaceous/Tertiary boundary clay. Science 1980; 209:921-923.
27. Jansa FA et al. Comets and extinctions; cause and effect? In Sharpton (31):223-232.
28. Marvin UB. Impact and its revolutionary implications for geology. In Sharpton (31):147-154.
29. Raup DM. Extinction, Norton WW 1991.
30. Kerr RA. Research News. Science 1991; 254:943.
31. Sharpton VL, Ward PD, eds. Global Catastrophes in Earth History; An Interdisciplinary Conference on Impacts, Volcanism, and Mass Mortality. Geological Soc Amer, Special Paper 1990; 247.
32. Johnson DR, Hickey LJ. Megafloral change across the Cretaceous/Tertiary boundary in the northern Great Plains and Rocky Mountains. 31:433-444.
33. Nichols DJ, Fleming RF. Plant microfossil record of the terminal cretaceous event in the western United States and Canada. 31:445-455.
34. Sheehan PM et al. Sudden extinction of the dinosaurs: latest cretaceous, upper Great Plains, USA. Science 1991; 254:835-839.
35. Kerr RA. Did a burst of volcanism overheat ancient Earth? Science 1991; 251:746-747.
36. Kerr RA. An about-face found in the ancient ocean. Science 1991; 253:1359-1360.

CHAPTER 3

THE PLAGUES OF EGYPT AND THE EXODUS

The books of Genesis and Exodus tell, and the Passover Haggadah recalls, how Joseph, who had been Pharaoh's chief counselor, brought his father Jacob and his brothers from their home in famine-stricken Canaan to Egypt, where the fields by the Nile were green and food and water were plentiful. There the children of Israel sojourned for some 430 years, probably in the 15th century B.C.E., and their numbers increased. A new and unfriendly Pharaoh, suspicious of the prospering Israelites, pressed them into servitude, treated them harshly, and ordered the death of their newborn males.

"And the children of Israel were fruitful, and increased abundantly, and multiplied, and waxed exceeding mighty; and the land was filled with them. Now there arose up a new king over Egypt, which knew not Joseph. And he said unto his people, Behold, the children of Israel are more and mightier than we:...let us deal wisely with them; lest they multiply, and it come to pass, that, when there falleth out any war, they join also unto our enemies, and fight against us....Therefore they did set over them taskmasters to afflict them with their burdens, And they built for Pharaoh treasure cities, Pithom and Raamses....And the Egyptians made the children of Israel to serve with rigour: And they made their lives bitter with hard bondage....And the king of Egypt spake to the Hebrew midwives...if it be a son, then ye shall kill him; but if it be a daughter, then she shall live." (*Exodus* 1:7-16)

God directed Moses, who now assumed his first historical role, to lead the Hebrews out of their bondage. When Pharaoh refused Moses' entreaties, the Almighty punished the Egyptians with plagues:[1]

"He sent darkness, and made it dark...

He turned their waters into blood, and slew their fish. Their land brought forth frogs in abundance, in the chambers of their kings.

He spake, and there came diverse sorts of flies, and lice in all their coasts.

He gave them hail for rain, and flaming fire in their land.

He smote their vines also and their fig trees; and brake the trees of their coasts.

He spake, and the locusts came, and caterpillars, and that without number,

And did eat up all the herbs in their land, and devoured the fruit of their ground,

He smote also all the first-born in their land, the chief of all their strength." (*Psalm* 105:28-36)

BLOOD

"...and he [Moses] lifted up the rod, and smote the waters that were in the river, in the sight of Pharaoh, and in the sight of his servants; and all the waters that were in the river were turned to blood. And the fish that was in the river died; and the river stank, and the Egyptians could not drink of the water of the river; and there was blood throughout all the land of Egypt."(*Exodus* 7:20-21)

The waters of the Nile are known to turn red from time to time as a result of pollution from various fungi, plants, and insects. The discoloration of the river that occurred in the middle of the second millennium B.C.E., however, was beyond anything the Egyptians had experienced.

It was just at this time, Velikovsky recalled,[2] that the planet Venus, a new member of the solar system, caused one of the Earth's major catastrophes. While still a comet, he reasoned, it approached the Earth from its perihelion, touching our planet with its gaseous tail. A fine dust of rusty pigment resulted, reddening the Earth and imparting a bloody color to its waters. Poisoned by the pigment in the rivers, the fish died and decomposed.

Humans and livestock were likewise affected by the dust — boils, sickness, and death resulting. Moses had warned Pharaoh: "For if thou refuse to let them go, and wilt hold them still, Behold, the hand of the Lord is upon thy cattle which is in the field, upon the horses, upon the asses, upon the camels, upon the oxen, and upon the sheep: there shall be a very grievous murrain...And the Lord did that thing on the morrow, and all the cattle of Egypt died." (*Exodus* 9:2-3, 6)

Moses and Aaron "took ashes of the furnace, and stood before Pharaoh; and Moses sprinkled it up toward heaven; and it became a boil breaking forth with blains upon man, and upon beast. And the magicians could not stand before Moses because of the boils; for the boil was upon the magicians, and upon all the Egyptians." (*Exodus* 9:10-11)

The passage of meteorites, Velikovsky explained, is known to result in a mantle of dust, best seen on snow surfaces, as on mountain tops and in polar regions. Others, it may be noted, including Pliny the Elder, in volume 2 of his *Natural History* (77 C.E.); his contemporary Plutarch, author of several physical as well as historical treatises; and the Babylonians, had also written of "blood" raining from the sky over limited areas: a red, water-soluble dust originating not in clouds but from volcanic eruptions or from outer space.

The Red Sea, modern scientists have suggested, is probably named after golden-brown algae, long thought free of toxicity, floating on the surface. Oceanographers have found them capable of making demoic acid, highly poisonous to humans and marine animals. In 1987 this neurotoxin was incriminated as the cause of death of three persons and illness in 100 others who had eaten mussels contaminated with the diatomaceous algae. In the same and the following year a red tide that had long plagued Florida's Gulf Coast spread northward as far as North Carolina, its flagellated algae releasing a neurotoxin that caused damage of $25 million to the shellfishing industry. Five years later this illness, named amnesic shellfish poisoning, from the same or a similar organism, left a number of its victims with short-term memory loss. In 1991 pelicans were found dying from demoic acid poisoning after feeding on anchovies offshore in California. Shellfish fisheries all along the Pacific Coast had to be closed because of high levels of demoic acid produced by a related species of the organism; and the following year saxitonin, a potentially lethal paralytic shellfish poison, was found in Dungeness crabs from Alaska.[3]

HAIL

The red dust was to presage a torrent of meteorites. God warned: "I will cause it to rain a very grievous hail, such as hath not been in Egypt since the foundation thereof even until now...for upon every man and beast which shall be found in the field, and shall not be brought home, the hail shall come down upon them, and they shall die." (*Exodus* 9:18-19)

Barad is the Hebrew word for hail, whether of ice or stone. God rained it down on the intransigent Pharaoh and his people. The Midrash and the Talmud, interpreting the Scriptures, suggest that the great stones that fell from the sky were meteorites: "And the Lord sent thunder and hail...and the Lord rained hail upon the land of Egypt. So there was hail, and fire mingled with the hail, very grievous, such as there was none like it in all the land of Egypt since it became a nation. And the hail smote throughout all the land of Egypt all that was in the field, both man and beast; and the hail smote every herb of the field, and brake every tree of the field." (*Exodus* 9:23-25) Torrents of fire and red-hot stones from the sky, Velikovsky recalled, are mentioned repeatedly in the cultures and mythology of various peoples.

Some 50 years later in the mid-15th century B.C.E., according to the Talmud and Jewish legend, in the days of Joshua when the sun and moon stood still for a full day (see chapter 2), hot hailstones that had remained overhead, stayed from their descent upon the Egyptians by the intercession of Moses, were now cast down upon the Canaanites. The comet that was to be Venus had returned, passing close to the Earth, with its shower of meteorites. In the words of the rabbis, "all the kingdoms tottered...the Earth quaked and trembled from the noise of thunder." Again, terrified mankind was decimated, carcasses were strewn like rubbish, in this Day of Anger.[4]

American geologists have now provided evidence, from impact craters in Western United States and the Yucatan, that the extinctions of 65 million years ago resulted from not one, but two major impacts, probably from a fractured comet whose pieces or debris struck the Earth at different times, variously estimated at 4 months to 120 years apart. The deposits resulting from the impacts always appeared in two distinct layers, the lower consisting of an inch or more of grayish clay with impact granules, showing the effect of prolonged exposure to the weather before the deposition above it of a thinner layer, also containing iridium and shocked quartz grains, apparently resulting from a separate, later impact. Microscopic examination of slices through the two layers showed in places traces of plant roots extending through the lower layer but not traceable into the upper, as if the plants had had time to grow on the surface of the lower layer before being smothered by the deposition of the upper. Astronomers have actually witnessed the breakup of more than 20 comets since the middle of the 19th century. Debris ending up on the Earth's orbital path would be brought into repeated contact with the planet.[5]

FIRE

Fire figures prominently in the devastation inflicted upon the Egyptians and the later desert wanderings of the Hebrews. *Exodus* 9:23 tells that "fire ran along the ground" while the Lord confounded Pharaoh's people with thunder and hail. When they refused to let the Israelites go He poured upon them streams of burning naphtha, together with hot stones, causing severe blisters and boils, according to several Midrashim. "He gave them...flaming fire in their land," states *Psalm* 105:32; Daniel saw that "a fiery stream issued and came forth from before him (*Daniel* 7:10); and the *Apocrypha* and *Pseudepigrapha* record that the Egyptians were "pursued with strange rains and hail...and utterly consumed with fire: for what was most marvelous of all, in the water which quencheth all things, the fire wrought yet more mightily." As the Israelites traveled from the Mountain of Lawgiving and displeased the Lord with their complaints, "his anger was kindled; and the fire of the Lord burnt among them, and consumed them that were in the uttermost parts of the camp." (*Numbers* 11:1) When the priests Korah, Dathan, and Abiram rebelled against the authority of Moses and Aaron, "the earth opened her mouth and swallowed them up..." (*Numbers* 16:32) "And a fire was kindled in their company; the flame burned up the wicked." (*Psalm* 106:18) Aaron's elder sons, "Nadad and Abihu died before the Lord, when they offered strange fire before the Lord, in the wilderness of Sinai." (*Numbers* 3:4)

Petroleum, now the major source of energy in the industrialized world, had not yet been recognized as a fuel; but, as Velikovsky pointed out, all the countries with historic traditions of fire from the sky, recalling the rain of a sticky fluid billowing heavy smoke, have rich deposits of oil underground (Mexico, the East Indies, Siberia, Iraq, Egypt). Just extinguished, at this writing (February 1992) were the fires in the oil wells of Kuwait, ignited by the Iraqis during the Persian Gulf War, one year ago.

Petroleum consists of two elements, carbon and hydrogen, trapped within the Earth's rock formations and subjected to heat and pressure over eons. The principal source of the carbon and hydrogen it is taught, was animal life, in the form of minute marine and swamp organisms. Roger Larson, University of Rhode Island geologist, attributes formation of half of the world's oil to the mid-Cretaceous volcanic activity of 120 million years ago, when gas-laden lava burst into the Pacific (see chapter 2). A newly formed warm and therefore buoyant ocean crust, he hypothesized, floating higher on the underlying mantle, reduced the available space in the ocean basins, with the result that the sea water rose up onto the land, forming inland seas. The inland seas of the mid-Cretaceous period were the most extensive of the past 500 million years. Their bottoms, Larson speculates, provided an ideal space for the accumulation of dead marine plankton and, with volcanically provided greenhouse warmth and nutrients, for the formation of oil and gas.[6]

Another possible source of the petroleum deposits in the Middle East, and an explanation for the conflagrations of Biblical times, has been suggested by Velikovsky:[7] The tails of comets, he pointed out, consist mainly of carbon and hydrogen. In the absence of oxygen the vaporous mixture does not burn; but upon entering the atmosphere part of the mixture would be set ablaze, binding all available oxygen. The part escaping combustion, in swift transition to a liquid state as it cooled, would fall to earth, sinking into the sand and the cliffs among the rocks, ultimately to supply mankind's energy needs. The Earth's petroleum may be, in part, a product of the comet of the Biblical Exodus.

DARKNESS

In Egypt, the scenario of the plagues and the comet's mischief continued: "And the Lord said unto Moses, Stretch out thine hand toward heaven, that there may be darkness over the land of Egypt, even darkness which may be felt. And Moses stretched forth his hand toward heaven; and there was a thick darkness in all the land of Egypt three days: They saw not one another, neither rose any from his place for three days." (*Exodus* 10:21-22)

Velikovsky explained the darkness and associated turbulence: "The earth entered deeper into the tail of the onrushing comet. This approach...was followed by a disturbance in the rotation of the earth. Terrific hurricanes swept the earth because of the change or reversal of the angular velocity of rotation and because of the sweeping gases, dust, and cinders of the comet."[8]

From numerous rabbinic sources he collated the following: "An exceedingly strong wind endured 7 days...On the fourth, fifth, and sixth days the darkness was so dense that they [the Egyptians] could not stir from their place....The darkness was of such a nature that it could not be dispelled by artificial means. The light of the fire was either extinguished by the violence of the storm, or else it was made invisible and swallowed up in the density of the darkness....Nothing could be discerned...nor could anyone venture to take food, but they lay themselves down...their outward senses in a trance. Thus they remained, overwhelmed by the affliction."

Confirmatory evidence of the plague of darkness is found in a hieroglyphic inscription on a granite shrine at El-Arish, in northeast Egypt, near the Israeli border: "The land was in great affliction," it reads. "Evil befell the earth....There was a great upheaval in the homes....No one could leave the palace for nine days, during which days of upheaval such a tempest raged that neither men nor gods [the royal family] could see the faces of those beside them." Scholars have noted but attached little significance to the variation from 3 days of darkness, as mentioned in the Bible, to the 7 days of storm described by the rabbis, to the 9 days of upheaval recorded in the hieroglyphics. For without the light of the sun, how could days be measured?

That the Egyptian tablet and the Biblical record both refer to the same event, Velikovsky persuasively points out, is attested by the reference in both to Pi-hahiroth, where Pharaoh's horsemen subsequently overtook the encamped Hebrews, departing from Egypt. (*Exodus* 14:9)

INSECTS

No culture or climate is without its insects. Many serve mankind, help maintain nature's balance, feed the planet's birds, and pollinate its fruit trees, vegetables, and flowers. Some become a seasonal nuisance; others, occasionally, a devastating pestilence.

When Pharaoh reneged on one of his several promises to free the Israelites, Moses warned, in the words of the Lord: "if thou wilt not let my people go, behold, I will send swarms of flies upon thee, and upon thy servants, and upon thy people, and into thy houses: and the houses of the Egyptians shall be full of swarms of flies, and also the ground whereon they are....And the Lord did so; and there came a grievous swarm of flies into the house of Pharaoh, and into his servants' houses, and into all the land of Egypt: the land was corrupted by reason of the swarm of flies." (*Exodus* 8:21, 24)

A modern version of the Egyptian plague of insects struck California's Imperial Valley late in 1991, in the form of a speck-sized invader dubbed "superbug." Clouds of the flies, believed related to a strain of sweet potato whitefly (*Bemisia tabaci*), also known as the "poinsettia strain," brought sudden disaster to the area, feeding on an estimated 500 varieties of plants including alfalfa, broccoli, cabbage, citrus, corn, cotton, melons, peanuts, sesame, sugar beets, and tomatoes, destroying more than $200 million worth of produce, and causing a state of emergency in two counties.[9] Sucking up the plants' leaf juices, they killed most before fruition. Surviving plants were stunted or spoiled by a secretion known as "honeydew," which encouraged growth of a black mold. Congregating on the undersides of leaves, the insects remained beyond the reach of aerial sprays and appeared resistant to common pesticides. A University of California entomologist commented: "It's difficult to walk among them...they get into your hair, eyes, mouth, nose. I've never seen anything like this in my 20 years in entomology."

LOCUSTS

Pharaoh remained obdurate. Again Moses warned, in the name of the Lord: "If thou refuse to let my people go, behold, tomorrow will I bring the locusts into thy coast: And they shall cover the face of the earth, that one cannot be able to see the earth: and they shall eat the residue of that which is escaped, which remaineth unto you from the hail, and shall eat every tree which groweth for you out of the field: And they shall fill thy houses, and the houses of all thy servants, and the houses of all the Egyptians; which neither thy fathers, nor thy fathers' fathers have seen, since the day that they were upon the earth unto this day....and the Lord brought an east wind upon the land all that day, and all that night; and when it was morning, the east wind brought the locusts. And the locusts went up over all the land of Egypt, and rested in all the coasts of Egypt: very grievous were they; before them there were no such locusts as they....For they covered the face of the whole earth, so that the land was darkened; and they did eat every herb of the land, and all the fruit of the trees which the hail had left: and there remained not any green thing in the trees, or in the herbs of the field, through all the land of Egypt." (*Exodus* 10:4-6, 13-15)

Nearly identical to that of the Egyptians was the plight of the Kansan pioneers in 1874. During their preceding 2 decades on the midwestern frontier the settlers had experienced minor annoyance by grasshoppers from time to time but were unprepared for the massive onslaught of the insects in 1874, which came to be known as "the Grasshopper Year." The crops had grown well during the summer and by the end of July a bountiful harvest appeared certain. On August 1, one of the settlers recorded, a great cloud of grasshoppers blanketed the sky and began their feast of destruction. "The sun was veiled almost like Indian summer," one woman wrote. "They began, toward night, dropping to earth, and it seemed as if we were in a big snowstorm where the air was filled with enormous-size flakes.

"Alighting to a depth of 4 inches or more, the grasshoppers covered every inch of ground, every plant and shrub. Tree limbs snapped under their weight, corn stalks bent to the ground, potato vines were mashed flat. Quickly and cleanly, these voracious pests devoured everything in their paths. No living plant could escape. Whole fields of wheat, corn and vegetables disappeared; trees and shrubs were completely denuded. Even turnips, tobacco and tansy vanished."

"When they came down," another recalled, "they struck the ground so hard it sounded almost like hail... There was a watermelon patch in our garden and the melons were quite large and long...by the evening of the second day they were all gone... In a few days they had eaten every green thing. They soon had every twig on every tree or bush eaten off and the trees were as bare as in midwinter."

"Desperate to save what little remained," a third chronicler noted, "the pioneers grabbed whatever coverings they could find to shield their crops and shrubbery. Out came the bed sheets, blankets, quilts and shawls. Even old winter coats and greasy burlap sacks were ripped apart to spread over precious vegetables. Yet these coverings proved useless; the grasshoppers ate straight through the cloth or wormed their way underneath...these creatures would stop at nothing."

The first lamented: "They went from the corn fields as though they were in a great hurry, and there was nothing left but the toughest parts of the bare stalks... They invaded our homes, and if our baking was not well guarded by being enclosed in wood or metal, we would find ourselves minus the substantial part of our meals; and on retiring to bed, we had to shake them out of the bedding . . .

"Within hours, no part of the countryside was left unscathed... Besides devouring the food left in cupboard, barrel and bin, they attacked anything made of wood, destroying kitchen utensils, furniture, fence boards and even the rough siding on cabins. Window curtains were left hanging in shreds, and the family's clothing was heartily consumed. Craving anything sweaty, the insects took a special liking to the handles of pitchforks and the harnesses of horses. Lumbering cattle stood by helplessly as the pests crawled all over their bodies... Young children screamed in terror as the creatures writhed through their hair and down their shirts."

Another settler recalled in her memoirs that the grasshoppers were so thick that the sun could scarcely be seen, and that in a nearby village the trains could neither stop nor start because the tracks were slick with crushed grasshoppers.

Even after the grasshoppers' departure, it was recounted, their devastation lingered on: "Everything reeked with the taste and odor of the insects. The water in the ponds, streams and open wells turned brown with their excrement and became totally unfit for drinking by either the pioneers or their livestock. Bloated from consuming the locusts, the barnyard chickens, turkeys and hogs themselves tasted so strongly of grasshoppers that they were completely inedible."[10]

Egypt revisited!

DEATH

One more plague was needed to persuade Pharaoh to release the enslaved Hebrews. The Lord spoke to Moses and Aaron: "I will pass through the land of Egypt this night, and will smite all the firstborn in the land of Egypt; and against all the gods of Egypt I will execute judgment... I will pass over you, and the plague shall not be upon you to destroy you, when I smite the land of Egypt... That ye shall say, It is the sacrifice of the Lord's passover, who passed over the houses of the children of Israel in Egypt, when he smote the Egyptians, and delivered our houses... And it came to pass, that at midnight the Lord smote all the firstborn in the land of Egypt, from the firstborn of Pharaoh that sat on his throne unto the firstborn of the captive that was in the dungeon; and all the firstborn of cattle...there was not a house where there was not one dead. And he [Pharaoh] called for Moses and Aaron by night, and said, Rise up, and get you forth from among my people, both ye and the children of Israel; and go, serve the Lord..." (*Exodus* 12:12-13, 27, 29-31)

The Earth, Velikovsky conjectured, forced from its orbit and normal movements by the approach of the body of the comet, forerunner of Venus, was convulsed by the shock of its lithosphere. The houses of the Egyptians were destroyed by the resulting earthquake. The selective demolition of the Egyptian dwellings and sparing of those of the Israelites he attributed to the different materials with which their homes had probably been built: the former with inflexible stone and brick; the latter, in marshy areas, with more resilient clay and reeds.[11]

Death was soon to overtake Pharaoh himself, in his final, futile effort to stay the Hebrews in their flight: "For the horse of Pharaoh went in with his chariots and with his horsemen into the sea, and the Lord brought again the waters of the sea upon them..." (*Exodus* 15:19)

A somewhat different version of Pharaoh's demise is narrated on the Egyptian shrine at El-Arish: "Now when the Majesty fought with the evil-doers in this pool, the place of the whirlpool, the evil-doers prevailed not over his Majesty. His Majesty leapt into the place of the whirlpool."

But lest it be thought that the Israelites remained unscathed while their Egyptian captors were afflicted with the plagues, rabbinic tradition tells that only a small fraction of the original population of Hebrews in Egypt survived, and that only one out of fifty was spared to leave.

THE EXODUS

On the night of the tenth plague, the Bible tells, a "mixed multitude" of Israelites and others, together with their livestock, began their hurried flight from Egypt, on foot (*Exodus* 12:37-38). The night, according to the Midrashim, was as bright as the noon of the summer solstice, lit up by the approaching comet. "The lightnings lightened the world: the earth trembled and shook." (*Psalm* 77:18) The children of Israel were being led "by a mighty hand, and by a stretched out arm, ...and with great terribleness, and with signs, and with wonders." (*Deuteronomy* 4:34; 26:8)

"The Lord went before them by day in a pillar of cloud, to lead them the way; and by night in a pillar of fire, to give them light..." (*Exodus* 13:21) Some scholars have suggested a volcano as a natural source of the cloud, comparing the Biblical description of the Exodus to the eruption of Mount Pelée on the Caribbean island Martinique, in 1902, when the town of St. Pierre was buried in mud, ashes, and stones spewed from the volcano, which killed the city's 30,000 inhabitants, while the sky was lit by flaming sulfuric gases; and an earthquake, occurring simultaneously, changed the level of the ocean.[12]

The precise route taken by the fleeing Hebrews is uncertain. The text of *Exodus* (13:17) tells us that "God led them not through the way of the land of the Philistines, although that was near;" and they probably avoided the route along the Mediterranean, which was fortified with Egyptian military posts, as recorded on an Egyptian tablet of about 1300 B.C.E.[13] "But God led the people about, through the way of the wilderness of the Red Sea.[14] (*Exodus* 13:18) Pharaoh, regretting his decision to release the Hebrews, set out with his warriors to recapture them.

As they approached the water, which was to be known as the Sea of Passage, "the children of Israel lifted up their eyes, and, behold, the Egyptians marched after them; and they were sore afraid...and the Lord caused the sea to go back by a strong east wind all that night, and made the sea dry land, and the waters were divided. And the children of Israel went into the midst of the sea upon the dry ground: and the waters were a wall unto them on their right hand, and on their left." (*Exodus* 14:10, 21-22)

If the term *suf* in the Biblical name *yam suf* (the Sea of Passage) is derived from *sufa*, Hebrew for "hurricane," one can visualize a cosmic upheaval resulting in the "dividing of the waters." Hurricanes of enormous force, described in the Talmud, may have resulted from rapid shifting of the Earth's atmosphere under the impact of the gaseous mass of the approaching comet, together with the inertial effect of a change in the Earth's rotation or polarity. The traditions of many peoples, the world over, recount that the waters were alternately dashed high and driven apart. According to the Mekhilta, a commentary on *Exodus*, the Great Sea (the Mediterranean) broke into the Red Sea in a huge tidal wave. A psalmist wrote: "The waters stood above the mountains. At thy rebuke they fled; at the voice of thy thunder they hasted away... They mount up to the heaven, they go down again to the depths..." (*Psalms* 104:6-7; 107:26)

The Bible recounts the devastation of Pharaoh's minions: "... and the Lord overthrew the Egyptians in the midst of the sea. And the waters returned, and covered the chariots, and the horsemen, and all the host of Pharaoh that came into the sea after them; there remained not so much as one of them." (*Exodus* 14:27-28)

Since neither reeds nor papyrus grow near the Red Sea, some recent scholars have interpreted *yam suf* not as the Red Sea but as Sea of Reeds, a marshy area or one of the lakes at the northern end of the Gulf of Suez, where these grasses are common. Two oceanographers, Doron Nof of Florida State University and Nathan Paldor of the Hebrew University of Jerusalem, have presented a scientific explanation of the parting of the waters based on a mathematical interpretation of the physical factors involved: the dimensions of the seas or lakes, the intensity and duration of the wind, and the resultant drag on the waters.[15] In the conceptual model of Nof and Paldor, of a shallow, narrow, and long channel, corresponding to the Gulf of Suez, connected to a larger body, corresponding to the Red Sea, a steady wind of 40 knots (72 kilometers per hour) blowing down the Gulf for 10 hours could have shifted its northern water line more than a kilometer south, the drop of 2.5 meters in its level exposing enough Gulf bottom for the Israelites' crossing. Further, they pointed out, if the Gulf bottom was slightly different in Biblical times and contained a ridge as a result of natural geologic processes, then crossing in "the midst of the sea," with water on both sides, would have been possible. With the sudden abatement of the wind, the displaced water would have returned within 4 minutes in a a massive wave, enough to drown the pursuing Egyptians.

The Bible continues: "Thus the Lord saved Israel that day out of the hand of the Egyptians; and Israel saw the Egyptians dead upon the sea shore." (*Exodus* 14:30) And the psalmist rejoiced: "He turned the sea into dry land: they went through the flood on foot...we went through fire and through water: but thou broughtest us out..." (*Psalm* 66:6, 12) But, Velikovsky suggests, many Israelites probably perished with the Egyptians at the Sea of Passage, as in the previous disasters wrought by fire, hail, and hurricane, according to the Lord's promise: "I will bring my people again from the depths of the sea." (*Psalm* 68:22)

An alternative view of the plagues of Egypt has been presented by Greta Hort, picturing them as a sequential scenario of events having a common origin in the flooding of the Nile.[16] The Blue Nile, the lesser of the river's two major components, with headwaters on the Abyssinian plateau, appears crystal clear throughout most of the year. Its color changes, however, with the melting of the snow in the mountains and with the summer rains, which wash particles of earth into it. Geologists have classified the soil in the entire basin of the Blue Nile as "tropical Roterde," or red earth, which is actually red or even carmine, consisting of unusually fine particles when dry, present in a thick covering layer. In a year with abnormally high precipitation the erosive force of the flow increases, the water reaching parts of the soil possibly unwashed for many years. Thus the greater the volume of water carried by the river, the redder it becomes, retaining its particulate suspension throughout its entire course. An abnormally high Nile inundates parts of the country which its waters usually fail to reach. This flooding would have taken place in September, when the Nile is at its highest. All Egyptians would have had to dig for water: those living close to the river, probably having no wells, to obtain the less polluted water that might filter through the earth; those who lived farther from the river, because their wells had been rendered useless from cave-ins and bursting dams and sluices.

The flagellates *Euglena sanguinea* and *Haematococcus pluvialis* and their associated purple bacteria, which inhabit the high mountain lakes, would have been washed down from Lake Tana by the high waters of the Blue Nile, imparting a stench to the water and intensifying its already red color to blood-red. The presence of the flagellates in the river, by disturbing its oxygen concentration, could also account for the death of its fish. The latter need a stable oxygen supply, at a fixed level. The flagellates, on the other hand, give off much oxygen to the water during the day, absorbing even more at night. In their presence, therefore, the fish would soon succumb, making the water impotable and adding to its stench.

Commentators on the Exodus make no mention of Goshen's having been exempted from this plague. Indeed, as Hort has portrayed it, all of Egypt must have been affected. The Biblical account, similarly, contains no reference to the plague's sudden cessation; for the Nile fell slowly, its sediment diminishing gradually. As the flagellates were swept out to sea the river again became habitable to the fish, and the water slowly regained potability. The first plague, having announced its onset with the rising of the Nile in July and August and peaking in September, probably came to a gradual end in October and November.

But more was to follow. The Nile is known for its large population of small frogs. The masses of dead and decomposing fish caught in the reeds and depostied along the river banks soon began to pollute the water and air of the frogs' normal habitat, forcing them to seek refuge on dry land but sheltered from the strong sun. Hence their mass invasion of the Egyptian houses and courtyards, carrying with them agents of disease acquired from the decaying fish. The disease that best fits the scenario, Horst believed, is anthrax. The *bacillus anthracis* is found along the Nile's banks, is spread by insects, and its spores survive well in dead animals. Having acquired the anthrax spores from the dead fish, the frogs would have died from the disease soon after reaching dry land. The stabled cattle would have been protected. Hort places the second plague, an indirect result of the first, in August.

Next, mosquitoes. In a year with an abnormally high Nile, their number must have greatly exceeded their normal seasonal fall peak. A single water-breeding mosquito, which has a life cycle of 16-20 days, can produce three 300-egg batches of eggs within a couple of days, most of which hatch. The mosquito's fly range extends up to 3 miles. Hort fixes the mosquito episode from early October to late November, during which period bloodthirsty mosquitoes must have plagued Egypt in astronomical numbers.

The sudden mass multiplication of flies in Upper Egypt, but not in Goshen, in early winter, is considered in conjunction with the sixth plague.

The "very grievous murrain" of the fifth plague fell upon all the cattle of the Egyptians in the field, so that "all the cattle of Egypt died: but of the cattle of the children of Israel died not one." The time when some of the cattle, but not all, were in the field, Hort points out, must have been early January; the rest of the cattle still remained stabled. The latter remained free of the anthrax which had infected the ground where the frogs had died; while the cattle in the field contracted the disease and succumbed to it. The cattle of the Israelites, in Goshen, in Upper Egypt, all of which remained stabled at the time, were likewise exempted from the murrain. By the time of their turning out to pasture, the rain squalls from the Mediterranean would have cleansed the ground surface of the remaining anthrax bacilli.

An apt description of skin anthrax is presented by the sixth plague, "a boil with blains." The lesions, confined mainly to the lower extremities, form initially as a large swelling of the skin, in the middle of which a bluish-red pustule with a central depression appears after a few days. When the latter dries up a new boil develops, swells, and finally peels. A principal vector of skin anthrax is the fly *Stomoxys calcitrans*, capable of sudden mass multiplication in warm climates. Each fly lays up to 800 eggs in about 2 months, in vegetable debris, a new generation appearing from each in about one month. The flies acquire the infection from the carcasses of animals dead of the disease and transmit it to the legs of its victims either by biting or by depositing the bacilli or spores through puncture wounds made by their feet. Large parts of Egypt, covered by rotting plant debris in October and November, when the Nile was falling, would have provided an ideal breeding ground for the fly. By the beginning of January their numbers would have been tremendous. It was then that the fourth plague began. When the field cattle died of internal anthrax in the fifth plague, *Stomoxys calcitrans* was present *en masse*, for transmission of the disease to the stabled cattle and to humans.

The hailstorm of the seventh plague, which came suddenly and vanished as it had come, destroyed the harvests of flax and barley, but spared the wheat and spelt. Flax, usually sown near the beginning of January, flowered in about 3 weeks. Barley, normally sown in August, was harvested in February. Wheat and spelt, sown in August, were usually harvested toward the end of March. In the year of the plagues, with flooding from the Nile, flax would have had to be sown 2 to 3 weeks later than usual because of sodden fields, and would thus have been endangered by hail in early February. The barley, also late in ripening, would have been sufficiently advanced at the beginning of February to be vulnerable to the hail and pelting rain. The wheat and spelt, on the other hand, would not have been threatened until much later. In the Mediterranean climatic zone hail-and thunderstorms occur in late spring and early autumn, rarely in summer, and almost never in late autumn, winter, and early spring. Goshen would therefore have been exempted from the plague if it occurred any time between November and March. That Goshen was indeed spared strengthened Hort's conviction in fixing the seventh plague in early February.

Invasions of locusts occur regularly in Egypt. The heavy precipitation in northern Abyssinia during the summer preceding the seventh plague had created ideal conditions for their breeding. During September the locusts deposit their eggs, which hatch during the winter; and in February and March the mature locusts bred from them migrate, invading Egypt. Wind is an important factor in their migration. A strong east wind, just as the Bible describes, blowing across the Sinai Peninsula, would have resulted in a mass invasion of locusts into northern Egypt, down the Nile Valley, and "throughout the land of Egypt."

The plague of darkness was ascribed by Hort to a khamsin, or duststorm, the first one of the year, early in March. The whole country had been flooded in the preceding September by the swollen Nile, which left behind an extensive thick deposit of fine *Roterde*. The land was subsequently laid bare by a violent hail-and thunderstorm and the invasion of munching locusts. With the strong sun of Egypt shining on the *Roterde* and with no vegetation to bind the soil, it was inevitably carried up with the sand and dust from the desert in the whirling winds of the khamsin, blotting out the sun. A khamsin in Egypt normally lasts 2 to 3 days; the Biblical ninth plague lasted 3 days. The Israelites, living in a circumscribed region of Goshen, probably the Wadi Tumalith, situated at right angles to the opening of the Nile Valley and with mountains lying to its south, would have been spared from the duststorm that raged through the rest of the country.

The tenth plague, Horst suggests, consisted not in the slaying of the first-born but in the destruction of the first-fruits, which would have been in Egypt at the month in which the feast of Passover is celebrated: the wheat and spelt harvests, or what the locusts had left of them. This destruction she viewed as a natural consequence of the ninth plague, which therefore did not extend to the Israelites but passed over them as had the ninth. Thus each of the ten plagues, except the seventh, Hort argues, followed directly or indirectly, but always necessarily, from the first plague, from the flooding of the Nile, and in the sequence described in the Bible. Each describes a natural phenomenon of known or possible occurrence in Egypt. Indeed, Egyptian records exist, although separated from the Biblical account by 2 1/2 millennia, telling of disaster caused by the Nile's superabundance. The first of several, dating back to 1359, tells that in that year the river rose abnormally high "and the people went into the desert to pray God for the waters to fall."[17]

Freed at last from Pharaoh, the surviving Hebrews began their 40-year odyssey in the desert. The Scriptures attest abundantly the darkness they endured during the early days and years of their wanderings—darkness attributable in part to disturbances in the Earth's movements (see chapter 2); in part to the clouds of dust, both vaporous and particulate, produced by the comet and the volcanoes it activated. "And when the cloud tarried long upon the tabernacle many days, then the children of Israel kept the charge of the Lord, and journeyed not... Or whether it were 2 days, or a month, or a year, that the cloud tarried upon the tabernacle, remaining thereon, the children of Israel abode in their tents, and journeyed not." (*Numbers* 9:19, 22)

With the darkness came death. A psalmist lamented: "Thou hast...covered us with the shadow of death: (*Psalm* 44:19); Isaiah spoke of "the people that walked in darkness...they that dwell in the land of the shadow of death" (*Isaiah* 9:2); and Job bemoaned: "because I was not cut off before the darkness, neither hath he covered the darkness from my face." (*Job* 23:17) A number of other documents, Velikovsky notes, describe years of darkness in Egypt corresponding to the period of the Israelites' wanderings in the desert; and the Ermitage Papyrus, in St. Petersburg, Russia, states: "None can live when the sun is veiled by clouds."[18]

WATER

The primary desideratum of desert travel is water. The Hebrews had none. The Bible recounts: "So Moses brought Israel from the Red Sea, and they went out into the wilderness of Shur; and they went 3 days in the wilderness, and found no water. And when they came to Marah, they could not drink the waters of Marah, for they were bitter... And the people murmured against Moses, saying, What shall we drink? And he cried unto the Lord; and the Lord shewed him a tree, which when he had cast into the waters, the waters were made sweet." (*Exodus* 15:22-25)

Oak bark is rich in tannin, which causes proteins to precipitate and settle out from solution. God had but to impart instructions to Moses, who then performed the "miracle," now widely understood.[19]

MANNA

On the fifteenth day of the second month after their departure from Egypt, their provisions having run low, the Israelites grumbled to Moses and Aaron: "Would to God we had died by the hand of the Lord in the land of Egypt, when we sat by the flesh pots, and when we did eat bread to the full; for ye have brought us forth into this wilderness to kill this whole assembly with hunger. Then said the Lord unto Moses, Behold, I will rain bread from heaven for you; and the people shall go out and gather a certain rate every day... And the Lord spake unto Moses, saying, I have heard the murmurings of the children of Israel: speak unto them, saying, At even ye shall eat flesh, and in the morning ye shall be filled with bread... And it came to pass, that at even the quails came up, and covered the camp: and in the morning the dew lay round about the host. And when the dew that lay was gone up, behold, upon the face of the wilderness there lay a small round thing, as small as the hoar frost on the ground. And when the children of Israel saw it, they said one to another, It is manna.... And Moses said unto them, This is the bread which the Lord hath given you to eat... And the house of Israel called the name thereof Manna: and it was like coriander seed, white; and the taste of it was like wafers made with honey." (*Exodus* 16:2-4, 11-15, 31) "And the people went about, and gathered it, and ground it in mills, or beat it in a mortar, and baked it in pans, and made cakes of it." (*Numbers* 11:8)

Similar traditions are recorded in other cultures. The mythology of the Greeks tells of their ambrosia, the food or drink of the immortals, resembling honey.

The Bible paints the appearance of manna as a miracle. Its natural counterpart, a product of the tamarisk (*Tamarix gallica*), a shrub that flourished in the western Sinai peninsula, has long been known to the Bedouin Arabs and called by them *man* or *man min sama*, meaning "manna from heaven." In late spring and early summer it falls to the ground in yellow granules or sticky droplets, depending on the temperature, in the early morning hours, when the Arabs gather it in leather gourds and preserve it. Sweet to the taste and slightly spicy, it provides the land's first delicacy of the growing season. Long believed to be a secretion or exudate of the tamarisk plant itself, it is now regarded by some as an excretion of a scale-insect (*Coccus manniparus*) that feeds on the tamarisk. Chemical analysis of the material has shown it to be a mixture of three sugars and pectin, which the insects obtain form the plant's high-carbohydrate sap.[20]

QUAILS

Meat for the hungry Israelites had been provided by the quails, flying along their migratory route. Quails served them less well at a later time in their desert wandering, at a site they named Taberah, which some think was south of Jebel Hellal, about 50 kilometers from the Mediterranean coast.[21] Tired of manna, they complained again: "There is nothing at all, beside this manna, before our eyes...and the anger of the Lord was kindled greatly..." Then did He say, through Moses: "The Lord will give you flesh, and ye shall eat. Ye shall not eat one day, nor two days, nor five days, neither ten days, nor twenty days; But even a whole month, until it comes out your nostrils, and it be loathsome unto you: because that ye have despised the Lord which is among you, and have wept before him, saying, Why came we forth out of Egypt?... And there went forth a wind from the Lord, and brought forth quails from the sea, and let them fall by the camp, as it were a day's journey on this side, and as it were a day's journey on the other side, round about the camp, and as it were two cubits high upon the face of the earth. And the people stood up all that day, and all that night, and all the next day, and they gathered the quails; he that gathered least gathered ten homers: and they spread them all abroad for themselves round about the camp. And while the flesh was yet between their teeth, ere it was chewed, the wrath of the Lord was kindled against the people, and the Lord smote the people with a very great plague. And he called the name of that place Kibroth-Hattaaveh [meaning 'graves of craving']: because there they buried the people that lusted." (*Numbers* 11:4, 6, 10, 18-20, 31-34)

Scholars have long pondered the poisoning of the Hebrews by the quail meat. Traditional explanations vary between gluttony and divine wrath. Interesting, if not persuasive, is a physical explanation based on observations by a Major C.S. Jarvis, who witnessed the two annual migrations of quails for the 14 years that he was stationed in the Sinai. "On the spring migration," he noted, "the quails are returning from Central Africa and also they travel back quite slowly. For instance in the Nile Valley some of them alight as far south as the Sudan border and work their way slowly northwards. They have the opportunity to eat of poisonous weeds on their way up. When they come south in the autumn they fly straight from the cornfields of Hungary, Roumania and Russia and are of course in very good condition to eat." The plants on which the returning quail feed include hellebore (*Aconitum napellus*) and hemlock (*Conium maculatum*), to the products of which the birds themselves are immune or resistant. Their flesh, however, becomes poisonous to higher animals, as shown in actual experiment.[22] Recent reports attribute toxicity of quail to the neurotoxin coniine.[23]

THE THEOPHANY AT MT. SINAI

"In the third month," according to Scripture, "when the children of Israel were gone forth out of the land of Egypt, the same day came they into the wilderness of Sinai." (*Exodus* 19:1) Physically emancipated, they were now to acquire a spiritual basis for their unity as a people, as they received the Law that was to govern their future existence.

"And it came to pass on the third day in the morning, that there were thunders and lightnings, and a thick cloud upon the mount, and the voice of the trumpet exceeding loud; so that all the people that was in the camp trembled... And mount Sinai was altogether on a smoke, because the Lord descended upon it in fire: and the smoke thereof ascended as the smoke of a furnace, and the whole mount quaked greatly. And when the voice of the trumpet sounded long, and waxed louder and louder, Moses spake, and God answered him by a voice... And God spake all these words..." (*Exodus* 19:16, 18-19; 20:1)

The song of Deborah and Barak tells of the theophany: "The mountains melted from before the Lord, even that Sinai from before the Lord God of Israel" (*Judges* 5:5); and the Midrash adds: "The sky and the earth resounded...mountains and hills were moved."

Electrical discharges from the comet made repeated contact with the Earth, Velikovsky believed, as the two bodies alternately approached and retreated. "For weeks now," he summarized, all [the Earth's] strata had been disarranged, its orbits distorted, its world quarters displaced, its oceans thrown upon its continents, its seas turned into deserts, its mountains upheaved, its islands submerged, its rivers running upstream —a world flowing with lava, shattered by meteorites, with yawning chasms, burning naphtha, vomiting volcanoes, shaking ground, a world enshrouded in an atmosphere filled with smoke and vapor. Twisting of strata and building of mountains, earthquakes and rumbling of volcanoes joined in an infernal din... It was a perfect setting," he concluded, "for hearing words in the voice of nature in an uproar."[24] Moses heard the trumpetlike blasts, followed by the words of God. "And God spake all these words, saying, I am the Lord thy God, which have brought thee out of the land of Egypt, out of the house of bondage..." (*Exodus* 20:1-)

Tangible evidence of one source of the havoc wrought during the Exodus is provided by today's terrain in the Middle East, over the plateau of the Sinai peninsula and wide stretches of the Arabian desert, from Palmyra (in present-day Syria) to Mecca (in present-day Saudi Arabia), where spent volcanoes that belched their innards a few thousand years ago dot the landscape and the ground glistens with basaltic lava.

JERICHO

The children of Israel, after 40 years in the wilderness and having received the teachings and commandments of God, approached the Promised Land, from the east bank of the Jordan. Ageing Moses had begun to share his leadership authority with Caleb and Joshua. Scouts, returning from their exploration of Canaan, reported it a land that "floweth with milk and honey" but held by strong inhabitants, "men of a great stature...which come of the giants." (*Numbers* 13:27, 32, 33)

Fearful at the prospect of an encounter with a more powerful adversary, again "all the congregation lifted up their voice and cried... Would God that we had died in the land of Egypt! or would God we had died in this wilderness! And wherefore hath the Lord brought us unto this land, to fall by the sword, that our wives and children should be a prey?" (*Numbers* 14:1-3) Again the Lord was angered. And again Moses interceded. Continuing through the desert, the Hebrews prevailed over the Canaanites, the Amorites, the Midianites, and Og, the king of Bashan. "Charge Joshua," the Lord commanded Moses, "and encourage him, and strengthen him; for he shall go over before this people, and he shall cause them to inherit the land which thou shalt see." (*Deuteronomy* 3:28)

"Hear, O Israel;" Moses exclaimed, "Thou art to pass over Jordan this day, to go in to possess nations greater and mightier than thyself." (*Deuteronomy* 9:1) And to Joshua he urged: "Be strong and of a good courage: for thou must go with this people unto the land which the Lord hath sworn unto their fathers to give them; and thou shalt cause them to inherit it." (*Deuteronomy* 31:7) Under Joshua's direction the priests led the people to the river's edge.

The Earth still trembled and its crust continued to crack in the quake's shocks and aftershocks. As Velikovsky viewed the scene, masses of the Jordan's banks fell away, into the river bed, blocking the stream's flow long enough to permit the tribe's crossing: "And it came to pass, when the people removed from their tents, to pass over Jordan, and the priests bearing the ark of the covenant before the people; And as they that bare the ark were come unto Jordan, and the feet of the priests that bare the ark were dipped in the brim of the water, (for Jordan overfloweth all his banks all the time of harvest,) That the waters which came down from above stood and rose up upon an heap...and those that came down toward the sea of the plain, even the salt sea, failed, and were cut off: and the people passed over right against Jericho. And the priests that bare the ark of the covenant of the Lord stood firm on dry ground in the midst of the Jordan, and all the Israelites passed over on dry ground, until all the people were passed clean over Jordan... And it came to pass, when...the soles of the priests' feet were lifted up onto the dry land, that the waters of the Jordan returned unto their place, and flowed over all his banks, as they did before." (*Joshua* 3:14-17; 4:18)

At last, the Promised Land!

But the people of Jericho feared the Hebrews and closed their gates to them: "Jericho was strictly shut up because of the children of Israel: none went out, and none came in." The Lord instructed Joshua: "Ye shall compass the city, all ye men of war, and go round about the city once. Thus shalt thou do six days. And seven priests shall bear before the ark seven trumpets of rams' horns; and the seventh day ye shall compass the city seven times, and the priests shall blow with the trumpets. And it shall come to pass, that when they make a long blast with the ram's horn, and when ye hear the sound of the trumpet, all the people shall shout with a great shout; and the wall of the city shall fall down flat...So the people shouted when the priests blew with the trumpets: and it came to pass, when the people heard the sound of the trumpet, and the people shouted with a great shout, that the wall fell down flat, so that the people went up into the city, every man straight before him, and they took the city." (*Joshua* 6:1, 3-5, 20)

Did the walls of Jericho succumb from the sympathetic vibration caused by the stomping feet of the marchers outside the city, as long taught in elementary science classes; or was the "sound of the trumpet" the rumbling of the Earth's crust? Excavations at Jericho suggest that its 12-foot walls were destroyed by an earthquake.[25]

SUMMARY

The plagues of Egypt, as recorded in the Book of Exodus, have been attributed by modern scholars to natural phenomena: the red discoloration of the Nile, to pollution by algae, plants, and insects, or to fine dust from gaseous eruptions from outer space, which dust might also have caused human boils and death of the Egyptian livestock; hail, of hot stones, from a shower of meteorites from the comet that was to become the planet Venus. Impacts from a fractured comet are now believed responsible for the extinctions, as of the dinosaurs, that occurred some 65 million years ago. The plagues of fire and darkness have likewise been attributed to the gases and dust of the onrushing comet Venus and the disturbance it might have caused in the Earth's rotation. A modern counterpart of the Egyptian plague of insects struck California's Imperial Valley in 1991, in the form of a tiny invader dubbed "superbug." An invasion of locusts that attacked the Kansan pioneers in 1874 was nearly identical to the plague of locust inflicted on the Egyptians. An ingenious analysis of the ten Biblical plagues by a recent scholar ascribes them all, sequentially, to a common cause, flooding by the Nile. Modern oceanographers have created a mathematical model of the Gulf of Suez and the winds to which it can be subjected, by which a scientific explanation is provided for the parting of the waters for the fleeing Israelites.

Moses made the bitter waters of Marah potable by casting into them wood from a tree that God had pointed out. Oak bark, we now know, is rich in tannin, which precipitates proteins from solution. The manna that fed the Israelites, the appearance of which the Bible paints as a miracle, has been identified as a mixture of three sugars and pectin, either an exudate of the tamarisk shrub of the Sinai peninsula or an excretion of an insect that feeds on the plant. Meat was provided the Hebrews by quails flying along their migratory route, some of which proved poisonous from having fed on hellebore and hemlock.

The spent volcanoes of the Sinai peninsula and the Arabian desert provide mute evidence of the havoc wrought during the Exodus, with the rsultant theophany at Mount Sinai. The Earth still trembled and its crust continued to crack as the Israelites crossed the Jordan into the Promised Land and approached Jericho. When the trumpets sounded and the people shouted, the city's walls fell down. Excavations at the site suggest their destruction by an earthquake.

NOTES AND REFERENCES

1. Some scholars believe that the plagues of Egypt are more a literary tour de force than historical phenomena, and that their recounting in the Bible and the Passover Haggadah is based on natural disasters antedating the time of the Exodus and recorded in earlier Egyptian compositions, notably the "Admonitions of Ipuwer," probably from about 2100 B.C.E. Excerpts: "The Nile is in flood, but no one plows for himself, because every man says: 'We do not know what may happen throughout the land!'

    Many dead are buried in the river. The stream is a tomb, and the embalming place has really become the stream.

    The river is blood. If one drinks of it, one rejects it as human and thirsts for water.

    The desert is spread throughout the land. The homes are destroyed. Barbarians from outside have come to Egypt.

    Such is our Water! Such is our welfare! What can we do about it? Going to ruin!

    Laughter has disappeared and is no longer made. It is wailing that pervades the land, mixed with lamentation." (Plaut, GW, ed. The Torah. New York: Union of American Hebrew Congregations 1981:372, 444)
2. Velikovsky I. Worlds in Collision. Garden City:Doubleday 1950:64.
3. Culotta E. Reed menace in the world's oceans. Science 1992; 257: 1476-1477.
4. Velikovsky I.Worlds in Collision. Garden City:Doubleday 1950:152.
5. Kerr RA. Extinction by a one-two comet punch? Science 1992; 255:160-161.
6. Kerr RA. Beyong a volcanic spasm. Science 1991; 251:747.
7. Velikovsky I. Worlds in Collision. Garden City:Doubleday 1950:69.
8. Velikovsky I. Worlds in Collision. Garden City:Doubleday 1950:74.
9. Culotta E. "Superbug" attacks California crops. Science 1991; 254:1445.
10. Stratton JL. Pioneer Women. New York: Simon and Schuster 1981: 102-105.
11. Moses had promised his people: "The Lord will pass over the door, and will not suffer the destroyer to come in unto your houses to smite you" (*Exodus* 12:23, King James version); but, as Velikovsky points out, more accurate is the translation: "The Lord will pass over the door, and will not suffer the destroyer to come and smite your houses."

12. Gressman H. Die Anfange Israels. Gottingen, Vandenhoek und Ruprecht 1914:58; cited by Plaut GW, ed. The Torah. New York: Union of American Hebrew Congregations 1981:482.
13. Plaut GW. ed. The Torah. New York: Union of American Hebrew Congregations 1981:483.
14. "Red Sea," an interpretive translation of the Hebrew *yam suf*, is the name given the Sea of Passage in the King James version, the Illustrated Jerusalem Bible, and the New English Bible. A more accurate translation, as appears in the Union of American Hebrew Congregations' The Torah, is "Sea of Reeds," possibly a now-extinct inland lake (?Lake Berdaouil). If it was indeed a sea of reeds, Velikovsky argues, its waters must have been fresh, not salt, for papyrus reed does not grow in salt water.
15. Nof D, Paldor N. Are there oceanographic explanations for the Israelites' crossing of the Red Sea? Bull Am Meteorological Soc 1992; 73:305-314.
16. Hort G. The plagues of Egypt. Ztschr f alttestamentliche Wissenschaft 1957; 69:84-103. 1958; 70:48-59.
17. Toussoun Prince Omar. Memoire sur l'histoire du Nil 2:481-482; quoted by Hort G. The plagues of Egypt. Ztschr f alttestamentliche Wissenschaft.
18. Velikovsky I. Worlds in Collision. Garden City:Doubleday 1950:141.
19. Plaut GW. ed. The Torah. New York: Union of American Hebrew Congregations 1981:497.
20. Plaut GW. ed. The Torah. New York: Union of American Hebrew Congregations 1981:502.
21. Sergent E. Les cailles empoisonneuses dans la Bible, et en Algérie de nos jours. Arch de l'Institut Pasteur d'Algérie 1941; 19:161-167.
22. Macht DI. An experimental pharmacological appreciation of Leviticus XI and Deuteronomy XIV. Bull Hist Med 1953; 27:444-450.
23. Van Veen AG. Toxicants occurring naturally in foods. Washington Nat Acad Sci 1973; 2:464-465.
24. Velikovsky I. Worlds in Collision. Garden City:Doubleday 1950:107-110.
25. Velikovsky I. Worlds in Collision. Garden City:Doubleday 1950:150 ff.

CHAPTER 4

MEDICINE IN THE BIBLE

The early Israelites attributed the power of healing solely to God, who reminded them after their delivery from Egypt: "I am the Lord that healeth thee." (*Exodus* 15:26) In the centuries that followed, medicine became a part of general knowledge. The prevention, diagnosis, and treatment of illness, which had been the province of God's agents, the priests,[1] were gradually transferred to the rabbis. In contrast to the early Egyptian, Arabian, and Greek scholars, who compiled their medical knowledge in special treatises, the Hebrew sages usually mingled their statements on health and medical matters with the codes of law and religious conduct.[2]

Prevention of disease is integral to Judaic doctrine. Although much of Jewish ceremonial is purely symbolic, many ritual acts are clearly based on hygienic principles. The Bible abounds with evidence of medical acumen. It describes diseases involving the various body systems: alimentary, integumentary, circulatory, sensory, skeletal, nervous, excretory, glandular, and reproductive;[3] and foretells some of the methods of modern medicine, such as antisepsis, incineration, and quarantine.

SANITARY CODE OF THE ISRAELITES

The camp life of the Israelites during their 40 years in the desert was that of a planned community, perhaps the first on record, numbered at 603,550 souls exclusive of the Levites, later counted at 22,000, all directed by Moses and Aaron (*Numbers* 2). "Every man of the children of Israel," the Lord instructed, "shall pitch by his own standard, with the ensign of their father's house: far off about the tabernacle of the congregation shall they pitch."

In the center of the enclave was the tabernacle of the congregation and the camp of the Levites, surrounding which was a double cordon of the tents of the 12 tribes pitched in a quadrilateral, the outer occupied by the military personnel and their families, the inner by noncombatants—all arranged for optimal civil, defensive, and ecclesiastical purposes.

Prominent were the provisions for sanitation. Persons with cutaneous ailments judged contagious were segregated outside the camp. Regulations were promulgated to ensure personal cleanliness, purity of the water supply, protection of food, prompt disposal of refuse, and avoidance of overcowding.[4]

The burial of excrement by shovel in a designated area outside the camp foretold the trench latrine of the recent military: "Thou shalt have a place...without the camp, whither thou shalt go forth abroad: And thou shalt have a paddle upon thy weapon; and it shall be, when thou wilt ease thyself abroad, thou shalt dig therewith, and shalt turn back and cover that which cometh from thee." (*Deuteronomy* 23:12-13) The blood of slaughtered animals was likewise to be covered: "And whatsoever man there be of the children of Israel, or of the strangers that sojourn among you, which hunteth and catcheth any beast or fowl that may be eaten; he shall even pour out the blood thereof, and cover it with dust." (*Leviticus* 17:13)

Through Moses the Lord instructed concerning the sanitary precautions to be taken by the priests: "What man soever of the seed of Aaron is a leper [suffers from a cutaneous eruption], or hath a running issue...and whoso toucheth any thing that is unclean by the dead, or a man whose seed goeth from him [with a urethral discharge]; or whosoever toucheth any creeping thing, whereby he may be made unclean, or a man of whom he may take uncleanliness...the soul which hath touched any such shall be unclean until even...unless he wash his flesh with water." (*Leviticus* 22:4-6)

For the leper whom the priest has examined and judged to be healed of his or her scaly affection Moses was told: "He that is to be cleansed shall wash his clothes, and shave off all his hair, and wash himself in water, that he may be clean: and after that he shall come into the camp, and shall tarry abroad out of his tent seven days. But it shall be on the seventh day, that he shall shave all his hair off his head and his beard and his eyebrows, even all his hair shall he shave off: and he shall wash his clothes, also he shall wash his flesh in water, and he shall be clean." (*Leviticus* 14:8-9)

The human corpse was considered hygienically as well as ritually unclean. Physical contact with the dead was to be avoided if possible. Speaking to Moses and Aaron, the Lord decreed: "He that toucheth the dead body of any man shall be unclean seven days. He shall purify himself with it [ashes[5]] on the third day, and on the seventh day he shall be clean....because the water of separation was not sprinkled upon him, he shall be unclean...when a man dieth in a tent: all that come into the tent, and all that is in the tent, shall be unclean seven days. And every open vessel, which hath no covering bound upon it, is unclean. And whosoever toucheth one that is slain with a sword in the open fields, or a dead body, or a bone of a man, or a grave, shall be unclean seven days. And for an unclean person they shall take of the ashes of the burnt heifer...and running water shall be put thereto in a vessel: And a clean person shall take hyssop, and dip it in the water, and sprinkle it upon the tent, and upon all the vessels, and upon the persons that were there, and upon him that touched a bone, or one slain, or one dead, or a grave: And the clean person shall sprinkle upon the unclean on the third day, and on the seventh day; and on the seventh day he shall purify himself and wash his clothes, and bathe himself in water, and he shall be clean at even....And whatsoever the unclean person toucheth shall be unclean; and the soul that toucheth it shall be unclean until even." (*Numbers* 19:11-19, 22)

Moses continued, providing further detail for the cleansing process after contact with the dead: "And purify all your raiment, and all that is made of skins, and all work of goats' hair, and all things made of wood." (*Numbers* 31:20) Eleazar the priest, speaking to the soldiers, gave additional instructions, for purification of all material that might have become contaminated in battle: "Every thing that may abide the fire, ye shall make it go through the fire, and it shall be clean...and all that abideth not the fire ye shall make go through the water. And ye shall wash your clothes on the seventh day, and ye shall be clean, and afterward ye shall come into the camp." (*Numbers* 31:23-24)

SEXUALLY TRANSMITTED DISEASE

Genital discharges in both men and women commonly result from but are not limited to venereal, or sexually transmitted, diseases. Some discharges are infectious; many are not. The instructions that the Lord ordered Moses and Aaron to convey to the Israelites, reminiscent of modern isolation techniques, did not distinguish among the discharges: "When any man hath a running issue out of his flesh, because of his issue he is unclean...Every bed, whereon he lieth that hath the issue, is unclean; and every thing, whereon he sitteth, shall be unclean. And whosoever toucheth his bed shall wash his clothes, and bathe himself in water, and be unclean until the even. And he that sitteth on any thing whereon he sat that hath the issue shall wash his clothes, and bathe himself in water, and be unclean until the even. And he that toucheth the flesh of him that hath the issue shall wash his clothes, and bathe himself in water, and be unclean until the even...And the vessel of earth, that he toucheth which hath the issue, shall be broken: and every vessel of wood shall be rinsed in water. And when he that hath an issue is cleansed of his issue; then he shall number to himself seven days for his cleansing, and wash his clothes, and bathe his flesh in running water, and shall be clean... This is the law of him that hath an issue...of the man, and of the woman..." (*Leviticus* 15; 2-7, 12-13, 32-33)

Implied if not stated in the Writings is a relation between disease and sexual indiscretion. Thus warned the psalmist: "Fools because of their transgression, and because of their iniquities, are afflicted. Their soul abhorreth all manner of meat; and they draw near unto the gates of death." (*Psalm* 107:17-18) Zophar, in the Book of Job, painted a similar picture of retribution for sexual adventure: "His bones are full of the sin of his youth, which shall lie down with him in the dust. Though wickedness be sweet in his mouth, though he hide it under his tongue; Though he spare it, and forsake it not; but keep it still within his mouth: Yet his meat in his bowels is turned, it is the gall of asps within him." (*Job* 20:11-14)

Solomon cautioned his son against the mischief of whoredom: "For the lips of a strange woman drop as an honeycomb, and her mouth is smoother than oil: But her end is bitter as wormwood, sharp as a two-edged sword. Her feet go down to death; her steps take hold on hell....Remove thy way far from her, and come not nigh the door of her house: Lest thou give...thy years unto the cruel...And thou mourn at the last, when thy flesh and thy body are consumed." (*Proverbs* 5:3-11) "Keep my words," Solomon urged, "that they may keep thee from the strange woman," for thus is the enticement of the irresolute. "He goeth after her straightway, as an ox goeth to the slaughter, or as a fool to the correction of the stocks; Till a dart strike through his liver [symbolized as an erotic organ in Biblical times]; as a bird hasteth to the snare, and knoweth not that it is for his life." (*Proverbs* 7:5, 22-23)

The Lord's command to Moses, that the non-virgins be killed, as the Israelites went into battle with the Midianites, may have been aimed at eradicating venereal disease: "Behold, these caused the children of Israel, through the counsel of Balaam, to commit trespass against the Lord...and there was a plague among the congregation of the Lord. Now therefore kill...every woman that hath known man by lying with him. But all the women children, that have not known a man by lying with him, keep alive for yourselves." (*Numbers* 31:16-18)

WATER FOR JERUSALEM

"Let thy fountains be dispersed abroad, and rivers of water in the streets." (*Proverbs* 5:16)

After their occupation of the Canaanite city of Jerusalem, which became to the Israelites the City of David, the ancient inhabitants ingeniously adapted the natural features of the land to ensure for themselves a water supply dependable in war as well as in peace. Repeated reference is made to this water source in the Bible, also in the Ecclesiasticus of Ben Sira:

"And the rest of the acts of Hezekiah, and all his might, and how he made a pool, and a conduit, are they not written in the book of the chronicles of the kings of Judah?" (*II. Kings* 20:20)

"Ye have seen also the breaches of the city of David, that they are many: and ye gathered together the waters of the lower pool." (*Isaiah* 22:9)

"And when Hezekiah saw that Sennacherib was come, and that he was prepared to fight against Jerusalem, He took counsel with his princes and his mighty men to stop the waters of the fountains which were without the city.... So there was gathered much people together, who stopped all the fountains, and the brook that ran through the midst of the land, saying, why should the kings of Assyria come, and find much water?... This same Hezekiah...stopped the upper watercourse of Gihon, and brought it straight down to the west side of the city of David." (*II. Chronicles* 32:2-4, 30)

"Hezekiah fortified his city, bringing water within its walls; he drilled through the rocks with tools of iron and made cisterns for the water." (*Ecclesiasticus* 48:17)

Gihon Spring, at the foot of the city's eastern slope, provided the only perennial source of water for ancient Jerusalem, which was built on a narrow spur of the Temple Mount. A complex system of subterranean channels permitted the spring's waters to be directed from outside the city's walls to an intramural pool, which served as a reservoir. Through these channels the spring could be approached from within the city. Completion of the system's original tunnel, directed by King Hezekiah about 700 B.C.E. in anticipation of attack by the Assyrians, was recorded in an inscription in ancient Hebrew on the tunnel's wall, now detached and in the custody of the Archeological Museum of Istanbul. It tells how two teams, working toward each other from opposite ends of the tunnel, made successful contact: "And on the day of the piercing through the stone-cutters struck through each to meet his fellow, axe against axe. Then ran the water from the spring to the pool for twelve hundred cubits, and one hundred cubits was the height of the rock above the head of the stone-cutters."

The history of the subterranean waterworks of Biblical Jerusalem has been recalled by Dan Gill, of the Geological Survey of Jerusalem, who has also shed new light on its origin.[6] The system's winding tunnels and conduits had long been considered man-made, but scholars had been puzzled by the numerous apparent mistakes in their design and the inadequate provision for ventilation. The surroundings of Jerusalem, Gill pointed out, are rich in karst, areas of limestone formations characterized by sinks, ravines, and underground streams, especially east of the regional water divide, where many caves, aquifers, and springs are found. Re-examination of the mineral constituents of the Jerusalem waterworks and their stratigraphic arrangement suggested its founding on a pre-existent natural karst system resulting from dissolution of the limestone and channeling by ground water in the dolomite hill on which the city was built. Obtaining ventilation through interconnecting existing conduits that opened to the atmosphere, Gill concluded, King Hezekiah's miners fashioned a functional water supply system not through their own planning but, guided by existing passageways, by skillful enlargement and integration of existing natural channels.

SKIN AILMENTS

Several poorly defined dermatologic disorders including discolorations, pustules, ringworm, burns, alopecia, leprosy, and skin cancer are considered in some detail in *Leviticus* 13, with instructions to the priest for differential diagnosis and management, quarantine, and criteria for ritual cleanliness or uncleanliness. The lesions described in verses 38 and 39 are probably those of psoriasis: "When a man or woman has inflamed patches on the skin and they are white, the priest shall examine them. If they are white and fading, it is dull-white leprosy that has broken out on the skin. The man is ritually clean." *Leviticus* 14 provides further instruction for ritual and animal sacrifice in the management of skin disorders and for the cleansing of clothing and domicile of persons with fungus infections.

LEPROSY

Known also as Hansen's Disease, leprosy, a chronic granulomatous infection that attacks superficial tissues, especially the skin, peripheral nerves, and nasal mucosa, is caused by the bacillus *Mycobacterium leprae*. The disease occurs predominantly in tropical countries, in some of which 1-2% of the population (probably 10-20 million persons the world over) are still affected. It has a long incubation period, ranging from 6 months to several decades. Crippling of the hands, plantar ulcers, and blindness are common complications.

Although this dread disease doubtless occurred in Biblical times it is likely that many other disorders with cutaneous manifestations were included under the rubric of leprosy. Witness, for example, Miriam's punishment: Miriam and Aaron had gossiped about an Ethiopian woman whom Moses may have taken as a wife in addition to the Midianite Zipporah. For this and for her questioning of Moses' prophetic standing the Lord chastised Miriam, "and, behold, Miriam became leprous, white as snow: and Aaron looked upon Miriam, and, behold, she was leprous." Whereupon Moses pleaded, saying: "Heal her now, O God, I beseech thee." And the Lord responded: "Let her be shut out from the camp seven days, and after that let her be received in again. And Miriam was shut out from the camp seven days: and the people journeyed not till Miriam was brought in again." (*Numbers* 12:1-15) Scarcely the clinical picture of leprosy!

More accurately, on the other hand, is the plight of the quarantined leper portrayed in *Psalm* 88, often termed the "Leper's Psalm":

"O Lord, God of my salvation, I have cried day and night before thee;

Let my prayer come before thee: incline thine ear unto my cry;

For my soul is full of troubles: and my life draweth nigh unto the grave.

I am counted with them that go down into the pit: I am as a man that hath no strength:

Free among the dead, like the slain that lie in the grave, whom thou rememberest no more: and they are cut off from thy hand.

Thou hast laid me in the lowest pit, in darkness, in the deeps.

Thy wrath lieth hard upon me, and thou hast afflicted me with all thy waves. Selah.

Shall thy loving kindness be declared in the grave? or thy faithfulness in destruction?

Shall thy wonders be known in the dark? and thy righteousness in the land of forgetfulness?

But unto thee have I cried, O Lord; and in the morning shall my prayer prevent thee.

Lord, why casteth thou off my soul? why hidest thou thy face from me?

I am afflicted and ready to die from my youth up: while I suffer thy terrors I am distracted.

Thy fierce wrath goeth over me; thy terrors have cut me off.

They came round about me daily like water; they compassed me about altogether.

Lover and friend hast thou put far from me, and mine acquaintance into darkness."

For the differentiation of leprosy from other diseases with cutaneous manifestations, such as boils, psoriasis, eczema, and alopecia of other causation, the Lord instructed Moses and Aaron: "When a man shall have in the skin of his flesh a rising, a scab, or bright spot, and it be in the skin of his flesh like the plague of leprosy...the priest shall look on the plague in the skin of the flesh: and when the hair in the plague is turned white, and the plague in sight be deeper than the skin of the flesh, it is a plague of leprosy...If the bright spot be white in the skin of the flesh, and in sight be not deeper than the skin, and the hair thereof be not turned white; then the priest shall shut up him that hath the plague seven days: And the priest shall look on him the seventh day: and, behold, if the plague in his sight be at a stay, and the plague spread not in the skin; then the priest shall shut him up seven days more: And the priest shall look on him again the seventh day: and, behold, if the plague be somewhat dark, and the plague spread not in the skin, the priest shall pronounce him clean: it is but a scab...but if the scab spread much abroad in the skin...he shall be seen of the priest again: and if the priest see that, behold, the scab spreadeth in the skin, then the priest shall pronounce him unclean: it is a leprosy...if the rising be white in the skin, and it have turned the hair white, and there be quick raw flesh in the rising; It is an old leprosy in the skin of his flesh...The flesh also, in which, even in the skin thereof, was a boil, and is healed, And in the place of the boil there be a white rising, or a bright spot, white, and somewhat reddish, and...it be in sight lower than the skin, and the hair thereof be turned white...it is a plague of leprosy broken out of the boil...But if the bright spot stay in his place, and spread not, it is a burning boil...If a man or woman have a plague upon the head or the beard...and, behold, if it be in sight deeper than the skin; and there be in it a yellow thin hair;...it is a dry scall [a scaly or scabby disorder], even a leprosy upon the head or beard...If a man also or a woman have in the skin of their flesh bright spots, even white bright spots...and, behold, if the bright spots...be darkish white; it is a freckled spot that groweth in the skin...And the man whose hair is fallen off his head, he is bald; yet is he clean...And if there be in the bald head, or bald forehead, a white reddish sore, it is a leprosy...And the leper in whom the plague is, his clothes shall be rent, and his head bare, and he shall put a covering upon his upper lip, and shall cry, Unclean, unclean...he shall dwell alone, without the camp shall his habitation be." (*Leviticus* 13:1-46)

Such was the treatment of the leper in Europe until the end of the Middle Ages.[7]

HEMORRHOIDS

Having overcome the Israelites, the Philistines took the ark of the covenant from Eben-ezer and set it in the house of their own god Dagon, in Ashdod. Infuriated, the Lord "smote them with emerods [hemorrhoids]...And when the men of Ashdod saw that it was so, they said, The ark of the God of Israel shall not abide with us: for his hand is sore upon us...They sent therefore and gathered all the lords of the Philistines unto them, and said, What shall we do with the ark of the God of Israel? And they answered, Let the ark of the God of Israel be carried about unto Gath. And they carried the ark of the God of Israel about thither. And it was so, that, after they had carried it about, the hand of the Lord was against the city...and he smote the men of the city, both small and great, and they had emerods in their secret parts...and the cry of the city went up to heaven." (*I. Samuel* 5:1-12)

PLAGUE

The term "plague" is generally used in the Bible in its generic sense, meaning any form of divine punishment, as in leprosy, the plagues of Egypt, the smiting of the complaining Israelites with poisoned quails, and the hemorrhoids inflicted on the Philistines; but as it appears in some places the term probably designates the specific, highly fatal infectious disease, bubonic plague, the "Black Death" of the 14th century, which is caused by the bacillus *Yersinia pestis*, affects rodents, and is transmitted to humans through the bite of infected parasites, especially the rat flea.

When Moses' scouts returned from their surveillance of the Promised Land, "and made all the congregation to murmur against him, by bringing up a slander upon the land, Even those men that did bring up the evil report upon the land died by the plague before the Lord." (*Numbers* 14:36-37)

Soon thereafter, when the children of Israel again provoked the Lord with their protests against the punishment of the rebellious Korah, Dathan, and Abiram, Moses directed Aaron to "make an atonement for them: for there is wrath gone out from the Lord; the plague is begun. And Aaron took as Moses commanded, and ran into the midst of the congregation; and, behold, the plague was begun among the people... Now they that died in the plague were fourteen thousand and seven hundred." (*Numbers* 16:46,47,49) Again the plague was inflicted upon them when the Israelites, abiding in Shittim, committed whoredom with the daughters of Moab and bowed down to their gods; "and those that died in the plague were twenty and four thousand." (*Numbers* 25:1, 9) Following pagan precedent, Zimri attempted to stay the plague's relentless course by cohabiting openly with a Midianite woman and urged his fellow Israelites to follow. (*Numbers* 25:6-8) Transmission of the infection by breath, however, only hastened its spread, producing the deadly pneumonic plague.

A serious pestilential disease strongly suggestive of bubonic plague was indeed endemic in the Near East during the period 1400-1000 B.C.E., and ancient narratives indicate a knowledge of its association with rodents. The relation between rats and plague was rediscovered early in the twentieth century.[8] From 1950 through 1991, 336 cases of plague were reported in the United States.

JOB'S DISEASE

Testing Job, Satan "smote Job with sore boils from the sole of his foot unto his crown. And he took him a potsherd to scrape himself withal; and he set down among the ashes...My flesh is clothed with worms and clods of dust," Job lamented; "my skin is broken, and become loathsome." (*Job* 2:7-8;3:5)

Job's affliction may have been yaws, or framboesia, a chronic infectious disease prevalent in tropical countries, caused by a spirochete, *Treponema pertenue*, probably transmitted by insects, and characterized initially by a skin eruption and later by destructive lesions of the skin and bones, especially the soles of the feet. The earliest reliable accounts of the disease date to the 17th century. In remote regions, unreached by modern medicine, natives still treat the sores of yaws in children by scraping with a rough stone.[9] Clinically related ulcerative conditions widespread in the tropics include tropical ulcer, of uncertain etiology, usually involving the foot or lower third of the leg; and Oriental sore, caused by *Leishmania tropica* and characterized by papular and ulcerating skin lesions.

SMALLPOX

Variola, or smallpox, is a severe, usually fatal viral infection, characterized by a vesicular and pustular eruption, fever, headache, abdominal and back pain, and vomiting. Complications include ocular inflammation, pneumonia, encephalitis, osteomyelitis, and joint effusion. Once widespread, the prevalence of smallpox began to decline after Edward Jenner's discovery of a method of prophylactic vaccination in 1798. By the end of 1975 endemic smallpox was confined to Ethiopia, where the disease was finally eradicated within a few years as a result of the World Health Organization's program of vaccination.

Smallpox may have been the subject of the lament in one of David's psalms:

"O Lord...thine arrows stick fast in me, and thy hand presseth me sore. There is no soundness in my flesh because of thine anger; neither is there any rest in my bones because of my sin...My wounds stink and are corrupt...I am troubled; I am bowed down greatly...For my loins are filled with a loathsome disease...I am feeble and sore broken...my strength faileth me: as for the light of mine eyes, it also is gone from me. My lovers and my friends stand aloof from my sore; and my kinsmen stand afar off." (*Psalm* 38:1-11)

COLITIS

Jehoram, eldest son of Jehoshaphat, after succeeding his father as King of Israel, promptly slew his brothers and performed other acts that were "evil in the eyes of the Lord." The prophet Elijah warned: "Because thou hast not walked in the ways of Jehoshaphat thy father...and hast made Judah and the inhabitants of Jerusalem to go a whoring...and also hast slain thy brethren of thy father's house, which were better than thyself: Behold, with a great plague will the Lord smite thy people...And thou shalt have great sickness by disease of thy bowels, until thy bowels fall out by reason of the sickness..." Soon thereafter, "the Lord stirred up against Jehoram the spirit of the Philistines, and of the Arabians, that were near the Ethiopians...and [they] carried away all the substance that was found in the king's house, and his sons also, and his wives..."

Psychic stress is frequently associated with the onset of ulcerative colitis, the major symptoms of which are bloody diarrhea, abdominal pain, fever, and weight loss. Anorectal complications are common. Jehoram apparently suffered from, and succumbed to, this bowel disorder and its resultant rectal prolapse in his reaction to situational stress: "and after all this the Lord smote him in his bowels with an incurable disease. And it came to pass, that...after two years, his bowels fell out by reason of his sickness: so he died of sore diseases." (*II. Chronicles* 21)

HEAT STRESS

Children and the elderly are particularly susceptible to the physiologic stress of excessive heat, which commonly produces prostration, headache, and nausea. The onset of heat exhaustion, or sunstroke, is usually sudden and may result in death within a few hours. Sunstroke may have been the fate of the Shunammite boy in the harvest field: "And when the child was grown, it fell on a day, that he went out to his father to the reapers. And he said to a lad, Carry him to his mother. And when he had taken him, and brought him to his mother, he sat on her knees till noon, and then died." (*II. Kings* 4:18-20)

Equally plausible as the cause of the boy's death is rupture of a saccular aneurysm, a frequent agent of cerebrovascular accidents. Saccular aneurysms, developmental arterial defects in the form of small, thin-walled blisters, commonly occur in the blood vessels at the base of the brain. They usually produce no symptoms until rupture occurs, when the subject may be stricken with severe headache; and if the resultant hemorrhage is massive, death may follow in minutes or hours.

More clearly was overexposure to the sun the cause of Jonah's malaise, after his loss of protective cover: "And the Lord God prepared a gourd, and made it to come over Jonah, that it might be a shadow over his head...So Jonah was exceeding glad of the gourd. But God prepared a worm when the morning rose the next day, and it smote the gourd that it withered. And it came to pass, when the sun did arise, that God prepared a vehement east wind; and the sun beat upon the head of Jonah, that he fainted, and wished in himself to die, and said, It is better for me to die than to live." (*Jonah* 4:6-8)

HYPOGLYCEMIA

An essential component of the circulating blood is glucose, a simple carbohydrate. Its concentration, commonly known as the "blood sugar," normally varies between 80 and 120 mgm per 100 cc in the fasting state. The level increases somewhat after a meal and may be markedly elevated in certain disease states, notably uncontrolled diabetes. A decline in the blood glucose concentration below normal levels, a condition termed hypoglycemia, may produce fatigue, confusion, hunger (especially craving for sweets), anxiety, rapid pulse, sweating, pallor, hyperactivity or even convulsions, and coma. The syndrome was defined by Dr. Seale Harris of Alabama in 1924. It may result from a variety of causes, such as insulin overdosage or overactivity, as from pancreatic tumor; excessive utilization of glucose by the body tissues, as by heightened metabolism or muscular exertion; and decreased secretion of glucose into the blood, as in starvation, chronic malabsorption, or liver damage.

Another cause of hypoglycemia, recognized only in the mid-twentieth century, is congenital adrenal hyperplasia, a condition in which the adrenal glands produce a surfeit of hormones that virilize the female and cause precocious development of secondary sexual characteristics in the male, including excessive hair growth.

The Torah notes, in the birth of twin sons to Rebekah, that Esau, the first-born, "came out red, all over like an hairy garment." (*Genesis* 25:25) When the twin boys grew up, Esau became a hunter; Jacob, his younger brother, a tiller of the soil. Their struggle for seniority, which had begun inside the womb, continued into adulthood. The first-born son was considered endowed with unique sanctity and was accorded special privilege as second to the head of the family. Ancient Near Eastern custom, nevertheless, permitted an heir to barter away his future inheritance.

My late colleague Dr. Robert Greenblatt, in a series of interpretive vignettes on the Scriptures,[10] interpreted Esau's hairiness as evidence of congenital adrenal hyperplasia, and the exhaustion and hunger that led to the barter of his birthright to his crafty brother as evidence of the associated hypoglycemia. Jacob was cooking a stew of lentils as Esau approached, fatigued and famished after foraging in the wilderness. "And Jacob sod pottage: and Esau came from the field, and he was faint: And Esau said to Jacob, Feed me, I pray thee, with that same red pottage, for I am faint...And Jacob said, Sell me this day thy birthright. And Esau said, Behold, I am at the point to die: and what profit shall this birthright do to me? And Jacob said, Swear to me this day; and he sware unto him: and he sold his birthright unto Jacob. Then Jacob gave Esau bread and pottage of lentils; and he did eat and drink, and rose up, and went his way..." (*Genesis* 25:29-34)

ALCOHOL: ITS USE AND ABUSE

"Inflaming wine, pernicious to mankind,
Unnerves the limbs, and dulls the noble mind."
—Homer: *Iliad*, VI, 261 (translated by Alexander Pope)

Alcohol, an essential in many religious rituals and a social amenity in large segments of society, may alter the function of virtually every organ system. In addition to the highly publicized hazard of drinking and driving, alcohol use in the United States has been associated with 41% of deaths from unintentional falls, 47% of drownings in children under 15 years, 69% of deaths in boating accidents, 49% of episodes of interpersonal violence such as murder or attempted murder, 39% of partner batterings, 50% of reported rapes, and 39 to 58% of deaths in fires.[11] The specific hazards of alcohol for pregnancy are considered separately, in the next chapter.

The intemperate use of alcohol creates problems in three categories: psychologic, sociologic, and medical. All are dealt with in the Scriptures.

The abuse of wine is recorded early in the Torah, near the beginning of human history, with the inebriation of Noah and the ensuing sexual misbehavior of one of his sons: "And Noah began to be an husbandman, and he planted a vineyard: And he drank of the wine, and was drunken; and he was uncovered within his tent. And Ham, the father of Canaan, saw the nakedness of his father, and told his two brethren without...And Noah awoke from his wine, and knew what his younger son had done unto him. And he said, Cursed be Canaan; a servant of servants shall he be unto his brethren."[12] (*Genesis* 9:20-25)

Ten generations later, after the destruction of Sodom and Gomorrah, as Lot dwelt in a cave with his two daughters, drink encouraged their incest with him: "And the firstborn said unto the younger, Our father is old, and there is not a man in the earth to come in unto us after the manner of all the earth: Come, let us make our father drink wine, and we will lie with him, that we may preserve seed of our father. And they made their father drink wine that night: and the firstborn went in, and lay with her father; and he perceived not when she lay down, nor when she arose. And it came to pass on the morrow, that the firstborn said unto the younger, Behold, I lay yesternight with my father: let us make him drink wine this night also; and go thou in, and lie with him, that we may preserve seed of our father. And they made their father drink wine that night also: and the younger arose, and lay with him; and he perceived not when she lay down, nor when she arose. Thus were both the daughters of Lot with child by their father." (*Genesis* 19:31-36)

Repeated reference is made to the mood-enhancing effect of wine in moderation: "Wine that maketh glad the heart of man" (*Psalm* 104:15); "A man hath no better thing under the sun, than to eat, and to drink, and to be merry" (*Ecclesiastes* 8:15); and its soothing effect when diluted with water (mingled) was widely recognized. *Proverbs* (9:1-2;4-6) counseled in poem: "Wisdom hath builded her house...she hath mingled her wine; she hath also furnished her table...as for him that wanteth understanding, she saith to him, Come eat of my bread and drink of the wine which I have mingled. Forsake the foolish, and live; and go in the way of understanding." In a later verse King Lemuel recalled the words of his mother, counseling drink as a balm for the afflicted: "Give strong drink unto him that is ready to perish, and wine unto those that be of heavy hearts. Let him drink, and forget his poverty, and remember his misery no more." (*Proverbs* 31:6-7) But at the same time Lemuel's mother warned: "It is not for kings, O Lemuel, it is not for kings to drink wine; nor for princes strong drink: Lest they drink, and forget the law, and pervert the judgment of any of the afflicted." (*Proverbs* 31:4-5)

Soured wine, turned to vinegar, became the beverage of the field worker. Said Boaz to Ruth as she gleaned ears of corn with him: "When thou art athirst, go unto the vessels, and drink of that which the young men have drawn....At mealtime come thou hither, and dip thy morsel in the vinegar....and he reached her parched corn, and she did eat, and was sufficed..." (*Ruth* 2:9, 14)

More numerous and more ardent are the Scriptural admonitions against drink. Solomon prayed: "Blessed art thou, O land, when thy king is the son of nobles, and thy princes eat in due season, for strength, and not for drunkenness!" (*Ecclesiastes* 10:17) The prophets warned: "Woe unto them that rise up early in the morning, that they may follow strong drink; that continue until night, till wine inflame them! (*Isaiah* 5:11) Referring to "him that sitteth in judgment, and...them that turn the battle to the gate," Isaiah added: "But they also have erred through wine, and through strong drink are out of the way...they are swallowed up of wine...they err in vision, they stumble in judgment." (*Isaiah* 28:6-7) *Proverbs* warn: "Wine is a mocker, strong drink is raging: and whosoever is deceived thereby is not wise"(20:1); "Be not among wine-bibbers; among riotous eaters of flesh: For the drunkard and the glutton shall come to poverty..." (23:20-21); and "Who hath woe? who hath sorrow? who hath contentions? who hath babbling? who hath wounds without cause? who hath redness of eyes? They that tarry long at the wine; they that go to seek mixed wine. Look not thou upon the wine when it is red, when it giveth his colour in the cup, when it moveth itself aright. At the least it biteth like a serpent and stingeth like an adder...They have stricken me, shalt thou say, and I was not sick; they have beaten me, and I felt it not: when shall I awake? I will seek it yet again." (23:29-32,35)

Jeremiah heard the words of the Lord: "Take the wine cup of this fury at my hand, and cause all the nations, to whom I send thee, to drink it. And they shall drink, and be moved, and be mad, because of the sword that I will send among them....Therefore thou shalt say unto them, Thus saith the Lord of hosts, the God of Israel; Drink ye, and be drunken, and spue, and fall, and rise no more...." (*Jeremiah* 25:15-16, 27)

Observed Hosea: "Whoredom and wine and new wine take away the heart." (*Hosea* 4:11) Of women and wine the Talmud warned: "One glass of wine makes the woman pretty; two glasses and she becomes hateful; at the third glass she lusts invitingly; at the fifth glass she becomes so excited that she will solicit an ass upon the streets."

NEURO-PSYCHIATRIC DISORDERS

ANXIETY SYNDROME

Among the curses for disobedience the Bible warns: "the Lord shall give thee a trembling heart, and failing eyes, and sorrows of mind: And thy life shall hang in doubt before thee; and thou shalt fear day and night, and shall have none assurance of thy life." (*Deuteronomy* 28:65-66)

Aphasia

Ezekiel apparently suffered temporary aphasia in his encounter with "the glory of the Lord...by the river of Chebar....Then the spirit entered into me," he recalled, "and spoke with me...and said unto me...I will make thy tongue cleave to the roof of thy mouth, that thou shalt be dumb...But when I speak with thee, I will open thy mouth..." (*Ezekiel* 3:23-27)

Hemiplegia

Zechariah threatened "the idle shepherd that leaveth the flock" with the curse of a stroke. "The sword," he warned, "shall be upon his arm, and upon his right eye: his arm shall be clean dried up, and his right eye shall be utterly darkened." (*Zechariah* 11:17)

Brachial Palsy

King Jeroboam was stricken for his defiance of the word of the Lord and his insistence on burning incense at the altar: "And, behold, there came a man of God out of Judah by the word of the Lord unto Beth-el: and Jeroboam stood by the altar to burn incense. And he cried against the altar in the word of the Lord...And he gave a sign the same day, saying, This is the sign which the Lord hath spoken; Behold, the Altar shall be rent, and the ashes that are upon it shall be poured out. And it came to pass, when King Jeroboam heard the saying of the man of God, which had cried against the altar in Beth-el, that he put forth his hand from the altar, saying, Lay hold on him. And his hand, which he put forth against him, dried up, so that he could not pull it in again to him." (*I. Kings* 13:1-4)

Trance or Petit Mal

Loss of consciousness, or a state of hypnosis, was commonly associated with the presence of God. When Balaam, traditional enemy of the Israelites, "saw that it pleased the Lord to bless Israel...and he saw Israel abiding in his tents according to their tribes...the spirit of God came upon him...He hath said, which heard the words of God, which saw the vision of the Almighty, falling into a trance, but having his eyes open: How goodly are thy tents, O Jacob, and thy tabernacles, O Israel!" (*Numbers* 24:1-5)

Psychoses

King Saul suffered from alternating bouts of exaltation, depression, and paranoia, and ended his life in suicide. Music, anticipating today's art therapy, apparently produced some temporary improvement in his condition. After being chastised for failing to execute the order of the Lord, to destroy all the Amalekites, Saul became depressed: "The Spirit of the Lord departed from Saul, and an evil spirit from the Lord troubled him. And Saul's servants said unto him, Behold now, an evil spirit from God troubleth thee." (*I. Samuel* 16:14-15) They suggested a remedy: "Let our Lord now command thy servants, which are before thee, to seek out a man, who is a cunning player on an harp: and it shall come to pass, when the evil spirit from God is upon thee, that he shall play with his hand, and thou shalt be well.

"And Saul said unto his servants, Provide me now a man that can play well, and bring him to me. Then answered one of the servants, and said, Behold, I have seen a son of Jesse, the Beth-lehemite, that is cunning in playing, and a mighty valiant man, and a man of war, and prudent in matters, and a comely person, and the Lord is with him. Wherefore Saul sent messengers unto Jesse, and said, Send me David thy son, which is with the sheep. And Jesse took an ass laden with bread, and a bottle of wine, and a kid, and sent them by David his son unto Saul. And David came to Saul, and stood before him: and he loved him greatly; and he became his armour bearer...And it came to pass, when the evil spirit from God was upon Saul, that David took an harp, and played with his hand: so Saul was refreshed, and was well, and the evil spirit departed from him." (*I. Samuel* 16:16-23)

But jealousy, suspicion, and fear of David were soon to overcome Saul. When David returned from his victory over the Philistines and was greeted with singing, dancing, and praise by his fellow Israelites, who proclaimed, "Saul hath slain his thousands, and David his ten thousands...Saul was very wroth, and the saying displeased him; and he said, They have ascribed unto David ten thousands, and to me they have ascribed but thousands: and what can he have more but the kingdom? And Saul eyed David from that day and forward. And it came to pass on the morrow, that the evil spirit from God came upon Saul...and there was a javelin in Saul's hand. And Saul cast the javelin; for he said, I will smite David even to the wall with it...And Saul was afraid of David...[and] Saul thought to make David fall by the hand of the Philistines...and Saul became David's enemy continually." (*I. Samuel* 18:6-29)

Jonathan, Saul's son and David's friend, warned of his father's ill intent, but David remained loyal to his master: "And Saul spake to Jonathan his son, and to his servants, that they should kill David." After renewed war with the Philistines, in which David "slew them with a great slaughter; and they fled from him...the evil spirit from the Lord was [again] upon Saul, as he sat in his house with his javelin in his hand; and David played with his hand. And Saul sought to smite David even to the wall with the javelin; but he slipped away out of Saul's presence, and he smote the javelin into the wall: and David fled and escaped that night." Saul sent messengers to capture David, so that he might slay him; but with his wife's collusion, David escaped. Whereupon Saul himself set out in quest of David, "And he went thither to Naioth in Ramah...And he stripped off his clothes...and he lay down naked all that day and all that night." (*I. Samuel* 19:1, 8-24)

David remained in hiding. When his place at the dining table remained empty and Jonathan attempted to explain his friend's absence, "Saul's anger was kindled against Jonathan, and he said unto him, Thou son of the perverse rebellious woman, do I not know that thou hast chosen the son of Jesse to thine own confusion, and unto the confusion of thy mother's nakedness?...And Saul cast a javelin at him to smite him...So Jonathan arose from the table in fierce anger...for he was grieved for David, because his father had done him shame." (*I. Samuel* 20:30-34)

Again the Philistines warred against Israel. "And the battle went sore against Saul...Then said Saul unto his armourbearer, Draw thy sword, and thrust me through therewith....But his armourbearer would not....Therefore Saul took a sword and fell upon it...So Saul died." (*I. Samuel* 31:1-6)

Death by suicide was also the fate of Ahithophel, aide to David's son Absalom. Ahithophel counseled the young warrior in his intrigue against his father: "let me now choose out twelve thousand men, and I will arise and pursue after David this night. And I will come upon him while he is weary and weak handed, and will make him afraid: and all the people that are with him shall flee; and I will smite the king only: And I will bring back all the people unto thee." But Absalom rejected Ahithophel's plan for that of Hushai the Archite. "And when Ahithophel saw that his counsel was not followed, he saddled his ass, and arose, and put his household in order, and hanged himself, and died..." (*II. Samuel* 17:1, 14, 23)

David himself, in his flight from Saul, had feigned insanity when seeking refuge in the court of Achish, king of Gath: "And the servants of Achish said unto him, Is not this David the king of the land? did they not sing one to another in dances, saying, Saul hath slain his thousands, and David his ten thousands? And David laid up these words in his heart, and was sore afraid of Achish the king of Gath. And he changed his behaviour before them, and feigned himself mad in their hands, and scrabbled on the doors of the gate and let his spittle fall down upon his beard. Then said Achish unto his servants, Lo, ye see the man is mad: wherefore then have ye brought him to me?" (*I. Samuel* 21:10-14)

Another king afflicted with manic, schizoid, and paranoid behavior was Nebuchadnezzar. He had made a golden image and decreed that all persons, on pain of death, fall down in worship before it. When the Israelites Shadrach, Meshach, and Abed-nego refused, Nebuchadnezzar ordered them bound and cast into "the burning fiery furnace"; but upon their bodies "the fire had no power, nor was an hair of their head singed, neither were their coats changed, nor the smell of fire had passed on them." Soon thereafter the king became troubled by dreams, which his magicians, astrologers, and soothsayers could not interpret. To Daniel he confided: "Thus were the visions of mine head in my bed; I saw, and behold a tree in the midst of the earth, and the height thereof was great. The tree grew, and was strong, and the height thereof reached unto heaven, and the sight thereof to the end of all the earth: The leaves thereof were fair, and the fruit thereof much, and in it was meat for all: the beasts of the field had shadow under it, and the fowls of the heaven dwelt in the boughs thereof, and all flesh was fed of it. I saw in the visions of my head upon my bed, and, behold, a watcher and an holy one came down from heaven; He cried aloud, and said thus, Hew down the tree, and cut off his branches, shake off his leaves, and scatter his fruit: let the beasts get away from under it, and the fowls from his branches: Nevertheless leave the stump of his roots in the earth...and let it be wet with the dew of heaven, and let his portion be with the beasts in the grass of the earth: Let his heart be changed from a man's, and let a beast's heart be given unto him..."

Daniel pondered an hour and responded: "It is thou, O king, that art grown and become strong: for thy greatness is grown and reacheth unto heaven, and thy dominion to the end of the earth...This is the interpretation...That they shall drive thee from men, and thy dwelling shall be with the beasts of the field, and they shall make thee to eat grass as oxen, and they shall wet thee with the dew of heaven....And whereas they commanded to leave the stump of the tree roots; thy kingdom shall be sure unto thee, after that thou shalt have known that the heavens do rule."

Twelve months later, as he walked in his palace in Babylon, Nebuchadnezzar heard "a voice from heaven, saying, O king Nebuchadnezzar, to thee it is spoken; the kingdom is departed from thee...The same hour was the thing fulfilled...and he was driven from men, and did eat grass as oxen, and his body was wet with the dew of heaven, till his hairs were grown like eagles' feathers, and his nails like birds' claws."

The king later recalled: "And at the end of the days I Nebuchadnezzar lifted up mine eyes unto heaven, and mine understanding returned unto me, and I blessed the most High...At the same time my reason returned unto me...mine honour and brightness returned unto me...and I was established in my kingdom..." (*Daniel* 3:1-27; 4:5-36)

DREAMS

Dreams figure prominently in several other Biblical narratives. Their interpretation, widely publicized through the twentieth-century writings of Freud and integral to the theory and practice of psychoanalysis, has been practiced by seers, prophets, and soothsayers from time immemorial.

Abram, later renamed Abraham, had sired no children in his marriage with Sarai, who was to become Sarah, and had voiced the fear that he would die childless, when the Lord reassured him. Abram then dreamed that his progeny would become mighty nations, but only after their Egyptian bondage: "After these things the word of the Lord came unto Abram in a vision, saying, Fear not, Abram: I am thy shield, and thy exceeding great reward. And Abram said, Lord God, what wilt thou give me, seeing I go childless...to me thou hast given no seed...and, behold, the word of the Lord came unto him, saying...out of thine own bowels shall be thine heir. And he brought him forth abroad, and said, Look now toward heaven, and tell the stars, if thou be able to number them: and he said unto him, So shall thy seed be....And when the sun was going down, a deep sleep fell upon Abram; and lo, an horror of great darkness fell upon him. And he said unto Abram, Know of a surety that thy seed shall be a stranger in a land that is not their's, and shall serve them; and they shall afflict them four hundred years. And also that nation, whom they shall serve, will I judge: and afterward shall they come out with great substance. And thou shalt go to thy fathers in peace; thou shalt be buried in a good old age. But in the fourth generation they shall come hither again: for the iniquity of the Amorites is not yet full. And it came to pass, that when the sun went down, and it was dark, behold a smoking furnace, and a burning lamp that passed between those pieces." (*Genesis* 15:1-5, 12-17)

Having settled in Gerar, Abraham told King Abimelech that Sarah was his sister, in order to protect himself from those who might covet his beautiful wife.[13] Whereupon "Abimelech king of Gerar sent, and took Sarah. But God came to Abimelech in a dream by night, and said to him, Behold, thou art but a dead man, for the woman which thou hast taken; for she is a man's wife. But Abimelech had not come near her: and he said, Lord, wilt thou slay also a righteous nation? Said he not unto me, She is my sister? and she, even she herself said, He is my brother: in the integrity of my heart and innocence of my hands have I done this. And God said unto him in a dream, Yea, I know that thou didst this in the integrity of thy heart; for I also withheld thee from sinning against me: therefore suffered I thee not to touch her. Now therefore restore the man his wife; for he is a prophet, and he shall pray for thee, and thou shalt live: and if thou restore her not, know that thou shalt surely die, thou, and all that are thine." (*Genesis* 20:1-7)

Paralyzed by the fear of the Lord, Abimelech had apparently become impotent with Sarah. Infertility was God's threat against his entire kingdom. The king atoned: "And Abimelech took sheep, and oxen, and gave them unto Abraham, and restored him Sarah his wife. And Abimelech said, Behold, my land is before thee: dwell where it pleaseth thee....So Abraham prayed unto God: and God healed Abimelech and his wife, and his maidservants; and they bare children. For the Lord had fast closed up all the wombs of the house of Abimelech because of Sarah Abraham's wife." (*Genesis* 20:14-18)

Joseph's dreams and his interpretations of dreams have provided abundant grist for the psychoanalyst's mill. Younger than his brothers, he competed with them as a boy by bearing tales of them to his father. "Now Israel [Jacob] loved Joseph more than all his children, because he was the son of his old age: and he made him a coat of many colours. And when his brethren saw that their father loved him more than all his brethren, they hated him and could not speak peaceably unto him."

Joseph retaliated against his brothers by recounting to them a dream he had had, with its possible sexual implications: "And Joseph dreamed a dream, and he told it his brethren: and they hated him yet the more. And he said unto them, Hear, I pray you, this dream which I have dreamed: For, behold, we were binding sheaves in the field, and, lo, my sheaf arose, and also stood upright; and, behold, your sheaves stood round about, and made obeisance to my sheaf. And his brethren said to him, Shalt thou indeed reign over us? or shalt thou indeed have dominion over us? And they hated him yet the more for his dreams, and for his words. And he dreamed yet another dream, and told it his brethren, and said, Behold, I have dreamed a dream more; and, behold, the sun and the moon and the eleven stars made obeisance to me. And he told it to his brethren: and his father rebuked him, and said unto him, What is this dream that thou hast dreamed? Shall I and thy mother and thy brethren indeed come to bow down ourselves to thee to the earth? And his brethren envied him..." (*Genesis* 37:2-11)

Some years later, while in Egypt, serving in the household of Potiphar, captain of Pharaoh's guard, Joseph again demonstrated his capacity for dream analysis. Pharaoh's cupbearer and baker had been put in Potiphar's custody and were imprisoned for having offended their master. Joseph was assigned to them. Seeing one morning that they were dejected, he asked the reason. "And they said unto him, We have dreamed a dream, and there is no interpreter of it. And Joseph said unto them...tell me them, I pray you. And the chief butler told his dream to Joseph, and said to him, In my dream, behold, a vine was before me; And in the vine were three branches: and it was as though it budded, and her blossoms shot forth; and the clusters thereof brought forth ripe grapes: And Pharaoh's cup was in my hand: and I took the grapes, and pressed them into Pharaoh's cup, and I gave the cup into Pharaoh's hand. And Joseph said unto him, This is the interpretation of it: The three branches are three days: Yet within three days shall Pharaoh lift up thine head, and restore thee unto thy place: and thou shalt deliver Pharaoh's cup unto his hand, after the former manner when thou wast his butler...When the chief baker saw that the interpretation was good, he said unto Joseph, I also was in my dream, and, behold, I had three white baskets on my head: And in the uppermost basket there was of all manner of bakemeats for Pharaoh; and the birds did eat them out of the basket upon my head.

And Joseph answered and said, This is the interpretation thereof: The three baskets are three days: Yet within three days shall Pharaoh lift up thy head from off thee, and shall hang thee on a tree; and the birds shall eat thy flesh from off thee. And it came to pass the third day, which was Pharaoh's birthday, that he made a feast unto all his servants: and he lifted up the head of the chief butler and of the chief baker among his servants. And he restored the chief butler unto his butlership again; and he gave the cup into Pharaoh's hand: But he hanged the chief baker: as Joseph had interpreted to them." (*Genesis* 40:7-13, 16-22)

Two years later Pharaoh dreamed that he was standing by the Nile. "And, behold, there came up out of the river seven well favoured kine [cattle] and fatfleshed; and they fed in a meadow. And, behold, seven other kine came up after them out of the river, ill favoured and leanfleshed; and stood by the other kine upon the brink of the river. And the ill favoured and leanfleshed kine did eat up the seven well favoured and fat kine. So Pharaoh awoke. And he slept and dreamed the second time: and, behold, seven ears of corn came up upon one stalk, rank and good. And, behold, seven thin ears and blasted with the east wind sprung up after them. And the seven thin ears devoured the seven rank and full ears. And Pharaoh awoke, and, behold, it was a dream." (*Genesis* 41:1-7)

When none of the wise men of Egypt could explain Pharaoh's dreams, his chief butler recalled the "young man, an Hebrew, servant to the captain of the guard," who had interpreted his and the chief baker's dreams two years before. Pharaoh summoned Joseph, recounted his dreams, and sought their meaning. "And Joseph said unto Pharaoh, The dream of Pharaoh is one: God hath shewed Pharaoh what he is about to do. The seven good kine are seven years; and the seven good ears are seven years...And the seven thin and ill favoured kine that came up after them are seven years; and the seven empty ears blasted with the east wind shall be seven years of famine...Behold, there come seven years of great plenty throughout all the land of Egypt: And there shall arise after them seven years of famine...and the famine shall consume the land...and God will shortly bring it to pass." (*Genesis* 41:25-32)

Joseph counseled Pharaoh accordingly: to stockpile grain during the good years to sustain the populace during the famine to follow. Pharaoh and his courtiers recognized the acuity of Joseph's interpretation and the soundness of his advice, "And Pharaoh said unto Joseph, Forasmuch as God hath shewed thee all this, there is none so discreet and wise as thou art. Thou shalt be over my house, and according unto thy word shall all my people be ruled: only in the throne will I be greater than thou...I have set thee over all the land of Egypt." (*Genesis* 41:34-41)

GIGANTISM

Pituitary tumors of a specific cell type known as eosinophiles, because of their affinity for the dye eosin, may produce excessive growth, acromegaly or gigantism, as a result of their uncontrolled secretion of the growth hormone. The Bible tells of two giants, Og king of Bashan and Goliath the Philistine: "For only Og king of Bashan remained of the remnants of giants; behold, his bedstead was a bedstead of iron...nine cubits was the length thereof, and four cubits the breadth of it"[14] (*Deuteronomy* 3:11); and Goliath of Gath, "whose height was six cubits and a span."

Remembered by every schoolchild is the tale of Goliath's encounter with David: "And he had an helmet of brass upon his head, and he was armed with a coat of mail; and the weight of the coat was 5000 shekels of brass. And he had greaves of brass upon his legs, and a target of brass between his shoulders. And the staff of his spear was like a weaver's beam; and his spear's head weighed six hundred shekels of iron [about 10 kilograms]...And all the men of Israel, when they saw the man, fled from him, and were sore afraid...And David said to Saul, Let no man's heart fail because of him; thy servant will go and fight with this Philistine. And Saul said to David, Thou art not able to go against this Philistine to fight with him: for thou art but a youth, and he a man of war from his youth. And David said unto Saul, Thy servant kept his father's sheep, and there came a lion, and a bear, and took a lamb out of the flock: And I went out after him, and smote him, and delivered it out of his mouth: and when he arose against me, I caught him by his beard, and smote him, and slew him...The Lord that delivered me out of the paw of the lion, and out of the paw of the bear, he will deliver me out of the hand of this Philistine. And Saul said unto David, Go, and the Lord be with thee...And he took his staff in his hand, and chose him five smooth stones out of the brook, and put them in a shepherd's bag...and his sling was in his hand: and he drew near to the Philistine...And David put his hand in his bag, and took thence a stone, and slang it, and smote the Philistine in his forehead...and he fell upon his face to the earth...Therefore David ran, and stood upon the Philistine, and took his sword...and slew him, and cut off his head therewith. And when the Philistines saw their champion was dead, they fled." (*I. Samuel* 17:4-51)

The genetic nature of Goliath's gigantism is suggested by a subsequent verse, which tells of a son of the giant, of tall stature with polydactyly (excessive digits): "And there was yet a battle in Gath, where was a man of great stature, that had on every hand six fingers, and on every foot six toes, four and twenty in number; and he also was born to the giant." (*II. Samuel* 21:20)

RESUSCITATION

"And the Lord God formed man of the dust of the ground, and breathed into his nostrils the breath of life; and man became a living soul." (*Genesis* 2:7)

Mouth-to-mouth resuscitation, still used in the absence of special equipment, was first described in the Torah, as Elisha ministered to the Shunammite lad, apparently dead after succumbing in the field: "And when Elisha was come into the house, behold, the child was dead, and laid upon his bed. He went in therefore, and shut the door upon them twain, and prayed unto the Lord. And he went up, and lay upon the child, and put his mouth upon his mouth, and his eyes upon his eyes, and his hands upon his hands: and he stretched himself upon the child; and the flesh of the child waxed warm. Then he returned, and walked in the house to and fro; and went up and stretched himself upon him: and the child sneezed seven times, and the child opened his eyes." (*II. Kings* 4:32-35)

The prone pressure method of artificial respiration, long recommended by the Red Cross, was anticipated by Elijah the Tishbite. Elijah, according to the word of the Lord, journeyed to Zarephath, where he met a widow who sustained him several days from her meager larder. "And it came to pass...that the son of the woman, the mistress of the house, fell sick; and his sickness was so sore, that there was no breath left in him...And he said unto her, Give me thy son. And he took him out of her bosom, and carried him up into a loft, where he abode, and laid him upon his own bed...And he stretched himself upon the child three times, and cried unto the Lord, and said, O Lord my God, I pray thee, let this child's soul come into him again. And the Lord heard the voice of Elijah, and the soul of the child came into him again, and he revived. And Elijah took the child, and brought him down out of the chamber into the house, and delivered him unto his mother: and Elijah said, See, thy son liveth." (*I. Kings* 17:10, 17-23)

Post-biblical techniques for restoring life to the limp and apneic newborn have included swinging, spanking, dipping the infant alternately into tubs of hot and cold water, and the administration of stimulant drugs. Henry R. Silvester introduced in 1858 a method of resuscitation of the apparently stillborn or drowned in which the subject was placed on its back, its shoulders elevated by a rolled towel, extending the neck. The arms were extended slowly over the head and held in this position through the count of 5. This maneuver elevated the ribs, expanding the chest and drawing air into the lungs. The arms were then carried back down and pressed against the chest, producing expiration.[15]

Bernhard Sigmund Schultze (1827-1919), distinguished German obstetrician, suggested a method of resuscitation in 1866 in which the infant was grasped by the shoulders and upper arms and swung upward, above the operator's head. The weight of the viscera, pressing against the diaphragm, helped expel fluid from the air passages. After being held in this position while the operator counted to 5, the infant was swung down again between the former's knees, where the drag upon the diaphragm aided inspiration.

Somewhat different in detail, but employing the same principles, was Dew's method of resuscitation, introduced a quarter-century later: "Grasp the infant with the left hand, allowing the neck to rest between the thumb and forefinger, the head falling far over backward...Then with the right hand...grasp the knees...This position will allow the back of the thighs to rest in the palm of the operator's hand...The next step is to depress the pelvis and lower extremities so as to allow the abdominal organs to drag the diaphragm downward, and with the left hand to gently bend the dorsal region of the spine backward. This enlarges the thoracic cavity and produces inspiration. Then, to excite expiration, reverse the movement...At the same time bring forward the thighs, resting them upon the abdomen. This movement...so bends the child upon itself as to crowd together the contents of the thoracic and abdominal cavities, bringing about a most complete and forcible expiration."[16]

All these mechanical methods of resuscitation have been superseded during the twentieth century by gentle handling, maintenance of a clear airway, supplementary oxygenation, and medicinal adjuvants.

SENILITY

"Old age hath yet his honor and his toil;
Death closes all; but something ere the end,
Some work of noble note, may yet be done."
—Alfred, Lord Tennyson: "Ulysses"

Unsurpassed in poetry or prose is the characterization of old age in the last chapter of Ecclesiastes, in which are depicted the depression, irritability, dementia, insomnia, phobias, tremors, arthritis, osteoporosis, loss of libido, urinary incontinence, and finally, heart failure, of senility:

"Remember now thy Creator in the days of thy youth, while the evil days come not, nor the years draw nigh, when thou shalt say, I have no pleasure in them; While the sun, or the light, or the moon, or the stars, be not darkened, nor the clouds return after the rain: In the day when the keepers of the house shall tremble, and the strong men shall bow themselves, and the grinders cease because they are few, and those that look out of the windows be darkened, And the doors shall be shut in the streets, when the sound of the grinding is low, and he shall rise up at the voice of the bird, and all the daughters of musick shall be brought low; Also when they shall be afraid of that which is high, and fears shall be in the way, and the almond tree shall flourish, and the grasshopper shall be a burden, and desire shall fail: because man goeth to his long home, and the mourners go about the streets: Or ever the silver cord be loosed, or the golden bowl be broken, or the pitcher be broken at the fountain, or the wheel broken at the cistern. Then shall the dust return to the earth as it was: and the spirit shall return unto God who gave it. Vanity of vanities,...all is vanity." (*Ecclesiastes* 12:1-8)

The dimming of Isaac's vision with aging is mentioned also in *Genesis* 27:1-2: "And it came to pass, that when Isaac was old, and his eyes were dim, so that he could not see, he called Esau his eldest son, and said unto him, My son...I am old, I know not the day of my death." Eli suffered similarly: "And it came to pass...when Eli was laid down in his place, and his eyes began to wax dim, that he could not see..." (*I. Samuel* 3:2) Abijah too "could not see; for his eyes were set by reason of his age." (*I. Kings* 14:4)

Barzillai the Gileadite had befriended King David but was too frail in his old age to accept the latter's hospitality: "Now Barzillai was a very aged man, even fourscore years old: and he had provided the king of sustenance while he lay at Mahanaim...And the king said unto Barzillai, Come thou over with me, and I will feed thee with me in Jerusalem. And Barzillai said unto the king, How long have I to live, that I should go up with the king unto Jerusalem? I am this day fourscore years old: and can I discern between good and evil? can thy servant taste what I eat or drink? can I hear any more the voice of singing men and singing women? wherefore then should thy servant be yet a burden unto my lord the king? Thy servant will go a little way over Jordan with the king: and why should the king recompense it me with such a reward? Let thy servant, I pray thee, turn back again, that I may die in mine own city, and be buried by the grave of my father and of my mother." (*II. Samuel* 19:32-37)

David himself, notorious for his amorous exploits in earlier years, was bereft of sexual ardor in later life: "Now king David was old and stricken in years; and they covered him with clothes, but he gat no heat. Wherefore his servants said unto him, Let there be sought for my lord the king a young virgin: and let her stand before the king, and let her cherish him, and let her lie in thy bosom, that my lord the king may get heat. So they sought for a fair damsel throughout all the coasts of Israel, and found Abishag a Shunammite, and brought her to the king. And the damsel was very fair, and cherished the king, and ministered to him: but the king knew her not." (*I. Kings* 1:1-4)

Wisely counseled the psalmist: "So teach us to number our days, that we may apply our hearts unto wisdom." (*Psalm* 90:12)

SUMMARY

The Bible abounds with evidence of medical acumen and foretells some of the methods of modern medicine, such as antisepsis, incineration, and quarantine. Modern geologic studies have documented the skill with which King Hezekiah's craftsmen created a water supply system for Jerusalem. Specific ailments are described and methods for their management prescribed. Sexual transmission of disease was recognized, but no distinction was made among types of genital discharge: any such issue rendered the subject unclean. The Bible provides a few criteria for the differential diagnosis of dermatologic disorders, but most were called leprosy. Hemorrhoids served as punishment to the Philistines for absconding with the ark of the covenant. The term "plague" is used not only in its generic sense, for any form of divine punishment, but also for a specific infectious disease, perhaps what was later designated "bubonic plague." Job's affliction may have been yaws, a chronic infectious disease still prevalent in remote tropical regions. Described also in the Bible are colitis, heat stress, hypoglycemia, alcohol abuse, gigantism, senility, and a variety of neuropsychiatric disorders including aphasia, hemiplegia, brachial palsy, petit mal, and psychoses. Dreams were interpreted by Joseph, as by today's psychoanalysts.

The Bible says little of therapy; but resuscitation by Elijah and Elisha foretells the mechanical methods of artificial respiration of the 19th and 20th centuries; and the latter prophet's successful resort to flour meal as an antidote against gourd toxins has been confirmed by modern pharmacologic experiment (chapter 14).

NOTES AND REFERENCES

1. Descendants of Levi, one of Jacob's sons.
2. The Talmud tells of a medical manuscript of King Solomon entitled *Sefer Refuah* ("Book of Health"), believed to have been hidden by King Hezekiah, and of a treatise on pharmacology, *Megilath Sammanim*, but both are lost.
3. Preuss J. Biblisch-Talmudische Medizin, 3rd ed. Berlin: Karger 1923; English translation by Fred Rosner: New York: Froben Press, 1936; Shepherd MB: The Bible as a Source Book for Physicians. Glasgow: MJ. 1955; 36:348-375.
4. Brim CJ. Medicine in the Bible. New York: Froben Press 1936:199-200.
5. Ashes from the fire of cedar wood, hyssop, crimson stuff from the scarlet worm, and a sacrificial heifer; perhaps serving as an abrasive in the ablution ritual.
6. Gill D. Subterranean Waterworks of Biblical Jerusalem: Adaptation of a Karst System. Science 1991; 254:1467-1471.
7. Garrison FH. Introduction to the History of Medicine. Philadelphia: WB Saunders 1929:67.
8. Mendenhall GE. The Tenth Generation. Baltimore: Johns Hopkins Press 1973:107.
9. Shepherd MB. The Bible as a Source Book for Physicians. Gasgow: MJ. 1955; 36:348-375.
10. Greenblatt R. Search the Scriptures. Philadelphia: Lippincott 1963:11-15.

11. JAMA 1992; 267:2289.
12. Ham was actually the middle of Noah's three sons. The Torah fails to make clear why Noah's curse was placed on Canaan, Ham's son, rather than on Ham himself, perpetrator of the sexual misdeed. Rabbinic authorities are divided as to whether Ham castrated his father or committed sodomy on him.
13. Abraham and Sarah did indeed have the same father, but different mothers.
14. The cubit is believed to have been measured from the tip of a man's middle finger to his elbow. Og's legendary bed is thus estimated at 13 to 16 feet in length and 6 to 7 feet in width.
15. Silvester HR. A new method of resuscitating still-born children, and of restoring persons apparently drowned or dead. Brit Med J 1858; 2:576.
16. Dew JH. Establishing a new method of artificial respiration in asphyxia neonatorum. Med Rec 1893; 43:289.

CHAPTER 5

BIBLICAL OBSTETRICS

FERTILITY AND INFERTILITY

"Children are an heritage of the Lord: and the fruit of the womb is his reward." (Psalm 127:3)

Among God's earliest words to humankind was the command to procreate: "Be fruitful, and multiply," He enjoined the first couple. (*Genesis* 1:28) Again, after the Flood, God repeated His blessing, to "Noah and his sons, and said unto them, Be fruitful, and multiply, and replenish the earth." (*Genesis* 9:1) Ten generations later, in God's covenant with Abraham, God promised: "I will make thee exceeding fruitful, and I will make nations of thee" (*Genesis* 17:6); and in reward for obeying His order to bind Isaac for sacrifice, God reiterated this commitment: "…because thou hast done this thing, and hast not withheld thy son…I will bless thee, and…I will multiply thy seed as the stars of the heaven, and as the sand which is upon the sea shore." (*Genesis* 22:16-17)

Abraham's grandson Jacob subsequently sired 12 sons[1] and a daughter, Dinah, of his two wives, Leah and Rachel, and their respective handmaids, Zilpah and Bilhah; and Rehoboam, son of King Solomon, "begat twenty and eight sons and threescore daughters," born of his 18 wives and 60 concubines (*II Chronicles* 11:21); but only one woman, it appears, Milcah, wife of Abraham's brother Nahor, produced more than seven offspring (*Genesis* 22:23): ("She that hath borne seven languisheth: she hath given up the ghost.") (*Jeremiah* 15:9). Nowhere was overpopulation a problem, and never was the need expressed for fertility control.

Infertility, on the other hand, was considered a curse from God. To Abraham Sarah explained: "The Lord hath restrained me from bearing." (*Genesis* 16:2) Hannah's infertility was likewise divinely ordained: "The Lord had shut up her womb." (*I Samuel* 1:5) And "the Lord had fast closed up all the wombs of the house of Abimelech," because of the king's treatment of Sarah. (*Genesis* 20:18) Jeremiah voiced the curse of God: "Write ye this man childless…" (*Jeremiah* 22:30)

Some characteristics of the infertile woman, indicative of hypoovarian or adrenogenital syndromes, are recognized in the Talmud: Any woman 20 years of age who has not produced two pubic hairs...without breasts and suffering pain during copulation...without a mons veneris like that of other women...or with a voice so deep as to be indistinguishable between male and female.[2]

To cure their sterility the Lord opened the wombs of Sarah (*Genesis* 18:10-14) and Leah. (*Genesis* 29:31)

Until the middle of the 19th century the male's biologic responsibility in procreation was believed to hinge solely on his ability to consummate the act of coitus. Potency was synonymous with fertility. This notion was dispelled only after the application of the microscope to the study of sterility and the observation of spermatozoa and their survivability within the female genital tract.[3] The Bible, however, had already suggested the role of man as well as woman in infertility: "There shall not be male or female barren among you..."(*Deuteronomy* 7:14)

The infertile woman became the subject of scorn and ridicule. When Sarah's handmaid Hagar realized that she had conceived while Sarah remained childless, "her mistress was despised in her eyes." (*Genesis* 16:4) Childless Rachel pleaded to Jacob: "Give me children, or else I die." (*Genesis* 30:1) Elkanah had two wives, Hannah and Peninnah, When Hannah remained childless, "her adversary...provoked her sore, for to make her fret, because the Lord had shut up her womb." (*I. Samuel* 1:6)

During her long period of infertility before conceiving Samuel, Hannah vowed: "O Lord of hosts, if thou wilt indeed look on the affliction of thine handmaid, but wilt give unto thine handmaid a man child, then I will give him unto the Lord all the days of his life..." (*I. Samuel* 1:11) Rebekah was slow to conceive after her marriage to Isaac. The patriarch "intreated the Lord for his wife, because she was barren: and the Lord was intreated of him, and Rebekah his wife conceived." (*Genesis* 25:21)

Not content with prayer alone, some resorted to teraphim, amulets, small idols or household gods, for help in procreation. When Rachel departed her father's household with her husband Jacob, she stole the images that it contained. (*Genesis* 31:19) Michal, Saul's daughter and David's wife, possessed an icon which, to cover her husband's escape from her enraged father, she placed in David's bed "and put a pillow of goat's hair for his holster, and covered it with cloth." (*I. Samuel* 19:13)

They sought other divinities also, in addition to the God of Israel. After the death of Joshua, while the children of Israel were dwelling among the Canaanites, some "forsook the Lord God of their fathers...and followed other gods, of the gods of the people that were round about them...and served Baal and Ashtaroth"[4] (*Judges* 2:12-13) Even wise King Solomon, who "loved many strange women...and had seven hundred wives, princesses, and three hundred concubines...went after

Ashtoreth the goddess of the Zidonians, and after Milcom the abomination of the Ammonites." (*I. Kings* 11:3,5)

When prayer and amulets failed, other means were sought to combat infertility. Immortalized in poetry and prose is the mandrake, or love apple, whose forked root, sometimes bearing a crude resemblance to the human form, suggested multiple medicinal virtues. A member of the tomato-nightshade family, it yields an alkaloid similar to belladonna.[5] Opinion was divided as to its primary effect being aphrodisiac or soporific. Shakespeare wrote:

"Not poppy, nor mandragora,
Nor all the drowsy syrups of the world,
Shall ever medicine thee to that sweet sleep
Which thou ow'dst yesterday."
(*Othello, III, iii*)
And Cleopatra pleaded:
"Give me to drink mandragora...
That I might sleep out this great gap of time,
My Antony is away."
(*Antony and Cleopatra, I, v*)

Dioscorides, famous herbalist of the first century C.E., told of other of the plant's effects: "Some do seeth the roots in wine...as much as half an Obolus, it expels ye menstrua, and ye embryo...The seed of the apples being drank purgeth ye matrix...Another sort called Morion...being drank as much as a dragm or eaten with Polenta, in Placetum, or Obsonium it doth infatuate." Some believed the mandrake so powerful in promoting conception that it needed only to be placed under a bedspread to produce its effect.[6]

To obtain the hand of his beloved Rachel, Jacob served his uncle Laban 7 years, only to be tricked into marriage with the latter's firstborn daughter Leah instead. Promising to serve Laban yet another 7 years, Jacob took Rachel to wife also. Bitter rivalry between the sisters resulted. Leah produced four sons (Reuben, Simeon, Levi, and Judah), then endured a period of infertility; while Rachel remained childless. Each provided her handmaid to Jacob, to augment their families; and each handmaid bore Jacob two children. Mandrakes were sought by the sisters for relief of their infertility:

"And Reuben went in the days of wheat harvest, and found mandrakes in the field, and brought them unto his mother Leah. Then Rachel said to Leah, Give me, I pray thee, of thy son's mandrakes. And she said unto her, Is it a small matter that thou hast taken my husband? and wouldest thou take away my son's mandrakes also? And Rachel said, Therefore he shall lie with thee tonight for thy son's mandrakes. And Jacob came out of the field in the evening, and Leah went out to meet him, and said, Thou must come in unto me; for surely I have hired thee with my son's mandrakes. And he lay with her that night. And God harkened unto Leah, and she conceived, and she bare Jacob the fifth son." (*Genesis* 30:14-17)

Rachel got the mandrakes. Leah got to sleep with Jacob. Both achieved pregnancy. But not until 3 years later did Rachel give birth to Joseph. Were the mandrakes to be credited for their tranquilizing effect or their power to directly enhance fertility? Or, as the Bible suggests, was the cure of Rachel's infertility God's handiwork?

CONCEPTION

Human conception, development, and birth were summarized in "The Wisdom of Solomon," vii: "I myself also am a mortal man, like to all, and the offspring of him that was first made of the earth, and in my mother's womb was fashioned to be flesh in the time of ten months, being compacted in blood, of the seed of man, and the pleasure that came with sleep. And when I was born, I drew in the common air, and fell upon the earth, which is of like nature, and the first voice which I uttered was crying, as all others do. I was nursed in swaddling clothes, and that with cares. For there is no king that had any other beginning of birth. For all men have one entrance into life, and the like going out."[7]

Embryology remained largely a mystery. The psalmist thus noted the fructification of man's seed within the womb: "My substance was not hid from thee, when I was made in secret, and curiously wrought in the lowest parts of the earth. Thine eyes did see my substance, yet being unperfect; and in thy book all my members were written, which in continuance were fashioned, when as yet there was none of them." (*Psalm* 139:15-16) Primitive also was Job's concept of human development: "Hast thou not poured me out as milk, and curdled me like cheese? Thou has clothed me with skin and flesh, and has fenced me with bones and sinews." (*Job* 10:10-11) The author of Ecclesiastes conceded: "As thou knowest not what is the way of the spirit, nor how the bones do grow in the womb of her that is with child: even so thou knowest not the works of God who maketh all." (11:15)

MIDWIVES

From earliest time and in every culture special attendants have proffered aid to the woman in labor, assuaging her pain, assisting her delivery, and tending her newborn. Reserved by tradition to females, the birth helper was known in Latin as *cummater*, in French as *sage-femme*, in German as *Hebamme*, in Spanish and Portuguese as *comadre*, in English as midwife. Prevalent until the 18th century was the view of Roderigo a Castro, expressed in 1594: *Haec ars viros dedecet* ("This art is not suitable for men"). Talmudic sages decreed that examination of Jewish women be carried out, never by male physicians, but by midwives or other female attendants, who in turn reported their findings to the physician or rabbi for diagnosis and treatment. In 1552 Wertt, a physician in Hamburg, was burned at the stake for having posed as a woman in order to attend a patient in labor.

The Biblical midwife was called *meyalledeth*, from the verb *yalad* (to bear, or bring forth), and in the Mishnah she is referred to as *hakhamah*, or wise woman. Special privileges were granted her, such as travel on the Sabbath or holidays in the practice of her profession; and she, in contrast to other women, could be introduced as a court witness in questions of establishing the rights of the firstborn.[8] "And it came to pass, because the midwives feared God, that he made them houses." (*Exodus* 1:21)

The Bible records the role of the midwife in Rachel's second labor: "Fear not," she reassured Jacob's wife, "thou shalt have this son also." (*Genesis* 35:17) In Tamar's pregnancy the midwife correctly predicted a twin birth and attended their delivery. (*Genesis* 38:27-30)

When the Hebrews were enslaved in Egypt and their high birth rate threatened Pharaoh's security, he ordered that the midwives Shiphrah and Puah destroy all the Jewish males at birth: "And he said, When ye do the office of a midwife to the Hebrew women, and see them upon the stools; if it be a son, then ye shall kill him: but if it be a daughter, then she shall live. But the midwives feared God, and did not as the king of Egypt commanded them, but saved the men children alive. And the king of Egypt called for the midwives, and said unto them, Why have ye done this thing, and have saved the men children alive? And the midwives said unto Pharaoh, Because the Hebrew women are not as the Egyptian women; for they are lively, and are delivered ere the midwives come in unto them. Therefore God dealt well with the midwives: and the people multiplied, and waxed very mighty." (*Exodus* 1:16-20)

Most of the later midwives received no training. Self-taught or instructed by older midwives, many were careless, dirty, and meddlesome. Their first formal training was instituted by Hippocrates in the 5th century B.C.E., but for several subsequent centuries efforts toward their education were halting and ineffectual. The celebrated text of Soranus (98-138 C.E.), the leading authority on obstetrics and gynecology of his era, provided a guide for midwives; but nothing furthered their education until 400 years later, when Eucharius Rösslin's *Rosengarten* appeared, a German language text based in part on the earlier work of Soranus. During the first half of the 18th century academic courses of instruction for student midwives were initiated in conjunction with several European medical schools and hospitals.

In America, despite the increasing role of the physician in obstetric practice during the 18th and 19th centuries, most labors were still attended by midwives. Commonly known as "granny midwives," the majority were untrained, illiterate, and superstitious; and their practices were reflected in the maternal and infant mortality statistics. In 1910 they were still reporting about half of all births in this country; but their numbers declined rapidly, as a result of governmental regulation. In New York City the last of the granny midwives retired in 1963, having performed her final delivery in 1961.

Superseding this unlamented guild of birth attendants, a new species of medically trained nurse-midwives appeared on the American scene, providing an ever-increasing proportion of obstetric care in both hospital and home, in cooperation with their physician counterparts.[9]

ANTENATAL CARE

"The pregnant woman is like a ship upon a stormy sea full of whitecaps, and the good pilot who is in charge must guide her with prudence if he is to avoid a shipwreck."
—François Mauriceau: *Traité des maladies des femmes grosses...*, Paris, 1668.

Antenatal care, introduced into medical practice by the nursing profession, is a product of the 20th century, perhaps its most important obstetric advance. Texts of earlier years contain scarcely a word on the subject. The accoucheur, midwife or physician, attended at labor and delivery, and was summoned earlier only if the woman had fits, bled, or suffered some other complication. Routine antenatal care as we now know it, with examination for pre-existing disease, hygienic and dietary counseling, measurement of weight and blood pressure, urinalysis, prophylactic immunization, and fetal surveillance, was nonexistent.

Early belief in maternal impression, the concept that exposure of the mother to specific sights, sounds, or other stimuli during pregnancy might result in marking or malformation of the fetus, is illustrated in the Biblical tale of Jacob and the speckled livestock. As Jacob was preparing to leave his uncle Laban, the two men agreed on an equitable division of their flocks, according to color: "And Jacob took him rods of green poplar, and of the hazel and chestnut tree; and pilled white strakes in them, and made the white appear which was in the rods. And he set the rods which he had pilled before the flocks in the gutters in the watering troughs when the flocks came to drink, that they should conceive when they came to drink. And the flocks conceived before the rods, and brought forth cattle ringstraked, speckled, and spotted." (*Genesis* 30:37-39) Jacob attempted to obtain the best animals for himself by placing the sturdiest in view of the marked staves while they mated. The coloring and markings of the offspring, he believed, would be influenced by the maternal visual impressions from the staves.

Traces of this belief are reflected among the ancient Greeks. Empedocles, philosopher of the 5th century B.C.E., remarked that women gave birth to infants resembling the statues that they had admired during pregnancy. The law of Lycurgus, of the 9th century B.C.E., required that Spartan wives look upon the representations of the strong and beautiful as, for example, statues of Castor and Pollux. Soranus of Ephesus (early 2nd century C.E.) spoke of ape-like children born to women who had looked at monkeys around the time of conception.

Such stories are repeated in the Talmud, together with indications of belief in the potency of sensory impressions on the mother after conception. Credence in the influence of maternal impressions on the fetus persisted into the 19th century before its complete rejection by the medical community.[10] For shelter against the evil machinations of Lilith, the embodiment of the devil, Jewish women for centuries wore during pregnancy amulets of the three protective angels Senoi, San-Senori, and Sammangelof.[11]

In the Bible's only example of antepartum hygienic counsel the wife of Manoah received dietary guidance: "And the angel of the Lord appeared unto the woman, and said unto her, Behold now, thou art barren, and bearest not: but thou shalt conceive, and bear a son. Now therefore beware, I pray thee, and drink not wine nor strong drink and eat not any unclean thing." And to Manoah the angel of God reemphasized: "Of all that I said unto the woman let her beware. She may not eat of any thing that cometh of the vine, neither let her drink wine or strong drink...And the woman bare a son and called his name Samson: and the child grew, and the Lord blessed him." (*Judges* 13:2-4,24) Not until the late 20th century was a scientific basis provided for the proscription of drink during pregnancy, with the demonstration of the "fetal alcohol syndrome."

The developing fetus has long been known to be particularly vulnerable to radiant energy. In one of my early researches I found that the rat fetus suffers stunting and increased mortality from intrauterine exposure to sulfanilamide administered in doses safe to the mother during pregnancy.[12] Phocomelia is a rare type of human malformation characterized by the absence of the proximal segment of one or more limbs, which thereby come to resemble seals' flippers. This anomaly attracted wide attention in the fall of 1961, when a great increase was noted in its occurrence and an association established between its appearance and the maternal ingestion of a newly introduced sedative drug, thalidomide. Since this observation a host of chemicals and drugs have been found to be specifically hazardous to the fetus, and all new medications are now studied for their teratogenic effects before being cleared for public use.

Maternal drinking during pregnancy had long been suspected of being injurious to the fetus. Medical evidence of the teratogenic effect of alcohol began to accumulate in the late 1960s, and within a few years the fetal alcohol syndrome was established as a definitive medical entity. Exposure of the fetus to alcohol appears to be the most frequent induced cause of mental deficiency in the Western world.[13] It results in fetal growth retardation and increased rates of abortion and of premature birth, hyperactivity at birth, diminished ability to suck well, and multiple physical defects including facial, cardiac, and cerebral abnormalities. In a study of 685 women, 32% of the infants born to heavy drinkers suffered these birth defects, 14% of the infants born to moderate drinkers were affected, while only 9% of those born to abstainers or women who drank but rarely showed congenital abnormalities.[14]

ABORTION AND MISCARRIAGE

Fully 10%, perhaps as many as 25%, of all pregnancies terminate in spontaneous abortion or miscarriage. Some early pregnancy failures result from maternal disease; other, from trauma or fetal exposure to noxious agents; the majority, from faulty germ plasm in the egg or sperm.

The Bible refers to abortion from trauma and prescribes punishment for the offender and recompense for the aggrieved: "If men strive, and hurt a woman with child, so that her fruit depart from her...he shall surely be punished, according as the woman's husband will lay upon him; and he shall pay as the judges determine." (*Exodus* 21:22)

The Prophets regarded abortion as a weapon of divine retribution. For their wickedness in idolatry and the worship of Baal-peor, Hosea threatened the Israelites: "Their glory shall fly away like a bird, from the birth, and from the womb, and from the conception....Give them, O Lord: what wilt thou give? give them a miscarrying womb and dry breasts....Ephraim is smitten, their root is dried up, they shall bear no fruit....yet will I slay the beloved fruit of their womb." (*Hosea* 9:10-16)

Pleading with Moses on behalf of their sister Miriam, who had been stricken with a cutaneous ailment that the Bible named leprosy, Aaron compared her lot to that of a macerated fetus: "Let her not be as one dead, of whom the flesh is half consumed when he cometh out of his mother's womb." (*Numbers* 12:12)

Job, in his anguish, cursed the day of his birth and bemoaned not having been aborted or having died a neonate: "Why died I not from the womb? why did I not give up the ghost when I came out of the belly?...Or as an hidden untimely birth I had not been; as infants which never saw light." (*Job* 3:11, 16)

The Apocrypha's optimistic prediction of fetal salvage still remains far beyond the reach of late 20th century science: "The woman with child shall bring forth untimely children of three or four months old, and they shall live, and be raised up." (*II Esdras* 6)

DURATION OF PREGNANCY

Although conception can sometimes be dated accurately from isolated coitus or artificial insemination, in the majority of cases the duration of pregnancy must be reckoned from the last menstrual period. William F. Montgomery, distinguished Irish obstetrician of the early-19th century, stated the difficulty in precise dating: "It can hardly be otherwise until we meet in society more numerous imitations of Zenobia, the beautiful Queen of Palmyra, who, if we are to credit Trebellius Pollio, 'never admitted her husband's embraces but for the sake of issue; if her hopes were baffled in the ensuing month, she reiterated her experiment'; but in the existing rarity of such instances of self-command, we are obliged to acknowledge, with regret, that 'as it is difficult to conceal the termination of pregnancy, so it is equally difficult to ascertain its commencement.'"[15]

Invoking Christian dogma, William Harvey, discoverer of the circulation of the blood, wrote in the early 17th century: "Unquestionably the ordinary term of utero-gestation is that which we believe was kept in the womb of his mother by our Saviour Christ, of men the most perfect; counting, viz. from the festival of the Annunciation, in the month of March, to the day of the blessed Nativity, which we celebrate in December [275 days]. Prudent matrons, calculating after this rule, as long as they note the day of the month in which the catamenia usually appear, are rarely out of their reckoning; but after ten lunar months have elapsed, fall in labour, and reap the fruit of their womb the very day on which the catamenia would have appeared, had impregnation not taken place."[15]

In actual practice the date of expected labor has long been estimated by the simple calculation: adding seven days to the date of the first day of the last menstruation and counting back three months, a crude formula known as Naegele's Rule, after Franz Carl Naegele (1778-1851), Professor of Obstetrics in the University of Heidelberg.[15]

Less precise were the authors of the Scriptures. In the account of Rebekah's pregnancy with twins Esau and Jacob we are told merely: "And when her days to be delivered were fulfilled, behold, there were twins in her womb." (*Genesis* 25:24) Solomon wrote of his having been "fashioned to be flesh in the time of ten months."[7]

Postterm pregnancy, of 42 weeks or more, resulting from failure of the woman to deliver within two weeks of the expected date of confinement, is a well-recognized obstetric complication, occurring in about 10% of pregnancies and carrying with it both maternal and fetal hazards, with a doubling of the perinatal mortality. The Prophet Esdras, recalling his conversation with God, denied its possibility: "So he answered me and said, Go thy way to a woman with child and ask of her when she hath fulfilled her nine months, if her womb may keep the birth any longer within her. Then said I, No, Lord, that can she not." (*II Esdras* 4)

LABOR

The cause of the onset of labor is still incompletely understood. Several factors are probably involved. Suspect in some cases is emotional trauma. Eli, a judge in Israel for 40 years and now an old man, hearing the news that his people had suffered defeat by the Philistines, that his sons had been killed, and that the ark of God had been captured, fell and broke his neck. "And his daughter-in-law, Phinehas' wife, was with child, near to be delivered: and when she heard the tidings that the ark of God was taken, and that her father-in-law and her husband were dead, she bowed herself and travailed; for her pains came upon her." (*I. Samuel* 4:19)

The rigors of labor can be ameliorated by training in relaxation and breathing exercises, techniques espoused by Dick-Read, Lamaze, and others; but parturition is inherently painful. After Eve's disobedience in eating the forbidden fruit in the Garden of Eden, God scolded: "I will greatly multiply thy sorrow and thy conception; in sorrow[16] shalt thou bring forth children . . ."(*Genesis* 3:16)

The pain of labor became a figure of speech. The Prophet Jeremiah, foretelling the destruction of Moab for the pride of its people and their contempt for God and the Israelites, predicted: "The mighty men's hearts in Moab at this day shall be as the heart of a woman in her pangs." (*Jeremiah* 48:41) Similarly did he judge the Edomites: "Behold, he shall come up and fly as the eagle, and spread his wings over Bozrah: and at that day shall the heart of the mighty men of Edom be as the heart of a woman in her pangs." (*Jeremiah* 49:22)

First labors are longer, on average, and more difficult, than those of multiparas. Jeremiah was clearly aware of this difference when he wrote: "For I have heard a voice as of a woman in travail, and the anguish as that of her that bringeth forth her first child...that bewaileth herself, that spreadeth her hands, saying, Woe is me now!" (*Jeremiah* 4:31) The Israelite women, however, were reported to be "lively, and are delivered ere the midwives come in unto them." (*Exodus* 1:19)

The identical account of uterine inertia, inadequate contractions leading to difficult labor, reported by King Hezekiah, appears in *II. Kings* 19:3 and *Isaiah* 37:3: "This day is a day of trouble, and of rebuke, and of blasphemy: for the children are come to birth, and there is not strength to bring forth."

POSITION FOR DELIVERY

The positions assumed by women in labor and at delivery, usually prescribed by local or tribal custom, have varied greatly, and their relative merits have been much disputed. A 19th-century obstetrician summarized: "According to their build, to the shape of the pelvis, [the parturients of different peoples] stand, squat, kneel or lie upon the belly; so do they vary their position in various stages of labor according to the position of the child's head in the pelvis....Primitive peoples have solved this problem by virtue of their instinct."[17] He enumerated 16 different postures for parturition among various races, and others expanded the list to 40. One student of the subject, in an effort to ascertain *the* natural position, surreptitiously observed a young primigravida, left alone during labor in a room containing a bed, chair, a couch, and obstetric stool. She assumed every possible position on each, finally giving birth while tossing about on the bed.

The Hebrew word *obnayim* means both "stones" and "stools." Thus Pharaoh's instructions to the midwives Shiphrah and Puah regarding the Israelite parturients can be translated either as "When ye...see them upon the stools" or "When ye...see them upon the stones." (*Exodus* 1:16) "To sit on stones" was synonymous in Egyptian hieroglyphics with "to give birth." When two stones on the sides of a stone trough were later connected by a transverse arm a type of birth-stool resulted.

Not to be confused as a posture for parturition is the symbolic gesture alluded to by Rachel when, acknowledging her childlessness, she urged Jacob: "Behold my maid Bilhah, go in unto her; and she shall bear upon my knees, that I may also have children by her." (*Genesis* 30:3)

In the cultures of the Near East and ancient Greece and Rome, the placing of a child upon the knees established its legitimation, whether in acknowledgment of actual parenthood or by adoption. Thus "Joseph brought them [his sons Ephraim and Manasseh] out from his knees..." (*Genesis* 48:12); and "Joseph saw Ephraim's children of the third generation: the children also of Machir the son of Manasseh were brought up upon Joseph's knees." (*Genesis* 50:23)

CESAREAN SECTION

One of the most frequently performed surgical operations in the late 20th century and the method of delivery in about one fourth of the births in urban America, cesarean section is not mentioned in the Bible. The origin of the operation remains unknown; but its name probably dates back to the 8th century B.C.E., when Numa Pompilius, a legendary king of Rome, decreed that the child be excised from the womb of any woman who died in late pregnancy. Known initially as the *lex regia*, or royal law, the mandate for postmortem abdominal section continued under the rule of the emperors or caesars, when it acquired the name *lex caesarea*.

Abdominal delivery was surely known to the Jews of the 2nd century C.E., for the Mishnah states that, in the case of twins, neither the first child brought into the world by an abdominal incision, nor the second, can receive the rights of primogeniture, either as regards the office of priest or succession to property. Children so born were known as *yotze dofen*. The operation may indeed have been performed on living women, for the Talmud prescribes laws of hygiene for survivors. The Niddah, one of its tracts, states that a woman delivered of a child by abdominal incision is not required to observe the days of purification in the puerperium. Also in the Talmud, rabbinic authority states that "if a woman who has been sitting on a birth-stool dies on a Sabbath, one may bring a knife and cut her womb open to take out the child."[18] Beyond these statements, however, there is no clear evidence that cesarean section was practiced on viable women until the early-17th century.[19]

MONSTERS

Deviations from the normal human form at birth have alternately bewildered, guided, frightened, and inspired mankind, but are not mentioned in the Bible. The *Apocrypha*, however, predicted that coitus during menstruation would lead to fetal deformity: "Menstruous women shall bring forth monsters" (*II Esdras* 5), a belief that was affirmed by Ambroise Paré in the 16th century and which is still not completely dead; and the Talmud attributed epilepsy, cretinism, and insanity to the same cause.[20]

MULTIPLE BIRTHS

The frequency of twinning varies among different races. It had long occurred in about one of 80 conceptions in the United States; but the incidence of multiple births of all orders has been rising since the late 1950s with the increasing use of fertility-enhancing agents, which often produce multiple ovulation. Twins are of two types. About one third are identical, always of the same sex, the result of the splitting of one egg fertilized by one sperm. Two-thirds of all twins are fraternal, of the same or opposite sexes, the product of two eggs and two sperm cells. A strong familial disposition exists with respect to fraternal twinning; identical twinning appears to occur by chance.

Some views of creation regarded the first human as a two-sexed being, joined at the back like Siamese twins: "Male and female created he them; and blessed them, and called their name Adam, in the day when they were created." (*Genesis* 5:2) Their subsequent division into separate beings, it was suggested, was the result of God's afterthought. In Hebrew folklore both of Eve's pregnancies were multiple, Cain being one of twins, Abel one of triplets; and each of Jacob's sons except Joseph was born with a twin girl sister.[21]

The Bible tells of but two twin pregnancies and births, none of higher order. After Isaac's entreaty to God because of his wife's barrenness Rebekah conceived. Her pregnancy was uniquely difficult in Biblical literature, as the lifelong rivals began their intrauterine strife: "And the children struggled together within her; and she said, If it be so, why am I thus? And she went to enquire of the Lord. And the Lord said unto her, Two nations are in thy womb...And when her days to be delivered were fulfilled, behold, there were twins in her womb." Although both were male, the twins were clearly fraternal, not identical: "And the first came out red all over like an hairy garment; and they called his name Esau. And after that came his brother out, and his hand took hold on Esau's heel; and his name was called Jacob." (*Genesis* 25:21-26) Details of the delivery are lacking. Presumably both births were by vertex (head) presentation, the membranes of Jacob's sac rupturing after Esau's birth and permitting prolapse of one of Jacob's hands, which grasped his brother's heel.

Judah, having finished mourning for his recently deceased wife, mistook for a harlot, in her veil, his daughter-in-law Tamar, lay with her, and impregnated her. In contrast to Rebekah's pregnancy, twins were not expected. Differing from the case of Rebekah, Tamar's labor apparently began prematurely, as is common in multiple pregnancy, for the Bible here states, not "when her days to be delivered were fulfilled," but rather: "And it came to pass in the time of her travail, that, behold, twins were in her womb."

More complicated than Rebekah's was Tamar's delivery: "And it came to pass, when she travailed, that the one put out his hand: and the midwife took and bound upon his hand a scarlet thread, saying, This came out first. And it came to pass, as he drew back his hand, that, behold, his brother came out...his name was called Pharez. And afterward came out his brother, that had the scarlet thread upon his hand: and his name was called Zarah." (*Genesis* 38:27-30) The twins were probably identical, for they apparently occupied a common amniotic sac. The mechanism of their birth remains conjectural. They presumably both lay in vertex presentation, with the hand of the second, later withdrawn, prolapsed alongside and extruding beyond the head of the first, when the midwife tagged it.

An alternative scenario presumes a transverse lie, or cross birth, the least favorable of all possible positions, for the presenting infant, whose arm prolapsed through the birth canal. Having received its scarlet tie, the hand returned into the uterus, as the infant withdrew or was pushed aside by its fellow twin, who then delivered by the vertex. The marked twin either followed in vertex presentation, having converted from the transverse lie, or underwent, through the rarest of labor mechanisms, spontaneous evolution, or *conduplicato corpore*, doubling upon itself, the head and thorax passing through the pelvic cavity at the same time. This mechanism has been observed in cases where the maternal pelvis is very large and the fetus very small, and occasionally in the birth of the second of premature twins.

MATERNAL DEATH

The Bible records two maternal deaths associated with childbirth.[22] No clue is given as to the cause of death of Phinehas' wife, whose labor was apparently precipitated by great emotional stress and who expired soon after delivery: "And about the time of her death the women that stood by her said unto her, Fear not; for thou hast born a son. But she answered not, neither did she regard it." (*I. Samuel* 4:20)

Only in the case of Rachel's parturition does the Bible mention that labor was hard, a feature emphasized by its repetition: As she journeyed with Jacob from Beth-el, "there was but a little way to come to Ephrath: and Rachel travailed, and she had hard labour. And it came to pass, when she was in hard labour, that the midwife said unto her, Fear not; thou shalt have this son also." Death apparently followed soon after delivery: "And it came to pass, as her soul was in departing, (for she died) that she called his name Ben-oni: but his father called him Benjamin." (*Genesis* 35:16-18)

The foremost diagnoses suggested by death in or soon after hard labor are uterine rupture and amniotic fluid embolism. The former may occur in cases of obstruction, from disproportion between the fetus and the maternal pelvis, or abnormal presentation of the fetus; or in cases of previous uterine surgery, with dehiscence of the incisional scar, when the uterine tear is commonly but not invariably associated with external bleeding. Labor often comes to a halt upon rupture of the uterus. More likely in Rachel's case is the diagnosis of amniotic fluid embolism, a highly fatal accident of labor in which amniotic fluid, which contains fetal skin cells and other particulate matter, is infused into the maternal uterine veins, causing mechanical blockage of the small blood vessels of the lungs, with resultant shortness of breath, chest pain, shock, and often death, sometimes within minutes. Only in 1941 was the syndrome recognized as a clinical entity and its mechanism explained. Amniotic fluid embolism is now diagnosed as responsible for about 12% of the maternal deaths in the United States each year.[23] It may have caused the matriarch's demise.

PUERPERIUM

The 6 weeks that follow childbirth, known as the puerperium, comprise a period of rapid and profound readjustment and recuperation from the pregnant to the nonpregnant condition, when the uterus undergoes involution, and changes commensurate with those induced by pregnancy take place in every organ system of the body. Speaking to Moses, God prescribed laws of sexual abstinence for the puerperal woman: "Speak unto the children of Israel, saying, If a woman have conceived seed, and born a man child: then she shall be unclean seven days; according to the days of the separation for her infirmity shall she be unclean...And she shall then continue in the blood of her purifying three and thirty days...But if she bear a maid child, then she shall be unclean two weeks, as in her separation: and she shall continue in the blood of her purifying three-score and six days." (*Leviticus* 12:1-5)

The mucous membrane lining the uterus requires three weeks for regeneration after childbirth. Most obstetricians counsel against coitus during this period, to avoid infection. Sexual abstinence for six weeks, standard advice until the late-20th century, is no longer considered medically necessary.

CARE OF INFANT AT BIRTH

An ancient practice, long since abandoned, was swaddling, tight wrapping of the newborn in cloth bands, soon after the cutting of the umbilical cord. Galen, the great medical authority of the second century, thus described care of the neonate: "The newborn infant...should be powdered moderately and wrapped in swaddling clothes, in order that his skin may be made thicker and firmer than the parts within. For during pregnancy everything was equally soft, since nothing of a harder nature touched it from without and no cold air came in contact with it, whereby the skin would be contracted and thickened, and would become tougher and denser than it was before and than the other parts of the body. But when the baby is born, it is necessarily going to come in contact with cold and heat and with many bodies harder than itself. Therefore it is appropriate that his natural covering should be best prepared by us for exposure."[24]

Ezekiel compared the wretched state of Jerusalem to that of an infant neglected at birth: "And as for thy nativity, in the day thou wast born thy navel was not cut, neither wast thou washed in water to supple thee; thou wast not salted at all, nor swaddled at all." (*Ezekiel* 16:4)

SUDDEN INFANT DEATH SYNDROME

The Bible tells of the death of an infant of one of the two harlots who appealed to King Solomon for resolution of their dispute over the surviving child: "And this woman's child died in the night; because she overlaid it." (*I. Kings* 3:19)

Abrupt and unexplained death of apparently healthy infants (Sudden Infant Death Syndrome), the second leading category of infant mortality in the United States, was initially attributed, as in the Bible, to suffocation resulting from the mother's overlying the infant during sleep. Defined by the National Institute of Child Health and Human Development as "the sudden death of an infant under one year of age which remains unexplained after a thorough case investigation, including performance of a complete autopsy, examination of the death scene, and review of the clinical history," this syndrome (SIDS) accounted for the lost lives of 47,932 infants born to U.S. residents from 1980 to 1988. Although many risk factors have been associated with SIDS, the preponderance of recent evidence seems to have established a causal relationship to the prone sleeping position of the infants. Many pediatric associations and governmental health departments, the world over, now counsel against the prone positioning of infants; and in the wake of public campaigns to avoid the prone position, reductions of 20 to 67% in the occurrence of SIDS have been reported.[25,26]

WEANING

The infant is withdrawn from its source of sustenance at the maternal breast at various ages in various cultures. The Bible tells of Isaac's weaning but not at what age: "And the child grew and was weaned: and Abraham made a great feast the same day that Isaac was weaned." (*Genesis* 21:8) The age at weaning in Pharaoh's household is likewise unmentioned: "And the sister of Tahpenes [the queen] bare him [Hadad]

Genubath his son, whom Tahpenes weaned in Pharaoh's house." (*I. Kings* 11:20)

Lactation is one of the oldest methods of contraception in current use, and in some cultures it is still a common means of birth control. The continuation of lactation tends to inhibit the resumption of ovarian function, as evidenced by a delayed return of the menses; and the associated suppression of ovulation results in temporarily impaired fertility. The Prophet Hosea took cognizance of the relation between termination of lactation and conception when he told of his wife Gomer's pregnancy with Lo-ammi, her third: "Now when she had weaned Loruhamah, she conceived, and bare a son." (*Hosea* 1:8)

SUMMARY

The Bible regarded fertility as a reward for obedience to God; infertility accordingly, as divinely ordained. Prayer and amulets, but also herbals, prominent among which was the mandrake, were resorted to for its cure. The Talmud recognizes some characteristics of the infertile woman, interpreted by modern endocrinologists as signs of hypoovarianism or the adrenogenital syndrome. Embryology remained largely a mystery, concepts of human development primitive. Obstetric care was the exclusive domain of women. Antenatal care was nonexistent; the midwife attended only at labor and delivery.

The angel of God warned of the hazard of wine for the pregnant woman. Only recently have physicians recognized the fetal alcohol syndrome. The list of chemicals and drugs considered safe for the mother but specifically harmful to the fetus continues to grow.

The Prophets spoke of abortion as a weapon of divine retribution. The Bible, in addition, recognized trauma as a cause of miscarriage, and prescribed compensation for the aggrieved. Neonatology continues to improve in the late-20th century, with the salvage of smaller and smaller prematurely born infants; but far beyond present reach remains the Apocrypha's optimistic prediction of survival of "untimely children of three or four months."

Well described in the Bible are the pains of labor; and accounts are given of uterine inertia, twin pregnancy and birth, and maternal death. The narration of Rachel's death in childbirth suggests as its cause amniotic fluid embolism, a clinical entity unrecognized until mid-20th century. The laws of sexual abstinence prescribed through Moses for the puerperal woman find a biological basis in the 3 weeks required for regeneration and healing of the uterine lining after childbirth.

The Sudden Infant Death Syndrome, the abrupt and unexplained death of an apparently healthy infant under one year of age, described only recently as a distinct clinical phenomenon but recognized now as the second leading category of infant mortality in the United States, finds its counterpart in the Bible in the oft-told tale of the death of the infant of one of two harlots, who appealed to King Solomon for resolution of their dispute over the surviving child. The Bible ascribed the child's death to suffocation from having been overlaid by its mother; modern evidence points to the prone position of the sleeping infant as a causal factor in the Sudden Infant Death Syndrome.

Lactation, which tends to delay the resumption of ovarian function after childbirth, is one of the oldest and most widespread methods of contraception, still in use in many cultures. The Prophet Hosea apparently knew of this association, when he related his wife's third conception and pregnancy to the weaning of their second child.

NOTES AND REFERENCES

1. Reuben, Simeon, Levi, Judah, Dan, Naphtali, Gad, Asher, Issachar, Zebulun, Joseph, and Benjamin, leaders of the 12 tribes of Israel.
2. Steinberg W. Gynecology and obstetrics in the old testament and the Babylonian Talmud. Int Rec Med 1960; 173:756-769.
3. Speert H. Obstetric and Gynecologic Milestones. New York: Macmillan 1958; 271-276.
4. The Babylonian Ishtar, the Phoenician Astarte, and the Greek Aphrodite, goddess of fertility.
5. Krutch JW. Herbal. New York: GP Putnam's Sons 1965; 100,102.
6. Krutch JW. (ed) The Gardener's World. New York: GP Putnam's Sons 1959; 77.
7. The Apocrypha. New Hyde Park, University Books 1962; 92-93.
8. Steinberg W. Gynecology and obstetrics in the old testament and the Babylonian Talmud. Int Rec Med 1960; 173:756-769.
9. Speert H. Obstetrics and Gynecology in America: A History. Chicago: Amer Col Obstetr and Gynecol 1980; 9-21.
10. Ballantyne JW. Teratogenesis: An Inquiry into the Causes of Monstrosities. Edinburgh: Oliver and Boyd 1897.
11. Speert H. Iconographia Gyniatricia. Philadelphia: FA Davis Co 1973; 228-229.
12. Speert H. The placental transmission of sulfanilamide and its effects upon the fetus and newborn. Bull Johns Hopkins Hosp 1940; 66:139-155.
13. Clarren SK, Smith DW. The fetal alcohol syndrome. New Eng J Med 1978; 298:1063-1067.
14. Ouellette EM, Rosett HL, Rosman NP, Weiner L. Adverse effects on offspring of maternal alcohol abuse during pregnancy. New Eng J Med 1977; 297:528-530.
15. Speert H. Obstetric and Gynecologic Milestones. New York: Macmillan 1958; 169-172.
16. The Hebrew *etser* is also translated as "pain" and is commonly construed to include the rigors of parturition. The intense pain of childbirth is believed unique to the human species.
17. Engelmann G. Labor Among Primitive Peoples. St. Louis: JH Chambers and Co, 2nd ed; 1883.

18. Steinberg W. Gynecology and obstetrics in the Old Testament and Babylonian Talmud. Part II. Int Rec Med 1961; 174:101-121.
19. Some believe that Jane Seymour's delivery of Edward VI in 1537 was by cesarean section, on the basis of ballads describing the event; but the time at which they were written is questionable. Moreover, no official record of the operation exists, and the Queen is known to have survived the prince's birth by 12 days, unlikely had the delivery been by abdominal section.
20. Crawfurd R. Of Superstitions Concerning Menstruation. Proc Roy Soc Med 1915; 9:49-66.
21. Ginzberg L. Legends of the Bible. New York: Simon and Schuster 1956.
22. Difference of opinion exists as to whether Michal, David's wife, died in childbirth. The Authorized King James Version of the Bible states that "Michal the daughter of Saul had no child unto the day of her death." (*II. Samuel* 6:23) Identical wording appears in *The Illustrated Jerusalem Bible* (English Trans, M. Friedlander, ed. Jerusalem Bible Pub Co). *The New English Bible* (Oxford University Press, 1970) similarly states: "Michal, Saul's daughter, had no child *to* her dying day." Others,[18] however, have translated the passage as "Michal the daughter of Saul had no child *until* the day of her death," [all italics mine] in the belief that she did indeed give birth to a child on the day she died. The latter view is based on *I Chronicles* 3:3 which, listing David's sons, names Ithream as the daughter of "Eglah his wife," Eglah being taken as another name for Michal.
23. Speert H. Obstetric and Gynecologic Milestones, 2nd ed.; 447, in press.
24. Greene RM A Translation of Galen's Hygiene. Springfield, Ill: Charles C. Thomas 1951.
25. Guntheroth WG, Spiers PS. Sleeping prone and the risk of sudden death syndrome. JAMA 1992; 267:2359-2362.
26. Sudden Infant Death Syndrome—United States, 1980-1988. JAMA 1992, 268; 856-858.

CHAPTER 6

THE DISEASE OF THEORIES

Inscribed on plaques in the courtyard of the Chicago Lying-in-Hospital are the names of the great figures in the history of obstetrics,[1] with one space left vacant—for the discoverer of the cause of eclampsia. This, together with infection and hemorrhage, comprised the traditional triad of killers of parturient women. Eclampsia is a complication of late pregnancy, affecting primigravidas mainly, and characterized by hypertension, fluid retention, proteinuria, convulsions, coma, and often death. Its incidence in America has declined sharply during the 20th century, to the point that one wag expressed the "concern" that the disease might disappear with its cause still undiscovered. But his fear was groundless. Year in and year out preeclampsia, the prodromal syndrome, remains one of the leading causes of maternal morbidity, fetal growth retardation, and circumnatal mortality.

In the first edition (1903) of his celebrated textbook John Whitridge Williams, dean of American obstetrics during the early decades of the 20th century, summarized some of the many theories of the etiology of eclampsia, and in later editions these theories and the researches into the nature of the disease were grouped under 12 rubrics.[2] Every important contribution to medical knowledge has been applied to the study of eclampsia. It still remains "the disease of theories."

The cause and mechanism of eclampsia being poorly understood, treatment has been largely empiric: to reduce the blood pressure and control the convulsions. In the many cases in which the fetus dies undelivered, before term or during labor, maternal improvement is usually prompt and dramatic. Termination of the pregnancy has thus been an obvious resort, to remove the sine qua non of the disease; but the trauma this entails usually makes the procedure self-defeating. Nonsurgical efforts to control the convulsions have included drastic and diverse measures, as cold compresses, hot packs, chloroform, purging, blistering, bloodletting, and leeching. Most effective in the management of eclampsia, however, has been maternal sedation, exemplified by the "Stroganov regimen," introduced in 1899 and so named for the Russian obstetrician Vasili Stroganov (1857-1938).[3]

It has been suggested[4] that Phinehas' wife died of eclampsia, but I can find nothing in the brief Biblical account of her death (*I. Samuel* 4:20) to support this diagnosis. The Bible does, however, provide a possible clue to the etiology of the disease, in the directions to subsequent humankind after God's creation of Eve: "Therefore shall a man leave his father and his mother, and shall cleave unto his wife: and they shall be one flesh." (*Genesis* 2:24) The Psalmist, further, recognized the permeability of the body's membranes: "Let it come into his bowels like water, and like oil into his bones." (*Psalm* 109:18) A tractate of the Talmud (*Sabbath* 86 a), confirming the concept of cutaneous absorption, equated anointing the body with oil on Yom Kippur with taking water by mouth.[5]

Anaphylaxis is the state of unusual or exaggerated susceptibility to a foreign protein which often develops after a primary injection of that protein. A second injection of the same protein, after an intervening rest period, may produce a severe reaction, including shock and even death. It was shown by Sewell in 1925 that such sensitization could be produced in experimental animals by nasal insufflation of the test protein as well as by injection; thus, that the sensitizing agent can be absorbed through the nasal mucosa.[6] Might foreign proteins, Macht[7] asked, be absorbed also through other of the body's membranes—the lining of the vagina, for example, after sexual intercourse?

Macht instilled small quantities of horse serum into the vaginas of guinea pigs daily for 1 to 2 weeks, and after a rest period of 9 to 12 days injected them subcutaneously or internally with another small dose of the serum. In the test cases the sensitized animals reacted with the same manifestations of anaphylaxis, with muscular twitching, sneezing, nose rubbing, labored respiration, paralysis, convulsions, and sometimes death, as did animals sensitized initially by direct needle injection. These experiments proved that the foreign protein in the serum could be absorbed vaginally. Macht speculated: that in normal physiologic cohabitation, in addition to fertilization of the ovum, a "merging or union" of the mates results from the vaginal absorption of seminal protein.[8] Importantly, both he and Sewell found that by introducing very small quantities of serum into their animals for long periods of time, they could produce a protective capacity against anaphylaxis.

A sharp reduction in the incidence of eclampsia was noted in Central Europe during World War I. In a brief note in a German medical journal published a few years after war's end and long since forgotten, speculating on the cause of this aberration, Mayer suggested that certain elements of the semen are normally absorbed through the vaginal or uterine lining during or after coitus, sensitizing the woman, and that the frequent repetition of this absorption might lead to an anaphylactic-like reaction, namely preeclampsia or eclampsia. The dramatic diminution in this disorder during the war he attributed to the restricted opportunity for sexual intercourse.[9]

Fresh evidence, on the other hand, has been adduced that unprotected coital exposure before a first pregnancy may diminish the risk of subsequent preeclampsia-eclampsia syndrome: that the greater the exposure to the partner's semen, the less the likelihood of a woman's developing the disorder. Elements in the seminal plasma, absorbed by the woman, it was postulated, provide a molecular message leading to her immunoprotection. The specificity of this protection was suggested by the observation that a change of partners by a multiparous woman was associated with a marked increase in the occurrence of the syndrome in subsequent pregnancy.[10] Pregnancies resulting from artificial donor insemination, reflecting a change in paternity, were similarly affected by a several-fold increase in the incidence of preeclampsia.[11]

In a case-control study of the contraceptive and reproductive histories of 110 primiparous women with preeclampsia and 115 unaffected pregnant women, a team of epidemiologists in concert with an obstetrician at the University of North Carolina found that birth control methods that prevent contact with sperm and seminal fluid may play a role in the etiology of the eclamptic syndrome; that resort to condoms, diaphragms, spermicides, or withdrawal for contraception was associated with a 2.37-fold increased risk of the disorder, as compared with nonbarrier methods (oral contraceptives, intrauterine devices, rhythm, and nonuse of any method), which permitted greater exposure to the semen and freedom for the sperm to travel from the vagina, through the cervical canal, and into the uterus.[12]

"Therefore shall a man...cleave unto his wife: and they shall be one flesh."

SUMMARY

"Therefore shall a man... cleave unto his wife," the Bible commanded, "and they shall be one flesh." Herein may lie a clue to the etiology of eclampsia, a dreaded complication of pregnancy and long a leading cause of maternal death. Chemicals, drugs, and presumably seminal elements can be absorbed from the vagina, and thus produce sensitization and susceptibility to an anaphylactoid reaction on subsequent exposure to the agent. Protection, in experimental animals, can be provided by the administration of small quantities of the sensitizing agent over long periods of time. Recent observations in humans indicate that unprotected coitus may diminish the risk of the preeclampsia-eclampsia syndrome in a subsequent pregnancy; and that the greater the woman's exposure to her partner's semen the less likely she is to develop the disorder.

NOTES AND REFERENCES
1. Ambroise Paré, 1510-1590; Hendrik van Deventer, 1651-1724; Jean Palfyn, 1650-1730; William Smellie, 1697-1763; Jean-Louis Baudelocque, 1746-1810; Edoardo Porro, 1842-1902; Max Sänger, 1853-1903.

2. Williams JW. Obstetrics. New York: D. Appleton and Co 1903:702-705; 7th ed. Appleton-Century f1936:754-755. Eclampsia: Researches and theories: (1) Uremia, (2) Bacterial origin, (3) Auto-intoxication, (4) Biological reactions, (5) Entrance of fetal elements into the maternal circulation, (6) Fetal metabolic products, (7) Placental decomposition products, (8) Alterations in maternal metabolism, (9) Endocrine disturbances, (10) Mammary toxemia, (11) Effect of dietary alterations, (12) Physicochemical changes.
3. Speert H. Obstetric and Gynecologic Milestones, 2nd ed; in press, 583-586.
4. Mead KCH. A History of Women in Medicine, Haddam Conn: The Haddam Press 1938:27.
5. Macht DI. A Biblical Adventure in Pharmacology. Am J Pharmacy 1936; 108:227-230.
6. Sewell H. The role of epithelium in experimental immunization. Science 1925; 62:293-299.
7. Born in Moscow in 1882, David I. Macht came to Baltimore as a child, received his bachelor's and medical degrees from the Johns Hopkins University, and after postgraduate study in Berlin, Munich, and Vienna, returned to his alma mater in 1909, where he spent a quarter-century as a member of its Department of Pharmacology. He then assumed directorship of the Pharmacological Research Laboratory of Hynson, Westcott, and Dunning, a pharmaceutical firm in Baltimore; and in his later years served in a similar capacity and consultant in pharmacology in that city's Sinai Hospital, where he died in 1961. In addition to his distinguished career as a medical scientist he was widely known and respected as a Biblical and Shakespearean scholar. I was a frequent visitor in his laboratory and guest in his home; I dined at his table, and delivered some of his grandchildren.
8. Macht DI. Sensitization of Guinea Pigs per Vaginam. Am J Obst and Gynec 1928; 16:263-267.
9. Mayer. Ueber die Beziehungen der Geburtshilfe u. Gynäkologie zum Krieg und zu den Kriegsverhältnissen. Cited in Williams Obstetrics,[2] 5th ed, 1927; 612,633.
10. Beer AE. Immunology, contraception, and preeclampsia. JAMA 1989; 262:3184.
11. Need J, Bell B, Meffin E. Preeclampsia in pregnancy from donor inseminations. J Reproduct Immunol 1983; 5:329-338.
12. Klonoff-Cohen HS, Savitz DA, Cefalo RC, McCann MF. An epidemiologic study of contraception and preeclampsia. JAMA 1989; 262: 3143-3147.

CHAPTER 7

THE CONJUGAL RELATIONSHIP

Humankind clings to the concept of monogamy as the ideal conjugal relationship, suggested by the words of God after His creation of Adam: "It is not good that the man should be alone; I will make him an help mate for him." (*Genesis* 2:18)

Solomon subsequently warned against adultery: "For the lips of a strange woman drop as an honeycomb, and her mouth is smoother than oil... To keep thee from the evil woman...lust not after her beauty in thine heart; neither let her take thee with her eyelids... Whoso committeth adultery with a woman lacketh understanding: he that doeth it destroyeth his own soul." (*Proverbs* 5:3; 6:24-25, 32)

Later, Job added: "The eye...of the adulterer waiteth for the twilight, saying, No eye shall see me: and disguiseth his face." (*Job* 24:15) And in his "Song of Songs" Solomon wrote: "My beloved is mine, and I am his... There are threescore queens and fourscore concubines, and virgins without number. My dove, my undefiled is but one; she is the only one of her mother, she is the choice one of her that bare her. The daughters saw her, and blessed her; yea, the queens and the concubines, and they praised her." (*The Song of Solomon* 2:16; 6;8-9)

But the hold of monogamy has been tenuous.

POLYANDRY

Most human societies have been male dominated. Perhaps also, because of the biological restraints of pregnancy and lactation and the domestic obligations of woman to her family and household, the formal concurrent union of a woman with more than one man has never received wide acceptance. Yet records exist of the practice of polyandry among many primitive societies throughout the world, including Tibet, South India, the South Sea Islands, the Himalayas, the Alaskan coast and Aleutian Islands, and among certain tribes of South America. The British Government prohibited polyandry in Ceylon about 1860.[1]

The mating of one female with more than one male, a common social arrangement in the animal kingdom, has been related among the primates to testicular weight in the males. As though to compensate for their competitive disadvantage, the males of those primate species in which several mate with the same female have larger testes than those in which the female limits herself, or is limited, to one male. The male chimpanzee, for example, whose female companions enjoy multiple mates, has testes much larger than a man's; while the bigger, domineering gorilla, who presides over a group of females, has tiny testes, scarcely visible even on dissection. In the plotting of testicular weight versus body size, the human lies on the borderline between polyandrous and monandrous species.[2]

No mention of polyandry is to be found in the Bible.

POLYGAMY

The Bible abounds, by contrast, with examples of polygamy. Not only was it not forbidden in Biblical law, but polygamy was apparently presupposed by the levirate provision (from *levir*, Latin for brother-in-law), which required a man to marry his deceased brother's widow, in order to preserve the brother's name and family line: "If brethren dwell together, and one of them die, and have no child, the wife of the dead shall not marry without unto a stranger: her husband's brother shall go in unto her, and take her to him to wife, and perform the duty of an husband's brother unto her." (*Deuteronomy* 25:5)

"Lamech [a sixth generation descendant of Cain[3]] took him two wives: the name of the one was Adah, and the name of the other Zillah." (*Genesis* 4:19) In the Generation of the Flood, soon to follow, each man took two wives, one for procreation and the other for sexual gratification, according to Midrashic narrative.[4] Jacob was married concurrently to two sisters, Leah and Rachel.[5] His brother Esau had at least three wives. David had four wives: Michal, Abigail, Maacah, and Bathsheba.

The Talmud specifically instructs that a man of learning should never be without a wife. According to legend, prophets detained from home for lengthy periods did indeed marry an additional woman. Mentioned in the Bible are the multiple wives of Samuel, Isaiah, Ezekiel, and Hosea.

CONCUBINAGE

The social institution permitting the maintenance of a surrogate wife without legal marriage had long existed among the ancient Babylonians. Concubinage is mentioned in the laws of Hammurabi, who reigned 2067-2025 B.C.E., but was restricted to specific circumstances, as when the wife was a priestess or had failed to produce offspring, in which case she was required to provide her husband with a slave-woman. The Bible tells of Sarah's resort to a concubine for her husband Abraham after a decade of childless marriage: "And Sarai said unto Abram, Behold now, the Lord hath restrained me from bearing: I pray thee, go in unto my maid; it may be that I may obtain children by her. And Abram harkened to the voice of Sarai. And Sarai Abram's wife took Hagar her maid the Egyptian, after Abram had dwelt ten years in the land of Canaan, and gave her to her husband to be his wife." (*Genesis* 16:2-3)

Two generations later Rachel found herself in a similar situation: "And when Rachel saw that she bare Jacob no children...she said, "Behold my maid Bilhah, go in unto her...that I may also have children by her. And she gave him Bilhah her handmaid to wife: and Jacob went in unto her." (*Genesis* 30:1-4)

Solomon, for his sexual pleasure, had some 300 concubines. The Bible mentions harlotry many times, always with deprecation.

Polygamy remained an accepted practice until the destruction of the first temple (586 or 587 B.C.E.). It came to be looked upon with disfavor among the Jews after the Babylonian exile (597-538 B.C.E.). Monogamy had become by then the custom as well as the ideal. Among the special requirements established for the High Priest by the Mishnah was that he be married, but to only one woman. In the *Targum*, a 4th century paraphrase of the Bible, the kinsman says, in the *Book of Ruth* (4:6): "I cannot marry her because I am already married; I have no right to take an additional wife lest it lead to strife in my home."[6] No instance of plural marriage is recorded among the more than 2000 sages of the Talmudic period.[7]

Long since abandoned in practice, polygamy was formally prohibited by the *Takkanah*, or ban, of a synod convened by Rabbi Gershom ben Judah of Mayence, about the year 1000. The Jewish settlements in Northern France and the Rhineland thus continued to be guided by the Jewish legal maxim of *Dina de-Malkuta Dina* ("the law of the land is the law of the Jew," except in matters of religious observance). Although Gershom's edict claimed only regional authority, it was embraced by almost all Jewish communities, far beyond the Rhineland. Among Sephardic Jewry in the Moslem countries of the Middle East however, plural marriage was considered lawful until 1960, when the Chief Rabbinate of Israel extended the ban on polygamy to them as well.

HOMOSEXUAL MARRIAGE

God's words to Moses regarding a male-male sexual relationship were unmistakable. "Speak unto the children of Israel," He said, "and say unto them... Thou shalt not lie with mankind, as with womankind: it is an abomination... If a man also lies with mankind, as he lieth with a woman, both of them have committed an abomination." (*Leviticus* 18:1-2, 22; 20:13) Homosexual relationships are thus condemned by Orthodox Judaism. The Reform movement has taken no position on the status of the increasingly visible and vocal segment of the gay membership in the community. At this writing (summer 1992) a rabbinic committee of the Conservative movement struggles with the question whether the union of homosexual couples should be sanctified, or even recognized. One member alleges that the Biblical prohibition of male-male sexual relations is "based on reasons which either no longer apply or were, in some cases, never applicable;" that "homosexuality is to be considered an halachically acceptable orientation, provided that this sexuality is expressed within the context of a mutually exclusive, committed, adult relationship;" and that the Torah's proscription against homosexual acts relates only to those that are "oppressive, coercive, or idolatrous." Another committee member insists, however, that since there "can be no legitimacy to the union, no matter how loving and caring, there can be no marriage."[8]

The Bible is silent on tribadism, or lesbian relationships. Shammai and Hillel, rabbinic scholars of the 1st century C.E., differed on this matter as on hundreds of other details of Jewish law. According to the school of the former, the Talmud relates, women who have engaged in a homosexual relationship are disqualified from marriage to a priest; whereas the school of the latter supported their eligibility for such a union.

MENSTRUATION AND COHABITATION

The Bible prohibits sexual union from the onset of menstruation through the 7 days following its cessation. The hygiene of the menstrual period is spelled out in God's words to Moses and Aaron, in *Leviticus* 15:19-28: "And if a woman have an issue, and her issue in her flesh be blood, she shall be put apart seven days: and whosoever toucheth her shall be unclean until the even. And every thing that she lieth upon in her separation shall be unclean: every thing also that she sitteth upon shall be unclean... And if any man lie with her at all, and her flowers be upon him, he shall be unclean seven days; and all the bed whereon he lieth shall be unclean. And if a woman have an issue of her blood many days out of the time of her separation, or if it run beyond the time of her separation; all the days of the issue of her uncleanliness shall be as the days of her separation: she shall be unclean... And whosoever toucheth those things shall be unclean, and shall wash his clothes, and bathe himself in water, and be unclean until the even. But if she be cleansed of her issue, then she shall number to herself seven days, and after that she shall be clean."

The subject is greatly expanded in the rabbinic law of the Talmud, the tractate *Niddah* of which establishes more rigid restrictions on sexual intercourse than those set forth in *Leviticus*. As a result the observant Orthodox Jewish woman often requires rabbinic consultation for guidance in her marital conduct.[9]

Prescribed also by the Talmudic rabbis was the ritual bath before the woman might resume her conjugal life. Immersion in "live," i.e. flowing, water, as a spring, stream, or the sea, was recommended; otherwise in a reservoir, or *Mikveh*, in which rainwater, as "the fountains of the great deep,"[10] was collected. The *Mikveh* continues in use by Orthodox Jewish women for ablution after menstruation and by brides just before their wedding; also by some men in preparation for the Sabbath and holy days. The laws of *Niddah* and ritual immersion have been regarded as purely religious and symbolic, without claim for any physical hygienic merit.

Menstruation, periodic, functional, non-organic bleeding from the uterus, is produced by hormonal factors of ovarian origin, and is associated with sloughing of the superficial layer of the endometrium, the uterine lining. Genital bleeding in women may have many other causes, including inflammations, trauma, or tumors of the vulva, vagina, and uterus. To none of these do the laws of *Niddah* apply, but only to menstrual bleeding. Definitive diagnosis for conjugal purposes might require medical consultation as well as rabbinic counsel. To differentiate between menstrual bleeding and that of vaginal origin the Talmud advocated, as a means of self-examination, the insertion high into the vagina of a metal tube containing a pledget of lint near its inner end. If blood appeared on the material after the tube's withdrawal, one could assume a uterine source; otherwise, a vaginal.

The laws of *Niddah* applied to the bleeding after an abortion as after a term gestation, if the pregnancy was of 40 days or more duration: 7 plus 33 days of abstinence after the delivery of a male; 2 weeks plus 66 days after a female (*Leviticus* 12:2-5). If the sex of the abortus could not be determined it was treated as female.

Neither the Bible nor the Talmud has anything to say about hydatidiform mole, a form of blighted pregnancy, or about ectopic pregnancy, conditions that commonly cause vaginal bleeding.

MENSTRUAL MYTHOLOGY

In every age and culture menstruation, the menstruous woman, and her menstrual blood have been the subject of myth and superstition. Pythagoras, in the 6th century B.C.E., called the menstrual discharge the froth of the blood, from "a superfluity in the aliment;" and Aristotle, 2 centuries later, explained menstruation as the process by which the body rids itself of the excess. The glance of a menstruating woman was thought possessed by an evil spirit which, residing in her blood, could harm the environment. Among the Kaffir tribes of South Africa, for example, she was forbidden to walk in parts of the kraal where the cattle wandered, for fear that any cow passing over even a drop of her blood might die. Pliny the Elder, in the 1st century C.E., wrote in his *Natural History*:

"If a woman strips herself naked while she is menstruating and walks round a field of wheat, the caterpillars, worms, beetles, and other vermin will fall off from the ears of corn... Seeds which are touched by her become sterile, grafts wither away, garden plants are parched up, and the fruit will fall from the tree beneath which she sits... Young vines, too...are injured irremediably by the touch of a woman in this state; and both rue and ivy, plants possessed of highly medicinal virtues, will die instantly upon being touched by her... All plants will turn of a yellow complexion on the approach of a woman who has the menstrual discharge upon her... A mare big with foal, if touched by a woman in this state, will be sure to miscarry."

As recently as the late-19th century menstruating women in Sumatra were excluded from the rice fields; they would damage the crop, it was feared, by their mere presence. In Northern France, similarly, they were forbidden to enter the sugar refineries during the boiling or cooling processes; for the presence of a menstruating woman, it was believed, would cause the sugar to blacken. They were also prohibited from picking mushrooms in regions of their culture. In Southern France women were furloughed from the great perfumeries during menstruation, and were not allowed to tend the silkworms. In canneries and florist establishments charts were kept of the menstrual dates of female workers, when they were not permitted to handle fruit or flowers, but were assigned to other duties. Neither were they allowed in wine cellars, lest they spoil the wine. Menstruating women were also cautioned against handling the yeast for bakery products or participating in the manufacture of sausage. In 1878 a correspondence dragged on for several months in the *British Medical Journal* on the dangers in the curing of meat during menstruation, before the editor closed its pages to further discussion of the matter, which he characterized as "an experimental example of the astonishing facility with which even among educated men superstitions, irrational and capable of easy disproof, retain their hold once acquired."[11]

Not only did the belief prevail that a powerful and noxious agent exists in the blood of menstruating women, but the menstruant herself was viewed by many as a semi-invalid, requiring special protection and additional rest. Edward H. Clarke, whose popular text *Sex in Education* went into 17 "editions" in 13 years, wrote in 1874: "A girl cannot spend more than four, or, in occasional instances, five hours of force daily upon her studies, and leave sufficient margin for the general physical growth that she must make... If she puts as much force into her brain education as a boy, the brain or the special apparatus will suffer."[12]

William J. Robinson's book *Woman: Her Sex and Love Life* continued to warn, well into the 20th century: "Rest is just as important during menstruation as cleanliness, if not more so... It is an outrage that many delicate, weak girls and women must stay on their feet all day or work on a machine when they should be at home in bed or lying down on a couch...there should be as much rest as possible. For delicate and sensitive girls it is always best to stay away from school during the first and second days... It is best that dancing, bicycle riding, horseback riding, rowing, and other athletic exercises be given up altogether during the menses. Automobile riding and railroad and carriage traveling prove injurious in some instances."[13,14]

The first attempt to study objectively the question of woman's need for extra rest during menstruation was made in 1876 by Mary Putnam Jacobi (1842-1906), one of the early female graduates from an American medical college, whose report won for her Harvard University's Boylston Prize. She called attention to statistics from various parts of the world attesting the work performed by women without provision for special rest during menstruation. In no country and at no time had women of the working classes confined themselves to their domestic chores, but had always entered eagerly into any type of remunerative employment that was open to them. Workshops for women existed in Europe before the 10th century. In convents the nuns manufactured everything needed for their own use and then for sale to others. Paris in 1861 contained 112,189 women known to be working outside the home, and in Great Britain 10 years later the textile industries were engaging 467,261 women, more than half the number of men employed in this field. The United States census for 1870 showed that one-sixth of the female population over age 10 was occupied in paid industry.

Using the meager technology of her era Mary Jacobi carried out a few simple experiments, making daily measurements of the urea excretion, pulse rate, body temperature, and muscular strength as gauged by a hand dynamometer; but she observed no significant variations related to menstruation among six subjects studied for periods up to 3 months. She submitted a list of 16 questions to 1000 young women. Thirty-five percent of the respondents reported that they had never suffered pain, discomfort, or weakness during menstruation. From her analysis of the questionnaire Jacobi concluded that no evidence could be found that rest during menstruation exerts any influence on pain. On the contrary, she maintained, "purely spasmodic pain of moderate intensity...is tolerated in an immense majority of cases, far better while the ordinary occupations are continued... There is nothing in the nature of menstruation to imply the necessity, or even the desirability, of rest, for women whose nutrition is really normal."[15]

Removal of the yoke of physiologic protectionism from women was but the first step toward their ultimate attainment of economic, political, and social equality with men. The concept that the menstruating woman was biologically inferior, handicapped, or even significantly different had been laid to rest. More remained to be learned, however, about her menstrual emanations.

On April 23, 1920 Dr. Béla Schick (1877-1967), Assistant in the Pediatric Clinic of the University of Vienna, who had achieved eponymic renown for his test for immunity to diphtheria a few years earlier, presented a paper before the Viennese Medical Society, which was published in abridged form in the Society's journal the following month.[16] Dr. Schick migrated to the United States in 1923, to join the staff of New York's Mount Sinai Hospital, where I knew him as an outstanding clinician and scientist in the early 1950s, when I served in that hospital's Department of Obstetrics and Gynecology. Because of his reputation for integrity within the medical community and the importance of his paper, reporting the first scientific investigation of a possible "menstrual toxin," I present in some detail the substance of my translation from his German.

On August 14, 1919, Schick reported, he received a bunch of about ten fresh, dark-red, long-stemmed, tightly budded roses, which he gave to a female assistant to put in water. The next morning he was astonished to find all the roses wilted, many of their petals having fallen off. When he asked the attendant if she could account for the flowers' demise, she answered that she knew this would happen and that she should not have handled them, because she was menstruating. Schick had heard of this phenomenon; and although he thought it probably a mere superstition, decided to test it by experiment.

On the second day of the woman's next menstruation she and a nonmenstruating woman, serving as a control, each obtained from the hospital gardener an anemone, a white chrysanthemum, and a yellow helianthus, which they held in their hands about ten minutes. Sixteen hours later the anemone held by the menstruating woman was streaked with brown lines; after another 24 hours it appeared quite withered; and by 48 hours it had dropped its petals. Comparable changes occurred in the other two flowers; least injured was the chrysanthemum. By contrast, the flowers held by the control woman still appeared completely fresh after 48 hours.

The experiment was repeated on the third day of the woman's menstrual period. She was given two white anemones, a white chrysanthemum, and a helianthus to hold for ten minutes. After only three minutes all the flowers began to wilt. Five hours later the anemones and the tips of the chrysanthemum were turning brown, but not the helianthus. The wilting of the anemones and chrysanthemum continued the next day.

On the fourth day of menstruation the woman's handling of the flowers seemed to have almost no effect on them; only their tips showed brownish discoloration. Some flowers indeed appeared fresher than the controls. After the fourth day of menstruation repetition of the experiment, conducted daily during the interval until the next period, no longer showed any damage to the flowers from handling.

In Schick's further investigations he found that many women failed to affect the test flowers during menstruation; and he assumed that these women produced lesser concentrations of the suspected menstrual toxin. Continuing his experiments with his original subject he learned that the damage to the anemones by handling during menstruation could be prevented or markedly reduced by her wearing rubber gloves.

Tobacco flowers handled during menstruation reacted similarly. Axillary sweat and blood obtained during menstruation, added to flasks of water holding the flowers, each produced the same effect.

Soon after the publication of Schick's paper, further investigation of the presumed menstrual toxin was taken up by David Macht[17] in the Johns Hopkins Medical School. Macht had been developing a method of testing the toxicity of fluids and tissue extracts by their effect on growing plants, an assay technique he termed "phyto-pharmacology," in which he used the seedlings of *Lupinus albus* as the test object.[18]

After soaking overnight in water, the seeds of the plant were embedded in sphagnum moss. Three days later the seedlings were placed in a nutrient solution in upright glass tubes, where their roots could be observed. Solutions to be tested were added to the tubes and their effect measured by the length of the roots after incubation for 24 hours. Quantitation of the toxicity was expressed by the "index of growth," the ratio of the length of the roots growing in the test solution to that of the seedlings in control tubes. Macht applied this technique to the study of the body fluids of menstruating women and, in later experiments, to the investigation of other problems.

SALIVA

Normal saliva, in a 1% mixture with the nutrient fluid, had a mild effect on the growth of the seedlings, producing an average growth index of 85%. Menstrual saliva, by contrast, usually from the same women, depressed the growth index to an average of 53%, specimens from the first day of or the day preceding menstruation manifesting greater toxicity than secretions from later days of the period.

BLOOD

Venous blood was obtained from 50 healthy women at the time of menstruation and again between their periods, and the serum tested in a similar manner for its effect on the *Lupinus* seedlings. The intermenstrual blood depressed the growth index slightly, to an average of 74%; whereas the serum during menstruation appeared significantly more toxic to the seedlings, as indicated by an average growth index of but 51%. Toxicity was greatest on the first 2 days of the period or the last premenstrual day, the growth index dipping as low as 35%. Whole blood proved even more inhibiting to the seedlings' growth than did the serum alone, lending support to Schick's view that the blood cells were the principal purveyors of the menstrual toxin, or "menotoxin".[19] Menstrual blood, extracted from perineal pads, was similar to systemic blood in toxicity to the seedlings.

OTHER SECRETIONS

Menstrual sweat proved even more toxic to the *Lupinus* seedlings than did saliva or blood. Lesser degrees of toxicity were observed in urine and milk secreted during menstruation.

CUT FLOWERS

Repeating Schick's experiments, but on the *Lupinus* seedlings, Macht confirmed the former's observations of the deleterious effect on cut flowers of the sweat of, or handling by, some menstruating women. Especially sensitive were roses, carnations, sweet peas, primroses, freesia, cineraria, and tulips. Hardy flowers, such as narcissus, appeared resistant to the menstrual factor.

OTHER EFFECTS OF MENOTOXIN

Plants normally grow in a specific direction. Thus the seed of *Lupinus albus*, germinating in a soft medium as sphagnum moss, normally sends its single straight root vertically downward (positive geotropism) and its stem straight upward (negative geotropism). Normal blood serum has but slight effect on this geotropic property of the plant. Both menstrual blood and saliva, by contrast, produced a marked disturbance in the geotropic behavior of the *Lupinus* seedlings, resulting in curvatures and deformities and causing both the roots and the stems to deviate from their normal vertical orientation.

The widespread belief that bread-dough kneaded during menstruation does not rise well was put to test with yeast paste added to a sugar solution. In tubes thus prepared and incubated, selective inhibition of the yeast activity, as evidenced by depressed gas production, occurred when the yeast was first rubbed on the hand of a menstruating woman, versus that of a non-menstruating control.

In other experiments menstrual serum appeared toxic to certain animals, including the unicellular paramecia and trypanosomes, goldfish, and guinea pigs; but their sensitivity to menotoxin was less than that of plants. The blood of menstruating rhesus monkeys, especially early in their period, was likewise found damaging to *Lupinus* seedlings. In experiments at the Fearing Research Laboratory in the Free Hospital for Women, an affiliate of the Harvard Medical School, the husband-and-wife team of George Van S. Smith and Olive Smith, he a gynecologist and she a biochemist, found menstrual discharge to be highly toxic to rats and rabbits, subcutaneous injections of the former with as little as 0.1 cc twice daily often resulting in death within 48 hours.[20] The Smiths associated the toxin in the discharge with the euglobulin fraction of the blood serum.[21] Macht found the postulated toxin to be soluble in alcohol and in chloroform, to a lesser extent in ether and in acetone; he believed it to be closely related chemically to oxy-cholesterin, a component of the fat in skin secretions and of fingernails and toenails.

Menstrual blood, systemic as well as uterine, does not clot as readily as blood of non-menstruating women. Menstrual serum, Macht showed, prolonged the coagulation time of both human and canine blood, a phenomenon he attributed to menotoxin.[22] Venous blood serum from menstruating women, the Smiths found, was consistently fibrinolytic;

that is, was able to dissolve a blood clot; whereas intermenstrual serum lacked this property.[23]

CONCEPTION AND THE LAWS OF NIDDAH

Until the 19th century little attention was paid to the timing of conception in the human. It had been commonly believed in the Talmudic era that women were fertile only around the time of menstruation, a view that prevailed for several centuries. Animal husbandrymen were familiar, of course, with the periodicity in the behavioral changes in female cattle and their sexual receptivity; and keepers of pets knew when a female animal was in heat and receptive to the advances of the male. In most primates, however, including monkeys, apes, and humans, in contrast to all other mammals, the female has no "heat" period. Menstrual bleeding is the only external manifestation of internal function; but its relation to the fertile period, the precise time of discharge of the egg from the ovary, remained unclear. In the mid-19th century T.L.W. Bischoff, a distinguished Austrian student of the physiology of reproduction, finding eggs in the genital tracts of female dogs in heat and with a bloody discharge, concluded that women too must be fertile at the time of their monthly flux. Nearly a century elapsed before proof of Bischoff's error was provided and the estrous bleeding in bitches was recognized as homologous not with menstruation but with the mid-cycle bleeding that occurs frequently in monkeys and occasionally in women.

The evidence that regularly menstruating women normally ovulate at mid-cycle was reviewed by Carl G. Hartman,[24] one of the 20th-century's foremost reproductive physiologists, at whose side in the Carnegie Laboratory of Embryology I was privileged to spend a year as a post-doctoral research guest. Many are the criteria of human ovulation, all in essential agreement:

Hormone Assays

Pituitary gonadotropins, hormones that stimulate ovarian secretions, are measurable in the blood in varying concentration in relation to the menstrual cycle, reaching their peak at mid-cycle (between days 12 and 17) in cycles between 24 and 33 days in length. Blood estrogen, the hormone of the enlarging ovarian follicle, also reaches its peak around the middle of the cycle, as the follicle approaches ovulation. Progesterone, the specific hormone of the ovary's corpus luteum, into which the follicle is converted after ovulation, is measurable in the urine as pregnanediol glucuronide, which is excreted in maximal concentration during the second half of the menstrual cycle.

Microscopic Analysis of Corpora Lutea

The age of the corpus luteum, and hence the time of ovulation, can be estimated by microscopic examination after surgical removal.

In one series, of 83 cases, ovulation was thus dated between the 16th and 12th day preceding menstruation. In another series, of 100 cases, the peak of ovulation occurrence was pegged at day 14 of the cycle.

The Endometrium

Like skin, liver, bone, and other organs, the endometrium had long been viewed as a tissue of specific histologic structure, variations from which were considered pathologic. Only at menstruation was the normal nonpregnant endometrium thought to undergo change. A meticulous study in 1908 of uterine specimens from 58 women at various stages of the menstrual cycle by Fritz Hitschmann and Ludwig Adler, assistants in Vienna's Universitäts-Frauenklinik, showed for the first time that the endometrium normally presents a continuously changing picture, repeated with each menstrual cycle, each picture characteristic of a specific phase of the cycle.[25] Thus the day-to-day histologic changes in the endometrium make possible dating of the stage of the menstrual cycle; and the secretory features associated with follicular maturation and rupture and the days that follow permit the confident diagnosis and timing of ovulation. All studies, based on biopsy, autopsy, and hysterectomy specimens, are in agreement: that the majority of women between ages 25 and 40 ovulate between 12 and 14 days before menstruation.

Vaginal Cytology

The lining of the vagina, like that of the uterus, being under the control of the ovarian hormones, also undergoes periodic changes—of build-up, breakdown, and sloughing of its cells. In specially stained preparations of vaginal smears ovulation can be diagnosed through specific cellular patterns and staining characteristics. A large study by this technique showed that when all the cycles were divided into percentiles of the whole and reduced to the conventional one of 28 days, the mode for the time of ovulation fell on day 14, exactly in the middle of the cycle.

Cervical Mucus

Also responsive to the changing levels of ovarian hormones are the cells lining the cervical canal which, in the course of their cyclic changes, produce an abundance of mucus at mid-menstrual interval. This outpouring of mucus constitutes one of the criteria of ovulation; but since it may precede ovulation by two or three days and may continue for several days thereafter, does not pinpoint the precise day of the event. Concurrent with the quantitative increase in the cervical mucus around the time of ovulation are physical changes in its character, including an increase in its threadability (*Spinnbarkeit*) and a fernlike pattern which the salts within the mucus form on drying.

Intermenstrual Pain

At about mid-cycle some women occasionally, and a few women repeatedly, experience pelvic pain, often on alternating sides from month to month, a phenomenon known as *Mittelschmerz*. The symptom is abolished by removal of the ovaries; and in cases in which the pain has led to surgical exploration and inspection of the pelvic organs, close correlation has been established with ovulation.

Basal Body Temperature

Early in the 20th century a Dutch gynecologist, in the course of recording the temperature of some of his patients, observed a drop in the temperature of one of them around the middle of her menstrual cycle, followed by a rise to a plateau, which was maintained almost to the onset of the next period. The physician casually suggested a relationship between the low point in the temperature readings and ovulation; but not until three decades later was the correctness of his surmise and the usefulness of basal body temperature recordings in the management of infertility demonstrated. About three-fourths of women with fairly regular cycles have typical biphasic temperature curves; the first phase, under estrogenic domination, one of gradually decreasing temperature to a low point at mid-cycle, when a "thermal shift" to the ascending leg occurs, under the influence of the corpus luteum, and a plateau is maintained to near the next menstrual period. Only rarely does such a temperature chart show the apparent sign of ovulation, the dip and thermal shift, at more than 4 days variance from 14 days before the onset of the next flow.

Artificial Insemination

Among women with cycles varying from 20 to 43 days in length who achieved pregnancy after a single artificial insemination, 98% conceived when inseminated between days 10 and 16.

Recovery of Eggs and Embryos

The age of young embryos can be estimated, within about half a day, by microscopic examination. With the cooperation of women who had to undergo hysterectomy for therapeutic reasons, the Harvard gynecologist-pathologist team of John Rock and Arthur Hertig secured a number of recently impregnated specimens, all of which confirmed the doctrine of mid-cycle ovulation and the greater consistency of the cycle's postovulatory phase, of about 14 days, than that preceding ovulation.

Remarkable agreement is found among all of the above criteria, indicating the time of ovulation and hence the optimal time for fertilization of the ovum and conception, at mid-cycle. More recent corroboration has been provided through monitoring of the growth of the developing ovarian follicle, destined for ovulation, by means of ultrasonography.

The Talmudic injunction of sexual abstinence for a minimum of 5 days, encompassing the time of the menstrual flow, followed by 7 blood-free days before marital relations could be resumed, thus brought first intercourse within a few days of ovulation for women with regular 28-day cycles, the ideal time for conception. Among women with significantly shorter cycles, on the other hand, observance of the laws of *Niddah* might serve in a contrary fashion, by delaying the resumption of coitus beyond the fertile days of the cycle.

NIDDAH AND THE SEX RATIO

The sex ratio in cattle, that is, the proportion of male to female births, increases, it is claimed, as mating takes place later and later in the estrous period. Cows mated early in heat produced calves with a sex ratio of 75; in the middle period, 116; late in heat, a sex ratio of 175.[26] Thus was apparent support given to Thury's theory of sex determination,[27] that ova that are over-ripe at the time of fertilization produce a preponderant number of male young.[28]

In a recently published novel[29] a woman begs Hannah the midwife for the secret for producing a male child, a secret she is confident the midwife carries because she is Jewish, and Jews "always have boys," allowing for a girl "now and then to keep your numbers growing." The sex ratio among viable infants in the general population is about 106; that is, 106 boys are born for every 100 girls. Prodded by her client's importuning, Hannah delved into the matter and learned that observant Jews of the early-19th century did indeed produce infants in a higher male-female ratio. Among the Jews of Prussia the sex ratio was reported at 113; of Breslau, 114; of Baltic Livonia, 120; as compared with a sex ratio of 104 among the non-Jewish segments of the population. The greater number of male than female births was ascribed by some to the laws of separation observed by Orthodox Jews, with coitus generally taking place late rather than early in the menstrual cycle; but others attributed the disparity to faulty registration data. In a sampling of Orthodox and presumably observant Jewish families in the east end of London in the early-20th century, however, the alleged preponderance of male over female births could not be confirmed.[30] My colleague Dr. Landrum B. Shettles has attributed the higher sex ratio among Orthodox Jews [if indeed a fact] to the competitive advantage that the faster swimming Y-chromosome-containing sperms have over those carrying the X-chromosomes, in the woman's alkaline cervical mucus around the time of ovulation.[31]

Conspicuously absent from medieval Jewish philosophy are attempts to rationalize the laws of *Niddah*. Only in the literature of the modern era have "reasons" been proposed in their justification, ranging from the medical, including cancer prophylaxis and fertility enhancement, to the psychological, under the rubric of "family purity." In the view of Rabbi Norman Lamm the cycle of abstinence and fulfillment provides for a recovery period for both husband and wife, with regulation of both male and female sexual rhythm and replenishment of the libidinal reservoir. "No voluntary separation," he insists, "can ever be as effective in providing this relaxation as one which is mutually accepted as religiously binding, and in which neither spouse may approach the other and, therefore, where neither need fear to decline and have his or her affection or ability suspect. Yet this, too, must not be mistaken for the purpose of these laws or as exhausting their full significance. Family Purity is a profoundly *spiritual, religious* institution. It may have...far-reaching psychological and beneficial consequences, but the appreciation of the meaning of these laws simply does not belong in the province of the psychologist or physician, nor of the anthropologist or sanitary engineer."[32]

SUMMARY

Polygamy, common in Biblical times, has been banned by Judaic law for 1000 years. The Bible considers male homosexual practice an abomination but has nothing to say about lesbian relationships.

The Bible and Talmud deal in detail with the conjugal restrictions during and following menstruation. The injunction of sexual abstinence for a minimum of 5 days, encompassing the duration of the menstrual flow, followed by 7 blood-free days before renewed conjugal relations, brings resumption of intercourse within what we now know to be the optimal time for conception; and may explain, in part, the legendary fertility of Jewish women.

The menstruating woman has ever been the subject of folklore and superstition. Widely prevalent was the belief that a powerful and noxious agent exists in her circulating blood. The concept that women are biologically inferior or handicapped during menstruation has long been laid to rest, but 20th-century observations, including pharmacologic experiments, attest the presence in the body fluids of some menstruating women of chemical agents toxic to certain plants.

NOTES AND REFERENCES

1. Encyclopaedia Britannica. 1953; 18:178.
2. Ackerman D. Wales. The New Yorker. Feb. 26, 1990:51.
3. It has been suggested that the identification of the first polygamist as a descendant of Cain might have implied a condemnation of the institution of polygamy. (Sarna, N.M., Ed: The JPS Torah Commentary: Genesis. Philadelphia, Jewish Pub Soc 1989; 37)
4. Feldman DM. Marital Relations, Birth Control, and Abortion in Jewish Law. New York: Schocken books 1974; 239.
5. This practice was banned by the Biblical edict of a later time, in God's instructions, through Moses, to the children of Israel: "Neither shalt thou

take a wife to her sister, to vex her to uncover her nakedness, beside the other in her life time." (*Leviticus* 18:18)
6. The Biblical original of *Ruth* 4:6: "I cannot redeem it for myself, lest I mar mine own inheritance: redeem thou my right to thyself; for I cannot redeem it."
7. Feldman DM. Birth Control in Jewish law. New York, New York University Press 1968; 36-37.
8. Ain S. Gay 'marriage'?: The Jewish Week, Dec. 27, 1991-Jan 2, 1992; 4,29.
9. Blasz E. The Code of Jewish Family Purity. Monsey, N.Y.: Committee for Preservation of Jewish Family Purity 13th ed. 1991.
10. *Genesis* 7:11.
11. Crawfurd R. Of superstitions concerning menstruation. Proc Roy Soc Med 1915; 9:49-66.
12. Clarke EH. Sex in Education, or a Fair Chance for Girls. Boston: James R. Osgood, 1874:156-157.
13. Robinson WJ. Woman: Her Sex and Love Life. New York: Eugenics Pub Co, 16th ed. 1928:80-81.
14. It would be interesting to correlate the performance of today's female athletes with their menstrual status.
15. Jacobi MP. The Question of Rest for Women During Menstruation. New York: GP Putnam's Sons. 1886.
16. Schick B. Das Menstruationsgift. Wien Klin Wochenschrift 1920; 33:395-397.
17. Born in Moscow in 1882, David I. Macht came to Baltimore as a child, received his bachelor's and medical degrees from the Johns Hopkins University; and after postgraduate study in Berlin, Munich, and Vienna, returned to his alma mater in 1909, where he spent a quarter-century as a member of its Department of Pharmacology and Experimental Therapeutics. He then assumed directorship of the Pharmacological Research Laboratory of Hynson, Westcott, and Dunning, a pharmaceutical firm in Baltimore; and in his later years served in a similar capacity and consultant in pharmacology in that city's Sinai Hospital, where he died in 1961. In addition to his reputation as a medical scientist he was widely respected as a Biblical and Shakespearean scholar. I was a frequent visitor in his laboratory and guest in his home; I dined at his table, and delivered some of his grandchildren.
18. Macht DI, Lubin DS. A phyto-pharmacological study of menstrual toxin. J Pharm and Exper Therap 1924; 22:213-220.
19. William Freeman and Joseph M. Looney, at the Worcester State Hospital and Memorial Foundation for Neuro-Endocrine Research, Worcester, Mass., failed to confirm these observations. (Studies on the Phytotoxic Index: II. Menstrual Toxin ("Menotoxin"), J Pharm and Exper Therap 1934; 52:179-183.
20. Smith OW, Smith GVS. Menstrual discharge of women. I. Its toxicity in rats. Proc Soc Exper Biol and Med 1940; 44:100-104.

21. Smith OW, Smith GVS. Menstrual discharge of women. II. Its progesterone-stimulating effect in mature rats. Proc Soc Exper Biol and Med 1940; 44:104-107.
22. Macht DI. Influence of menotoxin on the coagulation of blood. J Pharm and Exper Therap 1924; 24:213-220.
23. Smith OW, Smith GVS. A fibrinolytic enzyme in menstruation and late pregnancy toxemia. Science 1945; 102:253-254.
24. Hartman CG. The Time of Ovulation in Women. Baltimore; Williams and Wilkins, 1962.
25. Hitschmann F, Adler L. Der Bau der Uterusschleimhaut des geschlechtsreifen Weibes mit besonderer Berücksichtigung der Menstruation. Monatschr f Geburtsh u Gynäk. 1908; 27:1-82. (Translated in Speert H. Obstetric and Gynecologic Milestones, 2nd ed; in press, 283-310)
26. Pearl R, Parshley HM. data on sex determination in cattle. Biol Bull 1913; 24:205-225.
27. Thury M. Ueber das Gesetz der Erzeugung der Geschlechter bei den Pflanzer, den Thieren und dem Menschen. Leipzig, 1864.
28. It is now known that the sex of the mammalian offspring is determined not by the egg but by the sperm, half of which contain the X-chromosome (female) and half the Y-chromosome (male).
29. Courter G. The Midwife's Advice. New York: EP Dutton, 1992.
30. Pearl R, Salaman RN. The relative time of fertilization of the ovum and the sex ratio amongst Jews. Am Anthropologist 1913; 15:668-674.
31. Shettles LB, Rorvik DM. How to Choose the Sex of Your Baby. New York: Doubleday, 1989.
32. Lamm N. A Hedge of Roses. Spring Valley, New York: Feldheim Philipp 1977:44-45.

CHAPTER 8

FERTILITY AND ITS CONTROL

Most of the world's peoples, from tribes who have not yet learned to write, to the great historic civilizations of the past, have practiced some forms of population control.[1] Yet each year more than half of the more than 3 million pregnancies in the United States are unintended, 53% in the period 1985-1987.[2]

Were the words of God, to be fruitful and multiply, uttered to Adam and Eve, Noah and his sons, Abraham, and Jacob as a blessing or as a command? In postbiblical years, when men and women began to want babies only when they wanted them, and neither too few nor too many, the distinction became important. Some commentators have regarded the blessing of fertility as including the obligation of procreation. The majority of Biblical scholars, however, have viewed, in contrast to His charge to Adam and Eve, Abraham, and Jacob, only God's exhortation to Noah and his sons, after the Flood and the Earth's depopulation (*Genesis* 9:1 and its repetition in *Genesis* 9:7) as prescriptive; and further, as applying only to the men, for the women of Noah's household were not addressed in the mandate.[3,4] Interpretations of the commandment to reproduce and restrictions pertaining to contraception, abortion, and sterilization, all of postbiblical origin, are found in the Talmud and later law codes and their commentaries, and in the ever-growing body of *responsa*. Still in formation are Judaic attitudes toward artificial insemination, in vitro fertilization, sex selection, genetic counseling, and surrogate motherhood.

CONTRACEPTION

Linked with the commandment to man to procreate were his wife's conjugal rights; and on both was enjoined the pleasure principle, enunciated in 3rd-century Babylon by Rabbi Abba bar Aivu ("Rav"), founder of a number of early Talmudic academies. Renunciation of worldly pleasures he regarded as sinful ingratitude. "Man will have to render an account [to God]," he wrote, "for all the good things which his eyes beheld but which he refused to enjoy."[5] Sexual intercourse was thus viewed as involving two independent religious duties: reproduction and pleasurable marital union.

The ideal contraceptive would need be: acceptable to its users, safe and reliable, protective against sexually transmitted diseases, reversible when discontinued, free from side effects, convenient, and affordable. The over-riding principle governing all methods of contraception in traditional Judaic doctrine, however, has been the prohibition of *hash-hatat-zera* (improper emission of seed). Eligibility for contraceptive practice and the specific techniques and agents employed were judged by this standard.

The first example of *hash-hatat-zera* is related in the Biblical narrative of Onan, who refused to carry out the levirate obligation of inseminating his deceased brother's wife: "And Judah [his father] said unto Onan, Go in unto thy brother's wife, and marry her, and raise up seed to thy brother. And Onan knew that the seed should not be his; and it came to pass, when he went in unto his brother's wife, that he spilled it on the ground, lest that he should give seed to his brother. And the thing which he did displeased the Lord: wherefore he slew him also." (*Genesis* 38:8-10) Abhorrence of *hash-hatat-zera* was crystallized in the *Zohar*, the 13th-century text of Jewish mystic tradition, and codified in subsequent law, as the *Shulchan Arukh* of Joseph Caro.

In circumstances where pregnancy was viewed as hazardous to life or health, prevention of conception was not only permissible but mandated by Jewish law; but sexual abstinence would subvert not only one but both functions of the marital relationship. Recognized from the Talmudic era as categorically exempt from the procreational imperative, and to whom contraception was therefore permitted, was the triumvirate of women known as the *Baraita*: (1) a minor (between ages 11 and 12), because pregnancy, it was feared, might prove fatal;[6] (2) a woman already pregnant, whose conceptus might be compressed into a *fetus papyraceus* by a superimposed pregnancy;[7] and (3) a nursing mother, loss of whose milk might lead to death of her child.[8] Cognizant of differences of opinion among the rabbinate on details and on the precise interpretation of Talmudic passages, more recent scholars[9] have summarized the attitude of the early Talmudic authorities toward contraception: (1) that Talmudic-rabbinic law considers contraception inherently neither immoral nor illegal, but differentiates between birth control, which is permissible, and birth suppression, which is forbidden; (2) that the minimal reproductive requirement, incumbent upon every man, is the fathering of two children, in fulfillment of the Biblical command; and (3) that some circumstances may exempt a man from this duty, as (a) his engagement in religious work that might be hindered by familial responsibilities, or (b) impairment of his wife's health, making childbearing dangerous. In any case contraception was allowable only when acceptable to both parties.

Among the countless contraceptive substances that have been employed in various cultures for oral or intravaginal use are silphion,[10] okra seed pod, tannic acid, seaweed, root of spotted cowbane, lemon-juice, castor beans, marjoram, thyme, parsley, lavender, rosemary, crocus, myrtle, camphor, black hellebore, ball of opium, elephant dung, olive oil, cedar oil, copper sulfate, willow, fern root, cabbage blossoms, foam from a camel's mouth.[11]

Repeated reference is made in the Talmud to the "cup of roots," the ingredients of which are not specified, but the efficacy of which, both for the treatment of illness and as a sterilizing agent, was assumed to be widely known. "A man is not allowed to drink a cup of roots in order to become sterile," we are told (*Tosephta Yebamot*, viii, 4), "but a woman is allowed to drink a cup of roots in order to become sterile." In the time of the Great Flood, according to the *Midrash* (*Genesis Rabbah*, xxiii, 2) when it was customary for a man to have two wives, the wife for his sexual pleasure resorted to the cup of roots to prevent pregnancy. Rabbi Yohanan (d. 279 C.E.), respected for his medical knowledge during the Talmudic era, had his own recipe (*Shabbat*, 110 a): "Alexandrian gum [of the *Spina Aegyptia*], liquid alum, and garden crocus," he prescribed, "each in the weight of a denar, are mixed together… Two cups of beer with this medicine cure jaundice and sterilize." Three cups, it was believed, would be good for gonorrhea.[12]

Modern oral contraception had its origin in the late-19th century, when John Beard, an anatomist in Edinburgh, observed that ovulation is held in abeyance during pregnancy. Others soon found that this inhibition of ovulation was caused by a product of the corpus luteum, the ovarian structure into which the ovulated follicle is transformed. Fertile animals could be made infertile, it was shown, by injections or implants from corpora lutea. The physiologic basis for hormonal contraception was thus established.

The pharmaceutical industry led the way in its implementation, seeking synthetic compounds with longer action and greater oral potency than possessed by the natural hormones. By 1951 the agents for oral contraception were in hand. In May 1960 the U.S. Food and Drug Administration announced its approval of "Enovid," which had proved 100% effective in a 4-year test on 1500 women. Twenty pills a month provided women with a sure, easy method of contraception. This original contraceptive pill has since been replaced by a host of others which contain, in varying combinations, synthetic hormones that prevent ovulation by inhibiting the release of pituitary gonadotropin.[13] By 1982, 30 million women in the United States (55% of those aged 15 to 44 years) were using oral contraceptives.[14] With but few reservations, because of possible conflict with the doctrine of *p'ru ur'vu* (to be fruitful and multiply), the contraceptive pill has been approved in rabbinic *responsa*.[15]

Contraceptive protection for the three women of the *Baraita* was provided by the *mokh*, a spongy tampon that may have been adapted by the Israelites during their captivity in Egypt, from the lint used for vaginal occlusion by the Egyptian women. Rabbinic sages of the Talmudic period and later differed as to whether the use of the *mokh* was to be considered optional or obligatory by the three women; and some, following the most permissive opinion of Rabbi Joseph Caro in his 16th-century *Shulchan Arukh,* concluded that all women may use it. All agreed that it was preferable to the objectionable practice of *coitus interruptus,* for which Onan had been condemned. In the use of the *mokh* it was the woman, who was not committed to the duty of procreation, who performed the act of contraception, rather than the man.

Rediscovered, the moistened sponge was widely publicized as a contraceptive in England in 1823 through handbills disseminated by Francis Place and his assistants. The vaginal diaphragm was added to the contraceptive armamentarium by the Dutch Malthusian League in the early 1880s but received little recognition until early in the next century. Rabbinic *responsa* have been generally, but not universally, favorable to the diaphragm.[16]

A description of a linen penile sheath, for protection against venereal disease, was first published in 1564, by Gabriele Fallopio, the famous Italian anatomist for whom the uterine tubes are named. Not until the 18th century did the membranous condom, usually fashioned from an animal's cecum, become popular for contraception. With the vulcanization of rubber in 1884 contraception achieved explosive popularity because of the sudden cheapness of the new product, which virtually replaced its membranous antecedent. At mid-20th century the condom was the most widely used of all artificial contraceptives in the industrialized Western world. Eclipsed for several years by the diaphragm, oral contraceptives, and intrauterine devices, it has returned to the forefront at late-20th century as a result of heightened public concern over sexually transmitted diseases, especially acquired immunodeficiency syndrome (AIDS). The condom serves three functions: contraception, prevention of disease, and collection of semen for the investigation and treatment of infertility. Highly controversial is its current distribution to schoolboys in some communities. The traditional rabbinate stands together in opposition to the condom as a contraceptive because of its apparent incompatibility with the prohibition of *hash-hatat-zera.*

The earliest recorded mechanical agents for pregnancy prevention, the pastes and pessaries of animal feces described in the Kahun Papyrus of about 1900 B.C.E., served as contraceptives for 3 millennia. An intrauterine device for this purpose, consisting of a ring of silkworm gut bound by a spiral of aluminum bronze wire, was described by Richard Richter, a German physician, in 1909. Unaware of Richter's priority, his countryman Ernst Gräfenberg 2 decades later proposed a similar coil for contraception, which came to bear his name as the "Gräfenberg ring." Adapted in various new forms by American gynecologists, the intrauterine device enjoyed a meteoric rise in popularity in the 1970s but declined in favor in the closing decades of the century as an increasing number of complications came to light, especially menstrual disturbances and genital infections. Under the cloud of medicolegal liability the leading American manufacturer of intrauterine devices discontinued the sale of its two products in 1986; and the other major manufacturers also withdrew their uninsurable products from the market. In Feldman's analysis of rabbinic *responsa*,[4] in which the various methods of birth control were graded according to their degree of interference with the generative act, intrauterine devices, together with oral contraceptives, were ranked least objectionable.

Utilizing the physiologic principle that ovulation occurs about 2 weeks before the onset of a menstrual flow, Drs. Kayusaku Ogino of Japan and Hermann Knaus of Austria proposed a method of birth control in the early 1930s based on sexual abstinence between the 12th and 19th days before the expected next menses. In the course of abdominal operations on 83 patients whose cycles ranged from 23 to 45 days in length, Ogino noted whether the ovaries contained an unruptured follicle or a corpus luteum. Arranging his findings with reference to the last day of each patient's menstrual cycle rather than the first, he found that none of the women had ovulated after the 12th day nor before the 16th day *before* the end of the cycle. Allowing three days for the maximal survival time of the sperms, and convinced that the egg's survival time in measured in hours, not days, Ogino concluded that a woman is fertile from the 12th to the 19th day before the next expected menses. The remainder of the menstrual cycle was referred to as the "safe period," when no protection against conception was necessary. Ogino's teachings were extended and popularized by Knaus in a series of over 100 publications during the next 30 years.

Application of the Ogino-Knaus schedule of a "safe period" for coitus presented serious and obvious problems: (1) many women menstruate too irregularly to permit safe calculation of their fertile period; (2) the menstrual cycle is often disturbed by illness, pregnancy, psychic stress, or change in life routine. In short, a woman had no guarantee that her next cycle would follow the same pattern as the preceding cycles.

In actual practice the failure rate in reliance on the "safe period" for pregnancy avoidance was found almost triple that for mechanical and chemical methods of contraception.[17] In 1982 the International Planned Parenthood Federation concluded that "couples electing to use periodic abstinence should...be clearly informed that the method is not considered an effective method of family planning."[18] While emphasizing that reliance on the "safe period" provides inadequate safeguard when pregnancy is medically contraindicated, rabbinic *responsa* have condoned its practice for other than medical reasons, but only after the couple's procreative duty has been fulfilled. Like abstinence, traditional authorities point out, limitation to the "safe period" frustrates the commands of both *p'ru ur'vu* and of *onah* (sexual congress).[19]

STERILIZATION

Increasingly popular as a method of preventing conception has been interruption or mechanical blockage of the reproductive passages: the fallopian tubes in women and the vasa deferentia in men; but these procedures remain controversial on religious grounds. When the Fellows of the American Gynecological society, the nation's elite, debated the matter at its 21st Annual Meeting in 1896 Dr. Edward P. Davis argued: "I hold it to be the right of a woman...to make that choice... It is within the province of the accoucheur...to allow her the power of volition." Dissenting, Dr. H. J. Garrigues objected: "We must leave that to Nature or to God... I do not think that the woman has a right of that kind... The mere fact that she does not want to have more children should not decide the question."[20]

In a plea in 1921 for puerperal sterilization, John Whitridge Williams, obstetric chief at the Johns Hopkins medical institutions, lamented the rampant reproduction among Baltimore's prolific underprivileged: "It has always seemed to me," he wrote, "that one of the opprobia of medicine is...to advise the patient not to become pregnant again, and at the same time be morally certain that within a few months she will return in the same condition."[21]

On May 22, 1880 Dr. S. S. Lungren of Toledo, Ohio performed bilateral tubal ligation at the time of secondary cesarean section on a patient with a contracted pelvis, to preclude the possible need for another cesarean section, then highly dangerous.[22] According to the 1970 National Fertility Study almost three million married American women under age 45 or their husbands, living at that time, had opted for this method of pregnancy prevention. By 1980 sterilization was the method relied upon by most women over age 30, and the method of choice of 28% of women aged 15 to 44 years; and the proportion was continuing to increase.[23] More than one million sterilizing operations have been performed annually in the United States since then, the balance shifting from men to women as improved surgical and anesthetic techniques made the procedure easier for the latter. In 1970, for example, only 20% of the nation's 924,000 sterilizations were on women; whereas in 1975 they accounted for 51% of the 1,313,000 sterilizations performed. In that year more than one-third of tubal sterilizations in the United States were accomplished through the laparoscope; by 1993, the large majority. By 1979 a member of more than half of U.S. couples was undergoing sterilization within 10 years of the couple's last wanted birth.[14]

The basis for the traditional Judaic attitude toward sterilizing operations may be found in God's charge to Moses regarding offerings, from which all subsequent commentaries stem: "Ye shall not offer unto the Lord that which is bruised, or crushed, or broken, or cut; neither shall ye make any offering thereof in your land." (*Leviticus* 22:24) The Union of American Hebrew Congregations' edition of *The Torah* (W. G. Plaut, ed. New York: 1981; 916) gives the following version of the same passage: "You shall not offer anything [with its testes] bruised or crushed or torn or cut. You shall have no such practices in your own land." "No such practices" is interpreted as mutilations. *The New English Bible* (Oxford University Press, 1970; 135) reads: "If its testicles have been crushed or bruised, torn or cut, you shall not present it to the Lord; this is forbidden in your land."

Thus the Bible apparently prohibits sexual mutilation of male animals. The *Gemara*, however, views the verse as categorically forbidding castration of all animals, both male and female (*Shabbat* 110 b). Subsequent commentators on traditional Jewish law have extended this proscription to humans as well. Orthodox scholars agree that vasectomy for male sterilization is unacceptable,[24] but differ widely as to non-castrating sterilization of women. Some see such operations as a violation of Biblical law; others find no Biblical basis for prohibition of female sterilization. Many contemporary authorities maintain that only if pregnancy poses a threat to the life of the woman can sterilization be sanctioned.[25]

In summary, the Judaic attitude toward contraception is complex, reflecting a diversity of philosophies and of interpretations that defy reconciliation through the words of the Bible, the precepts of the Talmud, or the *responsa* of the rabbinate. The Reform and Conservative branches of Judaism have expressed approbation of contraceptive practice without serious qualification. The position of the former, first stated in 1931, was reiterated in 1960 by the Central Conference of American Rabbis. The Rabbinical Assembly of America, speaking for the Conservative movement, stated in 1934 that "Jewish tradition explicitly recognizes the desirability of the use of contraceptives... Proper education in contraception and birth control will not destroy, but rather enhance, the spiritual values inherent in the family and will make for advancement of human happiness and welfare." The Orthodox viewpoint, by contrast, as enunciated by the Rabbinical Alliance of America in 1958, condemned contraceptive measures used by the husband, while allowing for a diversity among the rabbinate in its restrictive attitude toward the practices of women. "In cases where the health of the female is jeopardized," the Alliance stated, "certain birth control measures are allowed, and then only through direct consultation between the medical and rabbinic authorities."

APPLIED GENETICS

The Account in *Genesis* 30 of Jacob's exposure of his mating flocks to streaked wooden rods and the speckled and spotted offspring that resulted was cited in chapter 5 as a possible example of the belief in maternal impressions: that stimuli to which the mother is exposed during pregnancy might affect the fetus. An alternative interpretation of the episode, embraced by some modern scholars,[26,27] credits Jacob with a knowledge of the principles of genetics some 4 millennia before the classical experiments of the Moravian Catholic abbot, Johann Gregor Mendel, in 1866. Mendel's observations on inheritance in garden peas, subsequently extended to all organisms that reproduce bisexually, led to the conclusion that the germ cells, male and female, contain paired factors now known as genes, which determine the organism's characteristics. When homozygous individuals with differing characteristics were crossed and their genes combined, the feature that prevailed in the genetically hybrid (heterozygous) offspring was called the dominant of the paired genes; the suppressed characteristic, the recessive. When members of the hybrid generation were now bred among themselves, half of the germ cells containing the dominant gene and half the recessive, one-fourth of the product, on average, were genetically pure (homozygous) for the dominant gene, one-fourth homozygous for the recessive gene, and half (heterozygous) had one of each. Thus three-fourths of the new generation showed the dominant physical characteristic, one-fourth the recessive.

Returning to the Biblical account of Jacob, who had worked 14 years in Haran for Laban, his devious uncle and now father-in-law, and was negotiating for compensation for his labor before returning to his homeland:

"And it came to pass...that Jacob said unto Laban, Send me away, that I may go unto mine own place, and to my country. Give me my wives and my children, for whom I have served thee, and let me go: for thou knowest my service which I have done thee. And Laban said... Appoint me thy wages, and I will give it. And he said unto him, Thou knowest how I have served thee, and how thy cattle was with me. For it was little which thou hadst before I came, and it is now increased unto a multitude; and the Lord hath blessed thee since my coming: and now when shall I provide for mine own house also? And he said, What shall I give thee? And Jacob said, Thou shalt not give me any thing... I will pass through all thy flock to day, removing from thence all the speckled and spotted cattle, and all the brown cattle among the sheep, and the spotted and speckled among the goats: and of such shall be my hire... And Laban said, Behold, I would it might be according to thy word."

The usual color of Syrian sheep is white; Syrian goats, black. Some of the former may have dark patches, and some of the goats white markings; but these comprise only a small minority of their respective flocks. Thus Laban readily accepted Jacob's proposal, in the belief that he was besting his son-in-law in the bargain. Nonetheless Laban promptly withdrew from the flocks all animals with the characters that would have destined them for Jacob's ownership and removed them a safe distance: "And he removed that day the he goats that were ringstraked and spotted, and all the she goats that were speckled and spotted, and every one that had some white in it, and all the brown among the sheep, and gave them into the hand of his sons. And he set three days' journey betwixt himself and Jacob: and Jacob fed the rest of Laban's flocks." (*Genesis* 30:25-36)

The battle of wits between Jacob and Laban continued: Jacob had probably noted, according to one suggestion,[26] that the mating of two white sheep occasionally resulted in a black offspring; and that the black goats sometimes produced a speckled animal. These anomalous young implied that the parent animals were heterozygous, carrying the recessive gene for the suppressed coloring. In such matings the recessive coat color would appear in a ratio to the dominant color of one to three.[28] By controlled breeding of the single-colored heterozygotes, which are detectable by a characteristic hybrid vigor known as heterosis, Jacob could have obtained the desired offspring.

Jacob credited to a dream his idea for thus breeding the animals, as he recounted the event to his wives Leah and Rachel: "And it came to pass at the time that the cattle conceived, that I lifted up mine eyes, and saw in a dream, and, behold, the rams which leaped upon the cattle were ringstraked, speckled, and grisled. And the angel of God spake unto me in a dream, saying... Lift up now thine eyes, and see, all the rams which leap upon the cattle are ringstraked, speckled, and grisled: for I have seen all that Laban doeth unto thee." (*Genesis* 31:10-12)

Thus ascribing to the grace of God his success in the selective breeding of the animals, Jacob achieved restitution for Laban's perfidy: "And Jacob took him rods of green poplar, and of the hazel and chestnut tree; and pilled white strakes in them, and made the white appear which was in the rods. And he set the rods which he had pilled before the flocks in the gutters in the watering troughs when the flocks came to drink, that they should conceive when they came to drink. And the flocks conceived before the rods, and brought forth cattle ringstraked, speckled, and spotted. And Jacob did separate the lambs, and set the faces of the flocks toward the ringstraked, and all the brown in the flock of Laban; and he put them not unto Laban's cattle. And it came to pass, whensoever the stronger cattle did conceive, that Jacob laid the rods before the eyes of the cattle in the gutters, that they might conceive among the rods. But when the cattle were feeble, he put them not in: so the feebler were Laban's, and the stronger Jacob's." (*Genesis* 30:25-42)

The three trees from which Jacob cut the rods were known to contain substances used for medicinal purposes in the ancient world.[29] The wooden stakes with peeled white stripes, erected in the watering troughs, may have stimulated the animals to copulate, either by acting as a visual aphrodisiac[26] or through chemical agents leeched from the wood into the water and hastening the females into estrus before their segregation.[29]

TAY-SACHS DISEASE

As it permitted Jacob to prevail over Laban, the application of genetic principles has made possible the elimination of a fatal disease to which Jews are particularly vulnerable. Tay-Sachs disease is one of at least 11 autosomal[30] recessive disorders that affect mainly Ashkenazi Jews.[31] Carriers can be detected for three: Niemann-Pick disease and Gaucher disease, lipid storage disorders, and Tay-Sachs disease, each caused by lack of a specific enzyme. Only for Gaucher disease has replacement of the missing enzyme given encouraging results.

In 1894 Warren Tay, a British ophthalmologist and surgeon, described the train of symptoms in a hitherto unrecognized syndrome: mental retardation, paralysis, blindness, and death. As he had noted previously in another infant in the same family, cherry-red spots were seen in the retinas of the eyes. Soon thereafter, unaware of Tay's report, Bernard Sachs, Bavarian-born New York neuropathologist, wrote an article on arrested cerebral development associated with a cherry-red retinal spot; and, recognizing the familial nature of the condition, called it "amaurotic familial idiocy." Known since as Tay-Sachs disease, the disorder usually becomes apparent by 5 months and ends in death by 4 or 5 years. It is now known to result from an abnormal accumulation in the brain of the metabolite ganglioside, caused by a deficiency in the enzyme hexaminidase A.

Tay-Sachs disease is the product of a defective recessive autosomal gene. Thus when both parents are carriers for it, each of their children bears a 25% risk of being affected. Carrier status can be determined by a blood test for the crucial enzyme. It is estimated that one in about 25 Ashkenazi Jews in the United States is a carrier; in some communities as many as one in 16. One New York rabbi watched four of his children succumb to the disorder. Among the non-Jewish population, by contrast, only one in 150 to one in 300 individuals has reduced hexasaminidase A activity consistent with Tay-Sachs carrier status.

A screening program for testing carriers, with centers throughout the United States and in Canada, Israel, South Africa, and Western Europe, has resulted in a dramatic decline in Tay-Sachs disease among Jews, to the extent that most new cases are now detected among non-Jews.[32] The traditional rabbinate emphasizes that such screening be done before marriage, so as not to frustrate a fertile union. Marriages should not be encouraged that are likely to lead to the birth of defective offspring; but once consummated, the marriage is bound to the obligation to "be fruitful and multiply."[25] The Committee on Obstetrics: Maternal and Fetal Medicine, of the American College of Obstetricians and Gynecologists, has recommended that among intermarried couples the Jewish partner be screened and if he or she is found to be a Tay-Sachs carrier, the other partner be screened also. If the woman is already pregnant both partners should be screened simultaneously, so that the results be received in a timely fashion. If both prove carriers genetic counseling should be recommended and amniocentesis for prenatal diagnosis offered.[33]

Management of pregnancies remains controversial, in which sampling of the amniotic fluid has shown the fetus to be affected with Tay-Sachs disease. In the view of Rabbi Eliezer Waldenberg abortion of such a fetus is permissible until the 7th month of pregnancy. Rabbi Moses Feinstein disagrees, on the ground that the fetus presents no threat to the life of the mother and its abortion is therefore forbidden by Judaic law. He advises, further, that observant Jewish physicians refrain from amniocentesis for testing for fetal Tay-Sachs disease, for fear that a positive diagnosis and the physician's subsequent constraint against pregnancy termination would lead to additional and unnecessary parental suffering. Moreover, in Rabbi Feinstein's opinion, the physician performing the amniocentesis would have to bear the onus for an abortion carried out by another.[34]

Since artificial termination of pregnancy is unacceptable to some, the Chevra Dor Yeshorim program was inaugurated in 1983 in an ultra-Orthodox community in Brooklyn, New York, permitting the computerized confidential screening, by number rather than name, of high school students, and the counseling of young men and women before marriage, with the halting of prospective matches in which both parties are Tay-Sachs carriers. In its first four years no births of Tay-Sachs affected infants occurred within the program. Similar programs have been instituted in several other major American cities and in Israel.[35]

ABORTION

Summarizing the attitude of the medieval rabbinate on the nature of ensoulment, acknowledged as a secret of God, Rabbi Meir Abulafia (d. 1244) concluded, in his oft-quoted Talmudic commentary, that the soul enters at conception but the embryo does not become a person until born. Fetocide thus came to be sharply differentiated from homicide in Judaic jurisprudence. Classic sources fail to provide a clear legal basis for the condemnation of voluntary abortion. No traditional authority, however, sanctions abortion for other than therapeutic purposes; and most frown upon the termination of pregnancy resulting from incest or rape.[25] A large segment of the liberal rabbinate, on the other hand, have taken a more permissive position on termination of early pregnancy, regarding as mere fluid, part of the mother, with no independent status, the fertilized ovum prior to 40 days after conception. In their view the slightest reason, including socioeconomic factors or family planning, might justify abortion.[36] The spiritual destinies of the fetus, state most *responsa*, are irrelevant to the abortion question.[37]

The Judaic attitude toward therapeutic abortion has evolved from the concept of the fetus as an aggressor. The *Mishnah* not only permits but requires abortion if necessary to save the life of the mother: "If a woman has [life-threatening] difficulty in childbirth, one dismembers the embryo within her limb by limb,[38] because her life takes precedence over its life. Once its head (or its greater part) has emerged, it may not be touched, for we do not set aside one life for another." (*Oholot:* 7,6) In a 19th-century *responsum*, paraphrased by Feldman,[37] Rabbi Yekutiel Teitelbaum (d. 1875) explained: "A pursuer or attacker may be killed in defense or self-defense even when disabling him *may* do the trick. Just as the law of pursuer applies even when such doubt exists, so a foetus whose threat to the mother's life is only doubtful (that is, the physicians see a strong *possibility* that her life is in danger), may, according to this reading, be aborted."

In another *responsum* a few years later Rabbi Shneur Zalman of Lublin (d. 1902) added: "A foetus is...like a pursuer in that, despite its innocence and because it is not yet a person, it must be sacrificed to save its victim... Thwarting a pursuer moreover, is fulfillment of a *mitzvah*;[39] hence Maimonides' distinctive citation of the commandment 'not to take pity on the life of the pursuer' in the matter of the foetus."

Judaism has never countenanced the destruction or neglect of the maimed, malformed, or weakling newborn, practiced in some other cultures. Sharp distinction exists in Jewish law, however, between a defective and a potentially defective infant, between a life in being and a life in prospect. Reasonable suspicion of disease or deformation of a fetus might justify its abortion, on the ground that the mere possibility of the birth of a defective is causing severe mental anguish to the mother. Feldman generalized from rabbinic *responsa*: "The fetus is unknown...the mother is known, present, alive, and asking for compassion."

Some environmental agents capable of frustrating normal development of the embryo were mentioned in chapter 5. Notorious among the drugs was thalidomide, causing phocomelia. Viruses, similarly, can damage the fetus. Cytomegalovirus, the viral agent acquired most frequently in utero, may result in hearing loss, mental retardation, and neurologic abnormality; but only a minority of infants are so affected by it. The large majority, although continuing to harbor and excrete the virus, grow up normally. Rubella (German measles) by contrast, a common childhood disease and almost always mild in the pregnant woman, produces devastating effects on the developing fetus in most cases, the congenital rubella syndrome, first recognized in 1941, including deafness, cardiac defects, and mental retardation. A pandemic of rubella in 1964 resulted in 20,000 to 30,000 affected infants in the United States alone. Preconceptual immunization is now available, but

10 to 15% of the adult U.S. population still has no detectable antibody to the virus and is thus considered at risk of infection. When rubella is diagnosed in pregnancy most rabbis, as most physicians, agree that abortion is justifiable.

EXECUTION IN PREGNANCY

When a woman known to be pregnant is charged with a capital crime, Talmudic law requires that her trial be postponed. If, on the other hand, a convicted woman is found to be pregnant only after the guilty verdict has been rendered and she has been sentenced to death, the *Mishnah*[40] ordains that execution not be delayed for her delivery, but proceed directly upon sentencing, in keeping with the basic obligation of the court embodied in *innui ha-din* (the law of suffering), which demands that unnecessary suffering of the convicted be avoided.

INTERVENTION DURING PREGNANCY

Responsibilities of the mother to the fetus during an ongoing pregnancy are tacitly implied, but not spelled out, in Jewish law. Some risk and some restraint must be assumed by the mother for the sake of the fetus. Her moral responsibility, however, does not necessarily imply legal obligation to accept recommended medical treatment or restriction, nor does it always coincide with religious doctrine. She may refuse to submit to cesarean section, for example, in a situation in which her physician urges the operation in the interests of the fetus. Or, as in the case with Jehovah's Witnesses, she may refuse blood transfusion, even in the face of clear medical indication. Current legal rulings emphasize the integrity of the individual and his or her right to refuse treatment.

No legal obligation exists requiring a person to render aid to another, especially when such an act imposes risk to the potential benefactor. The parent-child relationship is considered special under the Samaritan law, however, imposing a legal onus upon the parent.

The hazards to the fetus of maternal alcohol ingestion during pregnancy (see chapter 5) are now well known. Highly publicized also have been the fetal dangers of maternal addiction to other drugs and of tobacco smoking. Cocaine can cause spontaneous abortion and placental separation. Cocaine-exposed infants experience growth retardation, increased mortality, and a variety of physical abnormalities. Cigarette smoking likewise may result in spontaneous abortion, premature birth, low birth weight, and retarded development. The physician can only instruct and counsel in such matters, and cannot be held responsible for the patient's informed rejection of advice or refusal of medical care. Several state courts in the United States have ruled that existing statutes against child abuse and neglect do not apply to the mother-fetus relationship. The most effective method of preventing maternal behavior harmful to the fetus, concluded the Board of Trustees of the

American Medical Association, is through education and early medical and psychotherapeutic intervention.[41]

SEX SELECTION

Sex of the fetus, the ancients believed, could be influenced by prayer, but only up to the 40th day of pregnancy. Thereafter, according to the Talmud (*B'rachot*, 60a), supplication was in vain, for the sex of the infant was already determined. Sex, we now know, is fixed at conception. If the ovum is fertilized by an X-bearing sperm a female results; if by a Y-bearing sperm, a male. Recent research has shown that the male-determining gene begins to produce its effects in the developing embryo between days 43 and 49 after conception, in good agreement with the beliefs of the early Talmudists.[42]

The Talmud also tells how Leah's prayers during pregnancy resulted in the birth of Dinah, the only female among Jacob's 13 offspring. Jacob had already sired 10 sons: 6 by Leah and 2 by each of the maidservants Bilhah and Zilpah. Leah knew (whether through a voice or a dream we are not told) that Jacob was to be the father of 12 sons. Hoping to spare her sister Rachel, still childless, the humiliation of bearing fewer sons to Jacob than had each of the servant women, Leah prayed that the fetus already in her womb would be born a female, thus leaving the possibility to Rachel of producing two sons. Leah gave birth to Dinah; and Rachel, subsequently, to Joseph and Benjamin. According to the narrative in the Palestinian Talmud, Dinah's birth is to be seen as the result of an intrauterine sex reversal.[43] An alternative interpretation will be given in a later paragraph.

A long-held view relates fetal sex to the timing of orgasm, the sages teaching that if the woman emits her semen first she will bear a male child; if the man, a female. Rabbi Zadok saw recognition of this theory in the Biblical introduction to Leah's progeny: "These be the sons of Leah, which she bare unto Jacob in Padan-aram, with his daughter Dinah." (*Genesis* 46:15) The sons are thus ascribed to Leah, the daughter to Jacob.

The strength of manhood was seen as including the power of control in coitus and of restraint in orgasm. Scripture records that "the sons of Ulam were mighty men of valor, archers, and had many sons, and sons' sons, an hundred and fifty," (*I Chronicles* 8:40) an achievement attributed to the men's ability to hold back in intercourse so that their wives might be first to experience orgasm. Rabbi Kattina boasted: "I could make all my children to be males.[44]

Recent research by Dr. Landrum Shettles supports this ancient but still controversial belief. In his popular book on sex selection he explained: "The woman trying to conceive a boy should try to achieve orgasm just *before* the male orgasm. Female orgasm usually increases the quantity and flow of the natural alkaline secretions (more favorable to the male-producing sperm). And the orgasmic contractions of the female help rapidly transport sperm into the cervix, where the secretions are even more favorable for the male-producing sperm."[45]

Sex, in Jewish law, is determined irrevocably by the gonads at birth, whether external or internal; and is unaffected by subsequent situational factors, including surgical removal of the organs for therapeutic purposes, as in the treatment of tumors. Neither psychological considerations, as parental preference or sexual orientation, nor inability to function in one's biological gender role, justifies a change in sexual status.[46]

ARTIFICIAL INSEMINATION

So long as the husband could perform the conjugal act, infertility in a marriage was ascribed to the wife. Male potency implied virility. Only when coitus could not be consummated because of impotence or anatomic aberration was the husband's role in the reproductive process impugned. The obvious resort then was to artificial insemination, the deposition of semen into the female's genital tract without sexual intercourse. This was performed successfully with the eggs and sperm of fish in 1742 and in mammals in 1780, when the Italian anatomist Lazaro Spallanzani impregnated a bitch with the semen of a dog. At about the same time, the illustrious British surgeon John Hunter impregnated the wife of a man suffering from hypospadias, an anatomical penile defect, by vaginal injection of her husband's semen. For years Talmudic scholars had debated the possibility of a woman's conceiving by bathing in water into which a man had previously discharged his semen,[47] or by sleeping on a sheet stained with semen.[48]

Artificial insemination has become increasingly popular during the 20th century and is performed in tens of thousands of cases annually in the United States. In cases in which the husband's semen is used, the procedure is designated A.I.H.; when semen from a donor other than the husband, A.I.D. Both are fraught with serious halakhic difficulties. Orthodox rabbis have been unable to reach agreement as to whether A.I.D. should be looked upon as adultery, or as to the legitimacy of the resulting children. Jerusalem's Rabbi Eliezer Waldenberg and others termed the procedure an abomination, because it obscures the child's genealogy,[49] leads to the possibility of incest by subsequent marriage, and might permit wrongful inheritance after the donor's death. In addition, Rabbi Waldenberg continued, A.I.D. violates the Scriptural prohibition, even in the absence of the sexual act: "thou shalt not lie carnally with thy neighbor's wife, to defile thyself with her." (*Leviticus* 18:20)

The sages disagree also on the relationship of donor to offspring: whether the former should be considered its parent, and whether in his role he fulfills the Biblical commandment of procreation.[50]

More permissive has been the rabbinic attitude toward A.I.H., in which the objectionable features of A.I.D. are eliminated, but traditional authorities fail to agree whether the procedure may be carried out during the ritually unclean days of women with short menstrual cycles (see chapter 7). Rabbi Moshe Feinstein has argued that if a woman's ovulation is found to occur during her proscribed state of *niddah* and no other method has succeeded in producing conception, A.I.H. may be performed at any time during this period.[51]

Most agree that the procurement of semen for analysis, as well as for A.I.H., does not violate the proscription of *hash-hatat-zera* ("improper emission of seed"), for the semen is to be used for the prescribed purpose of procreation. Masturbation into a jar is recommended by most physicians for semen collection; but traditional rabbis sanction masturbation only when no other method can be employed for the purpose, such as *coitus interruptus*, or withdrawal, retrieval of semen from the vagina, or the Milex sheath (the latex rubber of ordinary condoms being toxic to sperm).

IN VITRO FERTILIZATION

The earliest account of fertilization of human ova outside the body dates back to 1946, when Drs. Miriam F. Menkin and John Rock, at Harvard, reported the development of two-cell and three-cell stages from ovarian eggs exposed to spermatozoa in an incubated glass dish. Widely heralded was the birth of Louise Brown, in London, 3 decades later, on July 25, 1978, the first resulting from in vitro fertilization and transplantation of the fertilized ovum into the woman's uterus, performed by Drs. Robert Edwards and Patrick Steptoe.[52] After a brief period of moral acculturation, medical institutions throughout the world rapidly embraced the procedure in their efforts to alleviate the barrenness of women without functional oviducts. By 1983 at least five in vitro fertilization clinics had been established in the United States as well as two in Australia. An international symposium on human in vitro fertilization was held in 1984, and a year later the American Fertility Society offered a course in in vitro fertilization at its annual meeting. The procedure had been recognized by the medical profession and approved by the community. The U.S. Office of Technology Assessment reported that some 14,000 attempts at in vitro fertilization were carried out in 1987 by 70 to 80 medical teams, and by the following year 160 in vitro fertilization clinics were in operation in the United States, with continually improving success rates.

Expressions of Judaic attitude toward in vitro fertilization were soon forthcoming, raising a number of moral and theological questions.[53] At the annual rabbinic convocation in Israel in the summer of 1978, soon after the birth of the Brown baby, Chief Sephardic Rabbi Ovadiah Yosef gave his qualified approval of the procedure; while his Ashkenazic counterpart, Rabbi Shlomo Goren, declared it "morally repugnant, although halakhically unobjectionable."

Initial moral reservations concerning in vitro fertilization were based largely on doubts of its safety. Although the original experimentation may have been unconscionable, ethicists pointed out, there would be no objection to the procedure once it was proved free of risk to the fetus. The safety of in vitro fertilization has since been amply demonstrated. "The history of medicine is full of instances," ethicist Dr. Daniel Callahan noted, "where things were done unethically but led to benefits for people."[54] "Jewish ethics knows of no Miranda principle," Bleich added, "which would bar the use after the fact of information obtained by illicit means."[55]

Traditional rabbis are in agreement that the sperm used for in vitro fertilization must be the husband's and collected within the same guidelines that apply to A.I.H.

OVUM TRANSPLANTATION

In vitro fertilization having proved feasible and safe, a variety of ovum transplant procedures soon followed, with the transfer of fertilized and unfertilized ova to fallopian tube or uterus, according to medical circumstance.[56] Ovum transplants figure in several of the eight methods of human reproduction listed by Fletcher:[57] (1) coital-gestational, (2) artificial insemination with husband's sperm, (3) artificial insemination with donor's sperm, (4) egg transfer from a wife inseminated by her husband, to another woman's womb for gestation (surrogate motherhood), (5) egg transfer from a donor to another woman, married or unmarried, before or after insemination ("prenatal adoption"), (6) egg obtained from a donor woman, inseminated by a donor male, and implanted into the uterus of another woman, (7) gestation of a fetus in an artificial womb with an artificial placenta, (8) cloning, in which the nucleus is removed from an egg (the subject's or a donor's), replaced with another nucleus from a body cell (from the same or another person, male or female), and the egg implanted into the subject's uterus. The developing fetus is thus genetically identical with the nucleus donor. Human pregnancy has been achieved through all but the last two of the above procedures.

Could the Talmudic sages have anticipated 20th-century technology in their legendary accounts of the gestations of Dinah and Joseph in the wombs of Leah and Rachel (*Genesis* 30:21-24)? Rachel, it will be recalled, got the mandrakes (see chapter 5), and her conception that ensued may have antedated that of Leah, although the former's delivery of Joseph did not occur until 3 years later. Leah, in the meantime, had given birth to Dinah. Rabbi David Bleich has pointed out that these pregnancies and births, as narrated in the Babylonian Talmud (*Berachot* 60a) and the Palestinian Talmud (*Berachot* 9:3), can be interpreted as resulting from in utero sex changes, or as embryo transfers: that Dinah was conceived by Rachel and transferred to Leah's womb, and that Joseph was later conceived by Leah and transplanted into Rachel.[58]

Jewish traditionalists regard the embryo of less than 40 days as a mere protoplasmic glob, without biologic identity; after 40 days, as a person in development. Accordingly, a child born from embryo transplantation more than 40 days after conception would be considered the legal offspring of the biologic parents; if born from an earlier transplant, the offspring of the host mother.[59]

SURROGATE MOTHERHOOD

In March 1986, in the nation's first legal opinion on the parentage of a child conceived from the egg and sperm of a married couple but carried through gestation and birth by a surrogate mother for a fee of $10,000, a Michigan judge declared the couple to be the legal as well as the biological parents.[60]

The issue was widely publicized the same year, when surrogate mother Mary Beth Whitehead, after a change of heart, unsuccessfully demanded custody of the child she bore after artificial insemination in contract with William Stern, the natural father;[61] but 2 years later the New Jersey Supreme Court ruled unanimously that such a contract violated state criminal laws against baby-selling. In another case of litigation over custodial rights, in September 1990, in which a couple's artificially inseminated egg was brought to term by a surrogate mother for a fee, a California judge awarded the child to the couple, the genetic parents.

On October 1, 1987 a 48-year-old woman in Johannesburg, acting as a surrogate for her 25-year-old daughter, who had previously undergone hysterectomy, gave birth to triplets from her daughter's ova that, as host mother, she had nurtured after they had been inseminated with her son-in-law's sperm. The grandmother was adjudged, under South African law, legal guardian of the three children whom, according to a law professor at the University of the Witwatersrand, the biological mother might have to adopt.[62] A similar case was reported in South Dakota in 1991.[63]

In the meantime for-profit programs for surrogate motherhood services were established by lawyers and physicians wherever permitted in the United States by state law. In 1993 only 15 states had laws dealing with surrogate births. In August 1989 the Infertility Center of New York announced the birth of the 300th baby under its auspices. The British Government, on the other hand, pursuant to its Warnock Commission's 1984 report proposing outlaw of all forms of surrogate motherhood, legislated to ban commercial surrogacy; and in 1992 New York State likewise enacted legislation declaring surrogacy contracts void. More aggressive was the Australian Commission for the State of Victoria, whose infertility laws in 1984 banned, in addition to all forms of surrogate mothering, the sale of human tissues including semen, ova, and embryos, and cloning.

Serious question exists as to the compatibility of surrogate motherhood with Jewish law. The Committee on Medical Ethics of New York's Federation of Jewish Philanthropies has judged host motherhood permissible within the framework of Judaism "only in the absence of an alternative";[64] but most rabbis who have commented publicly on surrogate parenthood have found it morally repugnant, without basis in Jewish law, and have recommended its ban. In the words of Britain's Chief Rabbi Immanuel Jakobovits, "to use another person as an 'incubator' and then take from her the child she carried and delivered for a fee is a revolting degradation of maternity and an affront to human dignity... Man," he insisted, "as the delicately balanced fusion of body, mind and soul, can never be the mere product of laboratory conditions and scientific ingenuity. To fulfill his destiny as a creative creature in the image of his Creator, he must be generated and reared out of the intimate love joining husband and wife together, out of identifiable parents who care for the development of their offspring, and out of a home which provides affectionate warmth and compassion."[65]

FROZEN EMBRYOS

Human blood, semen, bone, and eye corneas were being frozen and stored for future use; why not embryos? The viability of a fertilized ovum after preservation in the frozen state was demonstrated in 1984 by the birth of a child from a previously frozen embryo.[66] Only a year earlier, however, a morass of legal, ethical, and religious questions was created by the death in a plane crash of an American couple who had left two frozen embryos in the custody of a medical center in Melbourne, Australia for possible implantation at a later date, but without documented instructions for their disposition in this contingency.

In September 1989 a judge in Tennessee ruled in divorce proceedings that seven frozen embryos produced through in vitro fertilization were children, not property, and should go to the woman who might carry them to term, not to her estranged husband.[67] On appeal, however, the court reversed its opinion and found that the father had equal rights in the disposition of the oocytes. In 1992 the Tennessee Supreme Court upheld the decision of the court of appeals and ruled, in addition, that if no prior agreement exists concerning disposition of embryos, the right not to procreate ordinarily takes precedence over the right to procreate.

Infertility specialists have been freezing fertilized ova in quantity, for later implantation, since about 1986. In 1990 alone 129 American clinics froze 23,865 pre-embryos, according to the American Fertility Society. Tens of thousands, it is estimated, remain in storage. Authorities believe that, immersed in liquid nitrogen, the ova can be stored indefinitely.[68]

Conception is now possible without copulation; gestation can be postponed and birth delayed at will after the union of egg and sperm; children can be sired by fathers long dead; and the natural sequence of generations can be altered in the family's genealogy. A quarter-century after his popular projection of the future, Aldous Huxley reflected: "That we are being propelled in the direction of *Brave New World* is obvious. But no less obvious is the fact that we can, if we so desire, refuse to cooperate with the blind forces that are propelling us."[69]

SUMMARY

Interpretation of God's words to Adam and Eve, to be fruitful and multiply, repeated to Noah and his sons and to Abraham and Jacob, and the restrictions pertaining to contraception, abortion, and sterilization, all of the latter of postbiblical origin, are found in the Talmud, later law codes, and in the ever-growing body of *responsa*. Still in formation are Judaic attitudes toward artificial insemination, in vitro fertilization, sex selection, genetic counseling, and surrogate motherhood.

Linked with the commandment to man to propagate were his wife's conjugal rights, and on both was the pleasure principle enjoined. Sexual intercourse thus came to be viewed as embodying two religious duties: reproduction and pleasurable marital union. Contraception was sanctioned only to the extent that it did not violate the prohibition of *hash-hatat-zera* (the improper emission of seed). Jewish law mandated prevention of conception in circumstances where pregnancy was viewed as hazardous to life or health. The "cup of roots" prescribed by the Talmud for pregnancy prevention finds its modern counterpart in the contraceptive pill introduced in mid-20th century. Rabbinic *responsa* have given qualified approval to the vaginal diaphragm and intrauterine devices, but the traditional rabbinate opposes the use of the condom for contraception.

The Biblical account of Jacob's breeding of his uncle's livestock has been variously interpreted as a belief in maternal impressions and as a manifestation of Mendelian genetics. The application of genetic principles now makes possible the prevention of Tay-Sachs disease and other genetic disorders to which some Jews are particularly vulnerable.

According to an oft-quoted Talmudic commentary, the embryo does not become a person until born. Judaic jurisprudence thus sharply differentiates fetocide from homicide. Traditional Jewish authorities nonetheless sanction abortion only for therapeutic purposes; most frown upon termination of pregnancy even when resulting from incest or rape. Classic rabbinic sources fail, however, to provide a clear legal basis for the condemnation of voluntary abortion.

Recent research has provided some support for the long-held belief that fetal sex may be related to the timing of orgasm: the ancient sages having taught that if the woman experiences orgasm first, she will bear a male child; if the man comes to climax first, a female.

Artificial insemination with donor semen is rejected, on several grounds, by the traditional rabbinate; more permissive has been its attitude toward insemination with the husband's semen. Most agree that the procurement of semen for analysis, as in cases of infertility, as well as for artificial insemination, does not violate the proscription of *hash-hatat-zera*.

Since the widely heralded birth of Louise Brown in London in 1978, in vitro fertilization has achieved explosive popularity in the treatment of infertility of women without functional oviducts. A few traditional rabbis continue to find the procedure "morally repugnant," but most agree that it is halakhically unobjectionable, provided that the husband's sperm is used. Some modern scholars have read into the Talmudic accounts of the births of Dinah and Joseph a foretelling of the current practice of embryo transfer.

The Committee on Medical Ethics of New York's Federation of Jewish Philanthropies has judged surrogate motherhood permissible within the framework of Judaism, "in the absence of an alternative;" but New York State and a number of other legislative bodies have either banned it or declared surrogacy contracts void. Most rabbis find surrogate motherhood "an affront to human dignity."

NOTES AND REFERENCES

1. Newton N. Population limitation in cross-cultural perspective. I. Pattern of contraception. Lying-in: J Reproduct Med 1968; 1:343-354.
2. National Institute of Child Health and Human Development: Research Reports, November 1992.
3. Sarna NM. ed. The JPS Torah Commentary: Genesis. Philadelphia: Jewish Pub Soc 1989; 13,353.
4. Feldman DM. Marital Relations, Birth Control, and Abortion in Jewish law. New York: Schocken Books 1974; 46.
5. Feldman DM. Marital Relations, Birth control, and Abortion in Jewish law. New York: Schocken Books 1974; 82.
6. Rabbinic authority frowned upon the Oriental practice of marriage to child brides: but unable to stop it among the Jews, authorized contraception to mitigate its hazards.
7. Various other explanations, none convincing, have been suggested for the exemption of the second woman of the *Baraita*. Superfetation, which postulates ovulation during pregnancy, has never been proved in the human and was not widely accepted even in the Talmudic period.
8. The usual period for nursing was about 2 years, during which time interference with the maternal milk flow, as would result from a superimposed pregnancy, presented a threat to the nursling.
9. Rabbi Solomon Luria (1510-1574) and the late Dr. Jacob Lauterbach, Professor of Talmud in the Hebrew Union College, Cincinnati. See Gandz, S.: "The Bible and the Talmud," in Himes NE. Medical History of Contraception. New York: Gamut Press 1963 (1936):77-78.

10. An oral contraceptive from a species of *Ferula*, or giant fennel, that grew in antiquity in the hills near the Greek city-state of Cyrene in North Africa. After several centuries of cultivaiton, it was harvested into extinction. Experiments with extracts from its living relatives support the claims of the ancients that silphion was an effective contraceptive. (Riddle JM, Estes JW. Oral contraceptives in ancient and medieval times. Am Scientist 1992; 80:226-233).
11. Hardin G. The history and future of birth control. Perspect Biol and Med 1966; 10:1-2. citing Himes N. Medical History of Contraception. New York: Gamut Press 1963 (1936).
12. Himes N. Medical History of Contraception. New York: Gamut Press 1963 (1936); 76-77.
13. Speert H. Obstetrics and Gynecology in America: a History. Am Coll Obstetr and Gynecol. Chicago 1980; 164-166.
14. Bachrach CA. Contraceptive practice among American women: 1973-1982 Fam Plann Perspect 1984; 16:253-259.
15. Feldman DM. Marital Relations, Birth Control, and Abortion in Jewish Law. New York: Schocken Books 1974; 242.
16. Feldman DM. Marital Relations, Birth Control, and Abortion in Jewish Law. New York: Schocken Books 1974; 105, 235.
17. Hartman CG. Science and the Safe Period. Baltimore: Williams and Wilkins 1962.
18. IPPF International Medical Advisory Panel: Statement on Periodic Abstinence for Family Planning. IPPF Med Bull 1982; 18:2-3.
19. Feldman DM. Marital Relations, Birth Control, and Abortion in Jewish Law. New York: Schocken Books 1974; 248.
20. Speert H. Obstetrics and Gynecology in America: a History. Am Coll Obstetr and Gynecol. Chicago 1980; 68.
21. Williams JW. The problem of effecting sterilization in association with various obstetrical procedures. Am J Obst and Gynec 1921; 1:783-793.
22. Lungren SS. A case of cesarean section twice successfully performed on the same patient, with remarks on the time, indications, and details of the operation. Am J Obst 1881; 14:78-94.
23. Mosher WD. Contraceptive practice in the United States, 1982-1988. Fam Plann Perspect 1990; 22:198-205.
24. Amelar RD, Dubin L, Gordon J, Tendler MD. Male infertility practice and orthodox Jewish law. Urology 1977; 10:177-180.
25. Bleich JD. Judaism and Healing. Hoboken, New Jersey: Ktav Pub Co 1981:65,96.
26. Macht DI, Macht MB. A genetic appreciation of Jacob's wages (Genesis xxx). Synagogue Light 1939; 7:3-5, 14-15.
27. Flicks Y. Torsha Usevivah Bema'aseh Yaakov Batzon Laban (Heredity and Environment: Genetics in Jacob's Handling of Laban's Flock). Techumin 1982/5742; 3:461-472 (Hebrew).
28. The mode of inheritance of coat color in the goats may involve a modified two-factor ratio or other somewhat more complex mechanism. Macht

DI, Macht MB. A genetic appreciation of Jacob's wages (Genesis xxx). Synagogue Light 1939; 7:3-5, 14-15
29. Sarna NM. ed. The JPS Torah Commentary: Genesis. Philadelphia: Jewish Pub Soc 1989; 212.
30. Other than a sex chromosome; thus, disorders not sex-related.
31. Jews of central and northern European origin, as contrasted with Sephardic Jews, from Spain and the Mediterranean region.
32. Magil B. Progress in prenatal diagnosis of "Jewish" genetic diseases. Contemp OB/GYN 1978; 11:87-88.
33. ACOG Committee Opinion 93:March 1991.
34. Sinclair DB. Tradition and the Biological Revolution. Edinburgh: Edinburgh Press 1989; appendix A, 93.
35. Merz B. Matchmaking scheme solves Tay-Sachs problem. JAMA 1987; 258:2636,2639.
36. Rosner F. Modern Medicine and Jewish Ethics. Hoboken, New Jersey: Ktav Pub Co 1986:150.
37. Feldman DM. Birth Control in Jewish Law. New York: New York Univ Press 1968:262-292.
38. Maimonides, in "Laws of Homicide and Preservation of Life" in his code, the Mishnah Torah, about 1178, added: "either with drugs or surgery."
39. A commandment or precept.
40. Arakhin, I, 4 (7a).
41. Board of Trustees, American Medical Association: Legal Interventions During Pregnancy. JAMA 1990; 264:2663-2670.
42. Goldman AL. Religious Notes. New York Times July 28, 1990; 9.
43. Rosner F. Modern Medicine and Jewish Ethics. Hoboken, New Jersey: Ktav Pub Co 1986:121.
44. Rosner F. Modern Medicine and Jewish Ethics. Hoboken, New Jersey: Ktav Pub Co 1986:130.
45. Shettles LB, Rorvik DM. How to Choose the Sex of Your Baby. New York: Doubleday, 1989; 163.
46. Bleich JD. Judaism and Healing. Hoboken, New Jersey: Ktav Pub Co 1981:78.
47. According to legend, Ben Sira, son of Prophet Jeremiah's daughter, was conceived in a public bath by his mother's contact with sperm of a previous male bather, without sexual contact.
48. Rosner F. Artificial insemination in Jewish law. Judaism 1970; 19:452-464.
49. Medical ethics prevent identification of the donor, but concealment of paternal identity is prohibited by Judaic law. In adoption as well, natural parentage must be disclosed, either to the child or an intimate of the child, to permit avoidance of subsequent incestuous marriage. In a study of A.I.D. records at one hospital in the United States at least 500 pregnancies were attributed to semen donations by one intern. A similar study in Beersheba, Israel credited 73 births to a single donor. The resultant possibilities for close intermarriage are obvious, to say nothing of the eugenic contraindications to such a concentration of the gene pool. Rabbi

Feinstein suggested (Igrot Moshe: Even Haezer 10) that when A.I.D. is performed, although in the face of Judaic doctrine, records of paternity be kept and made available, and that the donor be preferably a non-Jew, to further reduce the risk of incestuous marriage. (Meir L. Ed. Jewish Values in Health and Medicine. Lanham Md: University Press of America 1991:166-167).
50. By 1985 about half of the states in the U.S. had enacted laws making the consenting husband the legal father of a child resulting from A.I.D. (Elias S, Annas GJ. Social policy considerations in noncoital reproduction. JAMA 1986; 255:62-68).
51. Amelar RD et al. Male infertility practice and orthodox Jewish law. Urology 1977; 10:177-180.
52. People magazine (March 5, 19484; 73) named Louise Brown one of the ten most prominent people of the decade "by simply being."
53. Bleich JD. Judaism and Healing. Hoboken, New Jersey: Ktav Pub Co 1981: 86.
54. New York Times July 27, 1978:A16.
55. Bleich JD. Judaism and Healing. Hoboken, New Jersey: Ktav Pub Co 1981: 86.
56. American College of Obstetricians and Gynecologists: ACOG Technical Bulletin 140, March 1990.
57. Fletcher J. The Ethics of Genetic Control. New York: Doubleday/Anchor 1974:40.
58. Rosner F. Modern Medicine and Jewish Ethics. Hoboken, New Jersey: Ktav Pub Co 1986:121.
59. Rosenfeld A. Generation, gestation and Judaism. Tradition 1971; 12:78.
60. New York Times March 18, 1986; April 17, 1986.
61. Kolbert E. Battle for baby M.: Fierce emotions and key legal issues. New York Times; August 23, 1986. After this case, in the wave of anti-surrogacy sentiment that followed, several countries including France, Germany, Japan, and Israel outlawed the procedure; two states passed statutes making surrogate brokering a crime; and nine others made surrogacy contracts unenforceable (Allen C. When motherhood is for sale. Wall St Journal Jan. 8, 1991).
62. Battersby JD. South African woman gives birth to three grandchildren, and history. New York Times Oct. 2, 1987.
63. Wall St. Journal, Aug. 6, 1991; 1.
64. Rosner F. Modern Medicine and Jewish Ethics. Hoboken, New Jersey: Ktav Pub Co 1986:120.
65. Jakobovits I. Eugenics in Jewish Medical Ethics. New York: Bloch Pub. 1975:261; quoted in Rosner F. Recombinant DNA, Cloning, Genetic Engineering, and Judaism. New York J Med Aug 1979; 1439-1444.

66. New York Times April 11, 1984, A16.
67. Int Herald Tribune Sept 22, 1989.
68. American College of Obstetricians and Gynecologists: ACOG Newsletter Aug. 1992; 6.
69. Huxley A. Brave New World Revisited. New York, Harper & Row 1958:24-25.

CHAPTER 9

CIRCUMCISION

A medical forebear of mine, a little over a century ago, envisaged the role of the foreskin in the life of Neanderthal man: "Nature," he wrote, "always careful that nothing should interfere with the procreative function, had provided him with a sheath or prepuce, wherein he carried his procreative organ safely out of harm's way, in wild steeplechases through thorny briars and bramble-brakes, or, when hardly pushed and not able to climb quickly a tree of his own choice, he was by circumstances forced up the sides of some rough-barked or thorny tree. This leathery pouch also protected him from the many leeches, small aquatic lizards, or other animals that infested the marshes or rivers through which he had at times to wade or swim; or served as a protection from the bites of ants or other vermin when, tired, he rested on his haunches on some mossy bank or sand hill."[1] The foreskin was thus grouped with other rudimentary organs of primitive man, including a climbing muscle, ear muscles, dilated and movable nostrils, and the appendix.

"In the far-off land of Ur," my 19th-century predecessor continued, "among the mountainous regions of Kurdistan, something over 6,000 years ago, the fathers of the Hebrew race, inspired by a wisdom that could be nothing less than of divine origin, forestalled the process of evolution by establishing the rite of circumcision."

"The Old Testament is for the study of circumcision," mused a scholar,[2] "what its story of creation was for the natural sciences, namely the point of departure instead of the terminus..."

The origins of circumcision lie buried in antiquity and in the ruins of the Alexandrian Library. In the view of Herodotus, Greek historian of the 5th century B.C.E., the Israelite rite was probably adopted by the Phoenicians, from Chaldea, in the mountains of Armenia and Kurdistan, whence it spread, through maritime enterprises, to foreign ports. The Egyptians adopted circumcision for the priesthood and nobility. Evidence of circumcision among the early Egyptians is found in their bas-reliefs[3] and their mummies. We can assume that Pharaoh was circumcised, from Ezekiel's warning to him, in the words of the

Lord: "To whom art thou thus like in glory and in greatness among the trees of Eden? yet shalt thou be brought down with the trees of Eden unto the nether parts of the Earth: thou shalt lie in the midst of the uncircumcised with them that be slain by the sword." (*Ezekiel* 31:18)

In the New World circumcision was practiced among the Aztecs, from whom the custom spread to the Incas and other tribes of the Americas.[4] A circumcision scene is clearly depicted in the Great Pyramid of Teotihuacán, near Mexico City, built before the Aztec civilization.[5]

The oldest of surgical operations, circumcision came to be the most widespread as well, practiced on every continent to the remote regions of the Earth, from Alaska to the South Sea Islands. It has been estimated that one-seventh of the world's male population is circumcised.[2] Year in and year out, it remains the most frequently performed surgical procedure in the United States,[6] usually done for hygienic or prophylactic purposes. In many cultures circumcision is a puberty ritual, a rite of passage.[5] It is traditionally practiced among peoples of the Islamic faith, but for other than religious reasons; circumcision is not mentioned in the Koran. The Arabs embraced it long before the birth of Mohammed.[7]

BIBLICAL BACKGROUND

For the Jews circumcision has been an indispensable religious ritual, the sign of the covenant, since God's command to Abraham; "This is my covenant which ye shall keep, between me and you and thy seed after thee; Every man child among you shall be circumcised. And ye shall circumcise the flesh of your foreskin; and it shall be a token of the covenant betwixt me and you. And he that is eight days old shall be circumcised among you, every man child in your generations, he that is born in the house, or bought with money of any stranger, which is not of thy seed. He that is born in thy house, and he that is bought with thy money, must needs be circumcised: and my covenant shall be in your flesh for an everlasting covenant." (*Genesis* 17:10-13)

The year has been reckoned as 2047 (1713 B.C.E.)[8] (some have put the date at 2107 of the Hebrew calendar[9]) when Abraham, at age 99 years, carried out God's command: "And Abraham took Ishmael his son, and all that were born in his house, and all that were bought with his money, every male among the men of Abraham's house; and circumcised the flesh of their foreskin in the selfsame day, as God had said unto him. And Abraham was ninety years old and nine, when he was circumcised in the flesh of his foreskin. And Ishmael his son was thirteen years old when he was circumcised in the flesh of his foreskin." (*Genesis* 17:23-25)

Although he was not to be born until the following year, the covenant, through the rite of circumcision, was intended for transmission to Isaac rather than his half-brother Ishmael, according to God's word to Abraham: "And God said, Sarah thy wife shall bear thee a son indeed; and thou shalt call his name Isaac: and I will establish my covenant with him for an everlasting covenant, and with his seed after him. And as for Ishmael... I have blessed him, and will make him fruitful...and I will make him a great nation. But my covenant will I establish with Isaac, which Sarah shall bear unto thee at this set time in the next year." (*Genesis* 17:19-21) Thus was established the principle of matrilineal inheritance of the covenant, still preserved among traditional Jewry.[10]

Whether Moses was ever circumcised is a matter of conjecture. Some commentators believe that he had undergone the ritual in infancy and was thereby identified as an Israelite when Pharaoh's daughter found him in a basket, hidden in the bulrushes: "And when she had opened it, she saw the child...and said, This is one of the Hebrews' children." (*Exodus* 2:3-6) Others, however, doubt that the leader of the Israelites was ever circumcised.

After 40 years' separation from his people, Moses left his father-in-law Jethro in Midian and, at God's command, returned with his wife Zipporah to the Israelites in Egypt, with the assigned mission of liberating the Children of Israel from their Egyptian bondage. God had warned, earlier, that "the uncircumcised man child whose flesh of his foreskin is not circumcised, that soul shall be cut off from his people; he hath broken my covenant." (*Genesis* 17:14) Understandable therefore was His anger at Moses' failure to circumcise his son:[11] "And it came to pass...that the Lord met him, and sought to kill him."[12] (*Exodus* 4:24)

At their encampment in the desert Zipporah saved the day in the enigmatic, cryptically related scene that followed, in which she used a traditional flint stone to fulfill the obligation of the covenant. The omission of essential details and the resultant multiplicity of versions of the event have been attributed by scholars to the belief that the full story was well known, either through oral tradition or in documents long lost: "Then Zipporah took a sharp stone, and cut off the foreskin of her son, and cast it at his feet, and said, Surely a bloody husband art thou to me." In an alternative translation[13] Zipporah "touched his legs with it, saying, "You are truly a bridegroom of blood to me. . . . A bridegroom of blood because of the circumcision."' (*Exodus* 4:25-26)

So important did circumcision become in Jewish culture and law that in later years one not circumcised, even though for medical reasons, was disqualified from participation in the Festival gatherings in Jerusalem and from entrance into the Temple. Neither an uncircumcised man nor his father was permitted to testify in a Jewish Court of Justice (*Beth Din*); nor were the usual laws of mourning observed for them.[9]

Nonetheless, after their Exodus from Egypt and during their 40 years in the wilderness the Israelites grew lax in observance of the circumcision ritual and may indeed have abandoned it, because of the rigors of desert life and travel and the extreme daytime heat: "Now all the people that came out were circumcised: but all the people that were born in the wilderness by the way as they came forth out of Egypt, them they had not circumcised." (*Joshua* 5:5)

Having arrived at the banks of the Jordan, the Israelites thus needed to be circumcised before their crossing over into the Promised Land. Joshua had succeeded Moses as their leader. The Bible explains: "At that time the Lord said unto Joshua, Make thee sharp knives, and circumcise again the children of Israel the second time. And Joshua made him sharp knives, and circumcised the children of Israel at the hill of the foreskins, And this is the cause why Joshua did circumcise: All the people that came out of Egypt, that were males, even all the men of war, died in the wilderness by the way, after they came out of Egypt... For the children of Israel walked forty years in the wilderness, till all the people that were men of war, which came out of Egypt, were consumed, because they obeyed not the voice of the Lord... And their children, whom he raised up in their stead, them Joshua circumcised: for they were uncircumcised, because they had not circumcised them by the way." (*Joshua* 5:2-7)

In later years circumcision was prohibited, from time to time, by rulers of the lands in which the Israelites lived. Proscription of the rite by Syrian King Antiochus, for example, helped fuel the Maccabean struggle, in the 2nd century B.C.E. Two hundred years later Roman Emperor Hadrian again prohibited the practice among the Jews.

Some of the circumcised, to facilitate their assimilation, attempted to obliterate evidence of the operation by lengthening the foreskin. The *Apocrypha* tells of the practice of *epispasmus* in the time of Antiochus Epiphanes: "In those days went there out of Israel wicked men, who persuaded many, saying, Let us go and make a covenant with the heathen that are round about us: for since we departed from them we have had much sorrow. So this device pleased them well. Then certain of the people were so forward herein, that they went to the king, who gave them license to do after the ordinances of the heathen: whereupon they built a place of exercise at Jerusalem according to the customs of the heathen: and made themselves uncircumcised, and forsook the holy covenant..."[14] Plastic operations for the purpose were described by Celsus (20 B.C.E.) and Galen (150 years later).

THE OPERATION

The early practice of circumcision consisted merely of amputation of the distal, redundant portion of the foreskin. "The Jewish rite," explained Briffault, "did not assume its present form until so late a period as that of the Maccabees (167 B.C.). At that date it was still performed in such a manner that the jibes of Gentile women could be evaded, little trace of the operation being perceptible. The nationalistic priesthood therefore enacted that the prepuce should be completely removed."[15]

The surgical requirements for ritual circumcision, as spelled out in the Talmud, entail three steps: (1) *milah*, amputation of the prepuce; (2) *priah*, tearing back of the mucous membrane and complete exposure of the glans; and (3) *mezizah*, application of the operator's lips to the wound and the sucking of a few drops of blood from it. (*Shabbath* 19:2)

Mezizah was decreed by the Talmudists as a hygienic adjunct, to prevent poisoning by the iron instruments; and was later elevated to a religious act.[16] Maimonides, in the 12th century, staunchly supported it as prophylactic against inflammation, through the healing power of saliva. Reports accumulated, however, of infection of a number of infants with tuberculosis and syphilis from the *mohel*, or operator. *Mezizah* fell under violent attack by both civil and ecclesiastic authorities in Germany, France, and England; and in the middle of the 19th century legislative reform movements for the standardization of circumcision procedures resulted in its abolition. To retain the symbolism of *mezizah* some traditional *mohelim* use a glass tube or pipette to aspirate a drop or two of blood from the fresh circumcision wound.[17]

The Talmudists recognized the hazard of hemorrhage from circumcision in families with bleeding tendencies. The tractate *Yebamoth* specifically forbids the procedure on the third son of a woman whose previous two male infants died of hemorrhage from it. Maimonides, in his *Mishneh Torah*, acknowledged the genetic basis of hemophilia and its transmission by the mother, in stating that the same prohibition applied even if the earlier sons were sired by different fathers. Additionally proscribed by the Talmud was the circumcision of an infant if two of his mother's sisters had lost a son from bleeding following the procedure.[18]

CIRCUMCISION IN THE UNITED STATES

The earliest recorded ritual circumcisions in America were performed in 1756 in New York by Abraham Isaac Abrahams, recently arrived from Brest-Litovsk, who served in a variety of religious capacities for the neighboring Jewish communities of New Jersey, Connecticut, and Rhode Island. By correspondence he instructed Moses Seixas, who became the *mohel* for Newport.[19] Not until the 20th century were measures undertaken in the United States to ensure the medical safety as well as the religious authenticity of the procedure. Each of the three major branches of Jewish observance now has its own Brith Milah Board, for certification and supervision of accreditated practitioners of the ritual. The Brith Milah Board of New York, organized in 1914 by the city's Jewish community, supervised by the New York Board of Rabbis, and supported by the Federation of Jewish Philanthropies, "produced a new type of mohel," in the words of Rabbi Leo Jung "one who is thoroughly acquainted with Jewish law and thoroughly familiar with the elements, methods and manner of hygiene and medicine."[20]

Together with New York's Mt. Sinai Hospital the Brith Milah Board of New York sponsored in 1968 a school for the formal training of *mohelim*, the first school of its kind, offering a 2-year program of instruction, with courses in anatomy, physiology, pathology, asepsis, microbiology, psychology, and circumcision technique and postoperative care, together with clinical seminars and a 1-year internship.

At that time, it was estimated, 100 *mohelim* were already practicing in the metropolitan New York area. Only a few were to be found, however, in some of the country's other major cities. Chicago and Boston, for example, had but three each. To meet the perceived need, the Brith Milah Board of New York and the New York Board of Rabbis helped establish the Brith Milah Board of America in 1978, for the purpose of instituting "programs, meetings and correspondence; to exchange experience, inform about problems...in a ceaseless process towards perfection," lest ritual circumcision "pass into oblivion in America."[20]

As a liberal alternative to the Orthodox school for *mohelim* in New York, the Reform Union of American Hebrew Congregations, together with the Hebrew Union College-Jewish Institute of Religion and the Central Conference of American Rabbis, in 1985 established a program for the training and certification of *mohelim* and *mohelot* (female). By Spring 1991, 86 Reform *mohelim* and *mohelot*, all medically licensed, had participated in the prescribed course of 14 2-hour instructional sessions, in nine major American cities, and received certification by the Brit Milah Board of Reform Judaism. In 1989 the National Organization of Mohelim and Mohelot was created, for the purpose of continuing their religious education.

That same year, the Conservative movement established its own training program for performers of ritual circumcision, in the form of a 6-day educational conference at the Jewish Theological Seminary in New York, co-sponsored by the movement's Rabbinical Assembly, to supplement the medical training in circumcision received by the participants in their home communities. As in the Reform movement, women were included in the program, eligible for certification as *mohelot*, in accordance with the Conservative interpretation of Jewish law.

TIMING OF CIRCUMCISION

The trend toward early discharge of mother and child after hospital births began during World War II. Only in cases of complications or medical necessity do they now remain in hospital as long as 8 days. Might the requirement that circumcision be carried out on the eighth day, many have asked, be liberalized to permit in-hospital performance of the ritual earlier? Its medical feasibility has been amply established. At one hospital, in Rochester, New York, for example, some 5000 infants were circumcised within an hour after birth without mishap.

Rashi (Rabbi Solomon ben Isaac), famous Talmudic scholar of Troyes, France during the late-11th and early-12th centuries, commented on the matter because of the difference in wording of verses 12 and 13 of *Genesis* 17. The former states, "he that is 8 days old shall be circumcised among you;" but the latter fails to specify age. In the *Mishnah*, Rashi pointed out, *Shabbath* 19:5 explains: "A child may be circumcised on the 8th, 9th, 10th, 11th, or 12th day, but never earlier and not later... If a child is sick it is not circumcised until it becomes well." The Talmud continues: that if one buy a female slave and her infant son, the latter is circumcised immediately upon purchase, even if not 8 days old. Similarly, if one have a female slave who converts to Judaism, her infant son is to be circumcised immediately upon his mother's conversion, regardless of his age.

Tractate *Shabbath* also refers to *Leviticus* 12:2-3, which says: "If a woman have conceived seed and born a male child...in the eighth day the flesh of his foreskin shall be circumcised." This specific wording, some scholars believed, excludes those who are not "born," as infants delivered by cesarean section;[21] but not all rabbis have agreed on this point.

Except in the case of the infants of slaves, circumcision before the eighth day is allowed, states *Yore Deah* (263:2), a section of the Jewish legal code, only when the child dies earlier. The rite is then performed at the grave, without recitation of the blessings. Modern authorities concur: according to a Reform *responsum* of 1953, circumcision before the eighth day "under ordinary circumstances" is not permissible.

PHYSIOLOGIC SIDELIGHTS

The newborn infant is at increased risk of localized or generalized hemorrhage.[22] The tendency of some newborns to bleed attracted the attention of the medical profession at least as early as 1694, when it was discussed by François Mauriceau in his obstetric text, *Observations sur la Grossesse...* Known by a variety of names during the years that followed, hemorrhagic disease of the newborn was attributed in 1912 to a deficiency of prothrombin, a blood factor essential for clotting. In this disorder umbilical, gastrointestinal, or diffuse cutaneous hemorrhage commonly occurs on the second or third day in apparently normal infants.

Subsequent investigations showed that the prothrombin concentration is normally low at birth, ranging between 14 and 39% of the normal adult level,[23] and declines even further in the first days of life.[24] Several other blood components, Vitamin K, and the blood platelet reactions, necessary for clotting, have also been measured at low levels in the newborn.[25] A remarkable rise in the Vitamin K level, as well as in other clotting factors, has been reported, however, between the time of birth and day 7.[26] Among a group of breast-fed infants the Vitamin K level rose from less than 0.02 nanograms (millionths of a milligram) per cc in the umbilical cord blood to 0.49 by day 7; Factor II, from 41 to 54%; Factor IIc, from 39 to 50%; Factor X, from 47 to 49%; Antithrombin III, from 59 to 72%; and the platelet count, from 204,000 to 357,000 per cu. mm. Among a group of formula-fed infants the chemical changes were even greater.

Bleeding is especially common in premature infants, who are born with fragile vessels, imperfect blood platelets, and low levels of nearly all clotting factors. Hemorrhage is now recognized as a major factor in a large proportion of neonatal deaths.[27] Since 1961 the Committee on Nutrition of the American Academy of Pediatrics has recommended the prophylactic administration of Vitamin K to all newborn infants, to combat any tendency to bleed.

PROS AND CONS OF ROUTINE CIRCUMCISION

Religious considerations aside, the medical profession has long debated the objective merit of routine circumcision of newborn male infants, but arguments have been obscured by bombast and hyperbole. One author,[28] a century ago, listed ten disadvantages of a long prepuce and, by implication, reasons for circumcision:

"1. A long foreskin causes constitutional as well as local irritation in infancy.

2. It predisposes to the accumulation of natural secretions, resulting in balanitis [inflammation of the glans] in boyhood.

3. A sore which occurs under the foreskin may result in phimosis [constriction of the foreskin so that it can not be retracted over the glans].

4. The foreskin may produce a mechanical impediment to the passage of urine.

5. It may be the cause of nocturnal incontinence.

6. Hernia or prolapse of the rectum may result from straining to urinate if the foreskin is tight.

7. If the foreskin is retracted and becomes fixed in the sulcus behind the glans, paraphimosis may result, with constriction, edema, ulceration, and slough.

8. A long foreskin means a moist glans, which is easily inoculated with the organism of syphilis and may be the starting point of cancer.

9. The foreskin may be a factor in some constitutional diseases such as hysteria, epilepsy, and chorea.

10. The foreskin makes cleanliness difficult, and the irritation may give rise to erotic stimulation and, consequently, masturbation."

Another,[1] about the same time, was less restrained in his indictment of the foreskin, writing: "The prepuce seems to exercise a malign influence in the most distant and apparently unconnected manner..,like some of the evil genii or sprites in the Arabian tales, it can reach from afar the object of its malignity, striking him down unawares in the most unaccountable manner; making him a victim to all manner of ills, sufferings, and tribulations; unfitting him for marriage or the cares of business; making him miserable and an object of continual scolding and punishment in childhood, through its worriments and nocturnal enuresis; later on, beginning to affect him with all kinds of physical distortions and ailments, nocturnal pollutions, and other conditions calculated to weaken him physically, mentally, and morally; to land him, perchance, in the jail, or even in a lunatic asylum. Man's whole life is subject to the capricious dispensations and whims of this Job's-comforts-dispensing enemy of man."

"Circumcision," the same author continued, "is like a substantial and well-secured life-annuity; every year of life you draw the benefit, and it has not any drawbacks or after-claps. Parents cannot make a better paying investment for their little boys, as it insures them better health, greater capacity for labor, longer life, less nervousness, sickness, loss of time, and less doctor bills, as well as it increases their chances for an euthanasian death."

Others not only viewed the operation as unnecessary but attributed a protective function to the foreskin and condemned routine circumcision.[29] Especially vitriolic was the late Joseph Lewis, Jew-turned-atheist. "Does anyone think for a moment," he quipped, "that a newborn babe, suddenly being pounced upon by a man with a knife, his flesh cut and torn in the tenderest part of his body, suffers no psychological reaction to this shocking brutality?"[30]

Local anesthesia, in the form of dorsal penile nerve block with lidocaine, has been advocated for neonatal circumcision;[31] but this procedure itself has been found not entirely innocuous.[32] In the performance of more than one thousand circumcisions over 4 decades of practice I have not been impressed with the pain it causes. Some infants cry upon mere handling or restraint, not necessarily because of pain. Properly performed, the operation is of but brief duration. The infant, given a nipple to suck, or a pledget soaked in wine or sugar solution, often drowses through it. I have never felt the need for anesthesia for newborn circumcision.

Of the several alleged benefits of neonatal circumcision, most persuasive is its prophylactic value against penile cancer. The evidence that the prepuce is a factor in the genesis of this form of cancer is incontrovertible.[33] It almost never occurs in men who have been circumcised early in life. Among the more than 1600 patients with penile cancer, in six major studies of the disease in the United States since 1932, none had been circumcised in infancy.[34] Jews provide the outstanding example of the immunity to penile cancer conferred by circumcision. All modern statistical studies confirm the clinical observation that cancer of the penis does not occur in Jews.[35-37] A review of 1103 cases, reported in 1932 from 205 hospitals including 26 Jewish hospitals, representing all parts of the United States, and in which the average Jewish population of the other hospitals was 4.4%, reported only one Jew with penile cancer; and he had never been circumcised.[38]

Further evidence of the protective value of circumcision is provided by the Mohammedans of India who, although not racially related to the Jews, are also relatively free of penile cancer. They thus present a sharp contrast to that country's Hindus, among whom the disease is common. During the years 1925 to 1930 carcinoma of the penis was recorded in some 1200 patients in four Indian hospitals. Mohammedans constituted an average of 21.2% of the hospital population but accounted for only 2% of the penile cancer cases. Mohammedans practice routine circumcision; Hindus do not. Failure of the procedure to provide complete protection of the Mohammedans has been explained by their delay in its performance to the third to tenth year of life, or even later; their incomplete removal of the prepuce in many cases; and their failure to retract the mucous membrane for complete exposure of the glans, as required in Judaic ritual.

Several reports in the 1940s pointed strongly to the probable etiologic association between phimosis and cancer of the penis. A constricted, non-retractable foreskin prevents easy removal of the smegma, a complex fatty material secreted by tiny glands in the sulcus beyond the glans. Large amounts of smegma are produced by the horse, in which species penile cancer is common;[39] and tumors have been produced in mice by application of smegma or its extracts.[40,41]

Cancer of the uterine cervix is likewise uncommon, if not rare, among Jewish women. In a mid-20th-century survey of ten American cities its occurrence was noted at 35.2 per 100,000 white women, 61.2 per 100,000 non-white. In Israel, by contrast, the rate was but 2.2 per 100,000, consistent with the infrequent diagnosis of this disease among Jews in the United States and Europe.[42] Among 1558 patients with cervical cancer at the New York City Cancer Institute during a 10-year period only three were Jewish. The same number of Jewish women were listed among 7000 cervical cancer patients in Sweden and among 999 at the Sloane Hospital for Women in New York. At the Mayo Clinic, in Rochester, Minnesota, not one of its 566 cervical cancer patients was Jewish.[43] Genetic factors are probably important in the relative immunity of Jewish women to cervical cancer.

In most of the Hispanic countries of the Western Hemisphere and among the Hindus of India cervical cancer accounts for about 40% of all malignant tumors in women. It almost never occurs in virgins. Coitus with uncircumcised sexual partners, with resultant exposure to smegma, or a viral agent, are strongly suspect as causative factors.

In an effort to evaluate the status of routine circumcision in modern medical practice I made a crude quantitative comparison, several years ago, of its complications, on the one hand, with its one universally acknowledged benefit, namely protection from penile cancer, on the other, based on statistics available at mid-20th century.[17] Complications of the operation fall into three categories: hemorrhage, infection, and surgical trauma. All are rare following circumcision by physicians, nurse-midwives, or certified *mohelim*. A death that occurred in New York in 1946, during my residency training, stimulated my interest in the subject.

The infant was born prematurely at 32 weeks. Circumcision was therefore postponed until 2 months later, when it was performed at home by an uncertified *mohel*. Persistent bleeding followed. Six and one-half hours later the infant was brought to the hospital's emergency room, where it died on arrival. No other death occurred in the city of New York, according to the records of its Department of Health, from the estimated more than one-half million circumcisions performed during the 13-year period 1939-1951.[44]

On my service in the Department of Obstetrics and Gynecology at New York's Columbia-Presbyterian Medical Center 10,802 newborn circumcisions were performed during the years 1933-1951 with six mishaps, one major. In one case an excessive amount of skin was removed by an intern performing his first such operation. Plastic repair achieved satisfactory correction. Postoperative infection occurred in another infant, but it was not clearly attributable to the circumcision. Bleeding followed the procedure in four other cases, but in only one was transfusion judged necessary.[45]

On the other side of the ledger are the cases of carcinoma of the penis, not a rare disease. Its frequency varies in different populations. Among the Chinese and Ceylonese, for example, it is quite common. In Puerto Rico penile cancer comprises 3.4% of the male cancer cases. During the years 1930-1932 death of 496 men resulted from this tumor in England and Wales. More than 1,000 cases are diagnosed each year in the United States, and 225 to 317 men die from it annually. The lifetime risk of penile cancer in an uncircumcised man in the U.S. is estimated at 1 in 600, by life-table analysis.[46] In New York City alone 224 deaths from penile cancer were recorded between 1939 and 1950, an average of 18.7 deaths per year.

On the basis of these data, in part, and similar observations from other sources, that circumcision prevents cancer of the penis, is associated with a reduced incidence of cervical cancer in sexual partners, and helps prevent phimosis and resultant local infection, the operation was widely accepted in the United States, until the mid-1970s, as a simple and safe hygienic measure. In the late 1960s, however, a number of pediatricians began to question the procedure as a routine, asserting that its benefits could be achieved by proper cleansing without the trauma of the operation. In 1971 and again in 1975 the Committee on the Fetus and Newborn of the American Academy of Pediatrics took a stand, in which it was joined in 1983 by the American College of Obstetricians and Gynecologists, opposing routine neonatal circumcision, with the statement that "no absolute medical indication exists for routine circumcision of the newborn."[47] Some third-party insurers refused to pay for the procedure.

Evidence has continued to mount, however, of the medical benefits of circumcision, especially in the prevention of urinary tract infection in boys and of sexually transmitted diseases in later life.[34] One study, in 1982, found that most of 109 infants up to 8 months of age with urinary infections were males, a reversal of the ratio in later life, almost all of whom were uncircumcised. A similar observation was made in 1985 among 5261 infants at an army hospital. Confirmation of these findings was provided by the records of 219,755 boys born in U.S. armed forces hospitals, which showed the frequency of urinary tract infections among uncircumcised boys to be ten times that among the circumcised.[48] Pyelonephritis (infection of the kidneys and upper urinary passages) would occur in at least 20,000 additional boys in the United States each year, according to an informed estimate, if no circumcisions were performed. It has been suggested that circumcision protects male infants from urinary tract infection by preventing bacterial colonization of the prepuce.[49]

More recent studies indicate a protective value of circumcision against balanitis[50] and urinary tract infections in young adult men as well as children,[51] and against infection with the AIDS virus and other organisms during heterosexual intercourse.[52] Virtually all sexually transmitted diseases occur more frequently among non-circumcised men than among circumcised men.[53]

Faced with an avalanche of such evidence the California Medical Association, by overwhelming vote in March 1988, endorsed neonatal circumcision as an effective health measure.[54] The following year, in a reversal of its previous stance, the American Academy of Pediatrics stated that "properly performed newborn circumcision prevents phimosis, paraphimosis [retraction of the constricted foreskin so that it cannot be replaced], and balanoposthitis [inflammation of the glans and prepuce] and has been shown to decrease the incidence of cancer of the penis," and cited the increased frequency of cervical cancer among the sexual partners of uncircumcised men infected with human papillomavirus.[55]

The *New England Journal of Medicine*, in 1990, editorialized: "As with other public health measures such as immunization, its disadvantages are short-term—any untoward effects occur during or shortly after the procedure—and its advantage is long-term—protection against future disease. The potential medical benefits of circumcision of newborns are seen over a lifetime and involve reducing the incidence of a number of diseases, ranging from urinary tract infections in early infancy to penile cancer in middle and old age, and the continued ease of genital hygiene and avoidance of balanoposthitis and phimosis...in experienced hands, infant circumcision involves a very low but not completely negligible risk... The benefits of routine circumcision as a preventive health measure far exceed the risks of the procedure."[34,56]

SUMMARY

The origins of circumcision lie buried in antiquity. Perhaps the oldest of surgical operations, it is practiced among many cultures, on every continent. It is estimated that one-fourth of the world's male population is circumcised. For the Jews it is purely a religious rite, the sign of the covenant between God and Abraham.

Recognizing the hazard of hemorrhage in families with bleeding tendencies, the Talmud forbade circumcision of the third son of a woman whose previous two male infants died from it, or if two of her sisters had lost a son following the procedure. Each of the three major branches of Judaism now has its own Brith Milah Board in the United States, for the training, certification, and supervision of practitioners of the ritual and to ensure its safety.

The Bible ordains that circumcision be performed on the eighth day, by which time, modern studies have shown, several of the blood coagulation factors, depressed at birth, have begun their rise toward adult levels. Circumcision before the eighth day, although proven safe, is not sanctioned by Jewish law.

The medical pros and cons of routine neonatal circumcision have long been debated. Its hazards are minimal. Among its benefits: protection against urinary tract infections in youth and against sexually transmitted diseases and penile cancer in later life, and reduction of the risk of cervical cancer in sexual partners. The operation is now endorsed as an effective health measure by the American Academy of Pediatrics.

NOTES AND REFERENCES

1. Remondino PC. History of Circumcision. Philadelphia: FA Davis 1891.
2. Bryk F. Die Beschneidung bei Mann und Weib. Neubrandenburg, Germany: Gustav Feller, 1931 (English translation by David Berger. New York: Amer Ethnol Press 1934.)
3. Speert H. Inconographia Gyniatrica. Philadelphia: FA Davis 1973:325.
4. Hand EA. History of circumcision. J Michigan State Med Soc 1950; 49:573-574.
5. Weiss C. Motives for male circumcision among preliterate and literate peoples. J Sex Research 1966; 2:69-88.
6. Wiswell TE. Routine neonatal circumcision: a reappraisal. Am Family Physician 1990; 41:859-863.
7. Bolande v JA. Les Rites de Passage. Paris: E. Mourry 1909.
8. Marx A et al. Seder Olam. Berlin:1903.
9. Asher A. The Jewish Rite of Circumcision, with the Prayers and Laws

Appertaining Thereto. London: Philip Vallentine 1873.
10. Not until the late-20th century did the Reform movement adopt patrilineal as an alternative to matrilineal inheritance of the covenant.
11. Moses had two sons, Gershom and Eliezer. The Bible does not specify which figures in the circumcision narrative; most commentators assumed it to be Gershom, the first-born.
12. The Biblical text fails to make clear whether it was Moses or the child whose life was imperiled.
13. The Torah, WG Plaut, ed. New York: Union of American Hebrew Congregations, 1981:412. The term "his legs" fails to distinguish between Moses and his son. Many interpret the Biblical reference as a euphemism for penis, and the brief statement to indicate that Zipporah smeared blood from her son's foreskin onto Moses' penis as a symbolic substitution for the circumcision he had never undergone.
14. The First Book of the Maccabees, 1. In The Apocrypha. New Hyde Park, New York: University Books 1962:171.
15. Briffault R. The Mothers, 3. New York: 1927; quoted by Will Durant: Our Oriental Heritage. New York: Simon and Schuster 1954:331.
16. Bergson J. Die Beschneidung. Berlin: Th. Scherk, 1844.
17. Speert H. Circumcision of the newborn: an appraisal of its present status. Obstet and Gynecol 1953; 2:164-172.
18. Rosner F. Circumcision. New York State J Med 1966:2919-2922.
19. Stern MH. Abraham, early mohel, in 1756 performed rite on son, Isaac. Jewish Week-Amer Examiner, Feb. 13-19, 1977:43.
20. Is Brith Milah in danger of disappearing? Jewish Week-Amer Examiner, Nov. 12, 1978.
21. Shakespeare also made an issue of mode of birth, in his *Macbeth*. Macbeth, having been assured by the Second Apparition that "none of woman born shall harm Macbeth" (IV, i, 79), taunted his assailant, Macduff:
    "As easy mayst thou the intrenchant air
    With thy keen sword impress, as make me bleed.
    Let fall thy blade on vulnerable crests;
    I bear a charmed life, which must not yield
    To one of woman born."
    Whereupon Macduff divulged his birth by cesarean section:
    "Despair thy charm;
    And let the angel whom thou still hast serv'd
    Tell thee, Macduff was from his mother's womb
    Untimely ripp'd." (V, vii, 38-45)
22. Buchanan GR. Neonatal coagulation: normal physiology and pathophysiology. Clinics in Haematology 1978; 7:85-108.
23. Brinkhous KM, Smith HP, Warner ED. Plasma prothrombin level in normal infancy and in hemorrhagic disease of the newborn. Am J Med Sci 1937; 193:475.
24. Owen CA, Hoffman GR, Ziffren SC, Smith HP. Blood coagulation during infancy. Proc Soc Exper Biol and Med 1939; 41:181.

25. Muntean W, Petek W, Rosanelli K, Muntz ID. Immunologic studies of prothrombin in newborns. Pediat Res 1979; 13:1262-1265.
26. Pietersma-de Bryn ALJM, van Haard PMM, Beunis MH, Hamulyak K, Kuijpers JC. Vitamin K$_1$ levels and coagulation factors in healthy term newborn till 4 weeks after birth. Haemostasis 1990; 20:8-14.
27. Bleyer WA, Hakimi N, Shepard TH. The development of hemostasis in the human fetus and newborn infant. J Pediat 1971; 79:838-853.
28. Clifford M. Circumcision: Its Advantages and How to Perform It. London: Churchill 1893.
29. Gairdner D. The fate of the foreskin: a study of circumcision. Brit M J 1949; 2:1433.
30. Lewis J. In the Name of Humanity. New York: Eugenics Pub 1949.
31. Stang HJ, Gunnar MR, Snellman L, Condon LM, Kestenbaum R. Local anesthesia for neonatal circumcision. JAMA 1988; 259:1507-1511.
32. Schoen EJ, Fischell AA. Dorsal penile nerve block for circumcision. JAMA 1989; 261:701-702.
33. Bleich AR. Prophylaxis of penile carcinoma. JAMA 1950; 143:1054.
34. Schoen EJ. The status of circumcision of newborns. New England J Med 1990; 322:1308-1312.
35. Howard HH, Holtham WH. Epidermoid carcinoma of the penis: a statistical study of 106 cases. Urol and Cutan Rev 1950; 54:45.
36. Melicow MM, Ganem EJ. Cancer and precancerous lesions of the penis: a clinical and pathological study based on twenty-three cases. J Urol 1946; 55:486.
37. Zausner J. Penile carcinoma: a review of 43 cases treated at Bellevue Hospital during the past twenty-five years. Radiology 1948; 50:786.
38. Wolbarst AL. Circumcision and penile cancer. Lancet 1 1932:150.
39. Sticker A. Ueber den Krebs der Thierre, insbesondere über die Empfänglichkeit der verschiedenen Hausthierarten und über die Unterschiede des Thier-und Menschenkrebs. Arch f Klin Chir 1902; 65:616.
40. Plaut A, Kohn-Speyer AC. The carcinogenic action of smegma. Science 1947; 105:391.
41. Auster LS. Genital cancer in Jews. New York State J Med, Jan. 15, 1965: 266-280.
42. Kennaway EL. The racial and social incidence of cancer of the uterus. Brit J Cancer 1948; 2:177-212.
43. The Doctors. Med World News, Nov. 12, 1965:141.
44. Reported from Jerusalem in 1991, among the more than 14,000 Ethiopian Jews airlifted to Israel in Operation Solomon, was another death from hemorrhage, in an 11-week-old boy after circumcision by his father with a razor blade (Jewish Week, June 21-27, 1991:8).
45. A similarly low complication rate was reported from the Huntington Memorial Hospital in Pasadena, California, where in 1949 and 1950, among 1844 newborn circumcisions the only mishap, in three cases, was bleeding requiring sutures but not transfusion (Hovsepian D. The pros

and cons of routine circumcision. California Med 1951; 75:359.
46. Kochen M, McCurdy S. Circumcision and the risk of cancer of the penis: a life-table analysis. Am J Dis Child 1980; 134:484-486.
47. Guidelines for Perinatal Care. Washington, D.C., Amer Coll Obstetr and Gynecol 1983.
48. Wiswell TE, Enzenauer RW, Holton ME, Cornish JD, Hankins CT. Declining frequency of circumcision: implications for changes in the absolute incidence and male to female sex ratio of urinary tract infections in early infancy. Pediatrics 1987; 79:338-342.
49. Roberts JA. Does circumcision prevent urinary tract infection? J Urol 1986; 135:991-992.
50. Fakjian N et al. An argument for circumcision: prevention of balanitis in the adult. Arch Dermatol 1990; 126:1046-1047.
51. Spach DH, Stapleton AE, Stamm WE. Lack of circumcision increases the risk of urinary tract infection in young men. JAMA 1992; 267:679-681.
52. Marx JL. Circumcision may protect against the AIDS virus. Science 1989; 245:470-471.
53. Parker SW, Stewart AJ, Wren MN, Gallow MM, Straton JA. Circumcision and sexually transmissible disease. Med J Australia 1983; 2:288-290.
54. California Medical Association. Resolution no. 305-88, March 8, 1988.
55. American Academy of Pediatrics. Report of the Task Force on Circumcision. AAP Policy Statement. Elk Grove Village, Ill. AAP 1989.
56. Poland RL. The question of routine neonatal circumcision. New Eng J Med 1990; 322:1312-1315.

CHAPTER 10

KASHRUTH: THE DIETARY LAWS

The Earth's first inhabitants were restricted vegetarians, permitted all the produce of the land—save the fruit of the tree of knowledge. To Adam and Eve "God said, Behold, I have given you every herb bearing seed, which is upon the face of all the earth, and every tree, in which is the fruit of a tree yielding seed; to you it shall be for meat... And the Lord God commanded the man, saying, Of every tree of the garden thou mayest freely eat: But of the tree of knowledge of good and evil, thou shalt not eat of it." (*Genesis* 1:29;2:16-17) The animals too were restricted by God to a vegetarian diet: "To every beast of the earth," the Bible records His words, "and to every fowl of the air and to every thing that creepeth upon the earth, wherein there is life, I have given every green herb for meat."[1] (*Genesis* 1:30)

Abel, son of the first couple, was a keeper of sheep. For what purpose they were kept we are not told—presumably for their wool, possibly for their hides. Milk would not have been permissible food in a strictly vegetarian subsistence economy.

Mankind remained herbivorous for ten generations, until the Flood. Noah and his entourage, having returned to dry land, added meat to their diet, according to God's word: "Every moving thing that liveth shall be meat for you; even as the green herb have I given you all things." (*Genesis* 9:3) Mankind was now omnivorous.

FORBIDDEN FOODS

Sixteen generations later, through Moses, the Israelites were to be told of the species of animals to be shunned; now, however, mankind was warned only that blood was prohibited, a restriction incumbent, through Noah, on all humanity; "But flesh with the life thereof, which is the blood thereof, shall ye not eat."[2] (*Genesis* 9:4) This proscription against blood, repeated in *Leviticus* (7:26; 17:10-14) and in *Deuteronomy* (12:16, 23; 15:23), and that against fat, are the only dietary restrictions for which a reason is given: "For the life of the flesh is in the blood," God said to Moses, "...therefore I said unto the children of Israel, No soul of you shall eat blood, neither shall any stranger that sojourneth among you eat blood...for it is the life of all flesh; the blood of it is for the life thereof." Nachmanides (Moses ben Nachman) argued, in the 13th century, that not only does the blood, which embodies the soul, belong to God, but combining the human soul with that of an animal, by eating its blood, would result in coarsening and denigration of the former.

God instructed Moses similarly concerning fat: "Speak unto the children of Israel, saying, Ye shall eat no manner of fat, of ox, or of sheep, or of goat. And the fat of the beast that dieth of itself, and the fat of that which is torn with beasts, may be used in any other use: but ye shall in no wise eat of it...all the fat is the Lord's." (*Leviticus* 7:23-24; 3:16)

Not until the mid-20th century did the medical community learn of the relation between fat consumption and the blood cholesterol level. Cholesterol and triglycerides are now universally recognized as major factors in the causation of narrowing and occlusion of arteries and resultant coronary heart disease. A clear association has also been established between high-fat diet and colon cancer. Enlightened cooks, nutritionists, and food processors have largely replaced animal fats, including butterfat, with vegetable oils. The demand for marbled meat has decreased; and hogs and beef cattle are being bred increasingly for less fatty carcasses.

Having known the pleasures of a carnivorous diet, the Israelites rapidly grew disgruntled when having to subsist without meat. During the second month after their departure from Egypt, for example, in the wilderness of Sin, "the whole congregation of the children of Israel murmured against Moses and Aaron... Would to God we had died by the hand of the Lord in the land of Egypt, when we sat by the flesh pots..." (*Exodus* 16:2-3) Whereupon God sent the miracle of the quails: "'I have heard the murmurings of the children of Israel,' He said, 'At even ye shall eat flesh' ...And it came to pass, that at even the quails came up, and covered the camp." (*Exodus* 16:12-13) Later in their desert wandering, tired of manna, "the children of Israel also wept again, and said, Who shall give us flesh to eat?" And God again sent them quails, "until it came out of their nostrils." (*Numbers* 11) (see chapter 3)

God's covenant with Noah, symbolized by the rainbow, was His covenant with all mankind: "And God said, This is the token of the covenant which I make between me and you and every living creature that is with you, for perpetual generations: I do set my bow in the cloud and it shall be for a token of a covenant between me and the earth. And it shall come to pass, when I bring a cloud over the earth, that the bow shall be seen in the cloud." (*Genesis* 9:12-14)

Different was God's covenant with Moses, which distinguished, for the first time, between clean and unclean animals. Promising Moses "land that floweth with milk and honey," He declared: "I am the Lord your God, which have separated you from other people. Ye shall therefore put difference between clean beasts and unclean, and between unclean fowls and clean: and ye shall not make your souls abominable by beast, or by fowl, or by any manner of living thing that creepeth on the ground, which I have separated from you as unclean." (*Leviticus* 20:24-25)

Speaking to Moses and Aaron, God laid down the criteria for separation of the clean animals from the unclean and specified among the two groups: "Whatsoever parteth the hoof, and is clovenfooted, and cheweth the cud, among the beasts, that shall ye eat. Nevertheless these shall ye not eat of them that chew the cud, or of them that divide the hoof: as the camel, because he cheweth the cud, but divideth not the hoof; he is unclean unto you. And the coney, because he cheweth the cud, but divideth not the hoof; he is unclean unto you. And the swine, though he divide the hoof, and be clovenfooted, yet he cheweth not the cud; he is unclean to you. Of their flesh shall ye not eat, and their carcass shall ye not touch; they are unclean to you." (*Leviticus* 11:1-8)

Pork has since been the ultimate symbol of forbidden foods, the pig an animal of special abhorrence. Antiochus Epiphanes, in his attack against Judaism, ordered its adherents to bring sacrifices of the animal's flesh.[3] In a notable example of martyrdom, Eleazer surrendered his life rather than eat, or even pretend to eat, the forbidden meat: At a birthday celebration for the Persian king, the *Apocrypha* relates, "Eleazer, one of the principal scribes, an aged man...was constrained to open his mouth, and to eat swine's flesh. But he, choosing rather to die gloriously, than to live stained with such an abomination, spit it forth, and came of his own accord to the torment, as it behooved them to come, that are resolute to stand out against such things... But they that had the charge of that wicked feast, for the old acquaintance they had with the man, taking him aside, besought him to bring flesh of his own provision, such as was lawful for him to use, and make as if he did eat of the flesh taken from the sacrifice commanded by the king; that in so doing he might be delivered from death... But he began to consider discreetly, and as became his age [90], and the excellency of his ancient years, and the honour of his gray head...and his most honest education from a child, or rather the holy law made and given by God: therefore he answered accordingly, and willed them straightways to send him to the grave... And when he had said these words, immediately he went to the torment... And thus this man died, leaving his death for an example of a noble courage, and a memorial of virtue...unto all his nation."[4]

The Talmudists, and most Biblical commentators, classified the proscription of pork, as most of the dietary laws, among the *chukim*, or unexplained laws, part of the moral and ethical code of Judaism, of no known practical value. Some anthropologists, including S. Reinach, Robertson Smith, and Sir James Frazer, have associated the prohibition of pork with the totemic worship of the pig (or wild boar) by the early ancestors of the Jews; its "worship" perhaps being a priestly device for making it taboo.[5] Maimonides, as the consummate physician as well as philosopher, conceived a medical basis for the food ban; and in agreement with an earlier 12th-century French commentator, Rabbi Samuel ben Meir (Rashbam), maintained in his *Guide for the Perplexed*,[6,7] that all the Biblically forbidden foods were unwholesome[8]—differing with the majority of scholars, who neither saw nor sought beyond faith in their acceptance of the word of God.

Rabbits and squirrels, we now know, are the principal vectors of tularemia, an infectious disease caused by the bacillus *Pasteurella tularensis*, so named because of its first recognition in Tulare County, California, in 1911, by G.W. McCoy of the U.S. Public Health Service. The disease, transmitted to humans by insect bite or by direct contact with an infected animal, is characterized by a localized skin lesion at the site of inoculation, lymph node enlargement, fever, gastrointestinal disturbances, and sometimes pneumonia. It commonly occurs among hunters, butchers, and handlers of infected rabbit carcasses. Untreated, tularemia carries a mortality of 6 to 7%; with antimicrobial therapy death is rare. An epidemic of the disease occurred in Vermont in 1968.

A hitherto unrecognized worm, seen encysted in a section of human muscle in 1835 by Sir James Paget and named *Trichinella spiralis* by English biologist Richard Owen, was found in American pork in 1846 by Joseph Leidy; and in 1860 the clinical characteristics of an acute disease caused by invasion of the parasite were described by Friedrich von Zenker.[9] Trichinosis is acquired through ingestion of raw or inadequately cooked meat, almost always pork, containing the encysted larvae of the worm. Soon after ingestion the larvae, released by the action of gastric juice, migrate from the stomach to small intestine, where they mate, producing young worms which enter the blood vessels and lymphatic channels and are distributed throughout the body. The prevalence of trichinosis in the United States was indicated by the encysted organism, identified in muscle specimens in 16.1% of routine autopsies throughout the country in the years 1936-1942.[10] Trichinosis may involve the skeletal muscles, heart, and central nervous system, producing a variety of symptoms including diarrhea, abdominal pain, nausea, prostration, fever, swelling of the eyelids, and signs of myocarditis and encephalitis. In most cases, however, the disease goes unrecognized. It carries a mortality of less than 2%.

Two other diseases directly or indirectly traceable to swine, both serious and occasionally life-threatening, are taeniasis and cysticercosis, from the pork tapeworm *Taenia solium*. Taeniasis results from the ingestion of raw or undercooked meat contaminated with cysts of the organism. In its adult stage the worm may live in the upper jejunum for decades. Taeniasis is common worldwide but of low prevalence in the United States.[11] Cysticercosis, on the other hand, which is acquired through the ingestion of taenia eggs shed in the feces of human carriers, is being diagnosed with increasing frequency in the United States, through pictures of the brain provided by computerized axial tomography (CAT) scans and magnetic resonance imaging. After the worm's eggs are ingested its larvae hatch in the small intestine, penetrate the bowel wall, enter the circulation, become encysted, and are deposited in various parts of the body including the brain, remaining in this stage for up to 10 years. The disease thus may occur in persons who eat no pork and have no contact with pigs. It is seen in the United States mainly, but not exclusively, in southern California and the other western states in which immigrants from Central and South America, especially Mexico, are numerous. Four cases in an Orthodox Jewish community in New York City, reported in 1992, were attributed to domestic help from Latin American countries.[12]

In His instructions to Moses God continued: "And whatsoever goeth upon his paws, among all manner of beasts that go on all four, those are unclean unto you... These also shall be unclean unto you among the creeping things that creep upon the earth; the weasel, and the mouse, and the tortoise after his kind, And the ferret, and the chameleon, and the lizard, and the snail, and the mole... And every creeping thing that creepeth upon the earth shall be an abomination; it shall not be eaten. Whatsoever goeth upon the belly...or whatsoever hath more feet among all creeping things that creep upon the earth, them ye shall not eat, for they are an abomination." (*Leviticus* 11:27, 29-30, 41-42)

Rodents, although not common dietary constituents, are major vectors of disease. Some 200 species of rodents, in various parts of the world, provide a vast reservoir for infection with the plague bacillus, *Pasteurella pestis*, cause of several major pandemics in the history if mankind, including the Black Death of the 14th century. The disease is transmitted from rodents, usually rats, to humans through the bite of infected fleas. Typhus, an acute febrile disease characterized by headache, rash, muscle pain, weakness, and neurologic disturbances, is transmitted similarly from mice, through the bites of fleas, lice, or mites.

Not only was the consumption of unclean animals forbidden, but, Moses instructed the Israelites, "neither shalt thou bring an abomination into thine house, lest thou be a cursed thing like it: but thou shalt utterly detest it, and thou shalt utterly abhor it; for it is a cursed thing." (*Deuteronomy* 7:26)

Moses listed the permitted animals: "These are the beasts which ye shall eat: the ox, the sheep, and the goat, The hart, and the roebuck, and the fallow deer, and the wild goat, and the pygarg [a type of antelope], and the wild ox, and the chamois." (*Deuteronomy* 14:4-5) The permitted quadrupeds thus restored, in a sense, the paradise of vegetarianism; for they themselves were obligate herbivores, both because of distinctive alimentary tracts and specialized digestive enzymes, and because of their hoofed extremities which, as Georges Cuvier, the distinguished French naturalist of the late-18th and early-19th centuries pointed out, could not serve for seizing prey.[13]

The toxicity of tissues from the quadrupeds named in *Leviticus* 11 and *Deuteronomy* 14 was investigated by David Macht[14] by his technique of phytopharmacology, previously described (see chapter 7). In his research laboratories in Baltimore he prepared fresh muscle extracts of the ox, calf, sheep, goat, and deer (Biblically clean species), and of the pig, rabbit, guinea pig (believed to be closely related to the coney), and camel (delivered by air from the Near East) (Biblically prohibited species). Extracts of horseflesh were also tested. Each was added, in a 2% solution, to a culture medium of *Lupinus albus* seedlings and the effect on their growth noted (Table 10.1). Toxicity to the seedlings was reflected in a depression of their "index of growth" (the ratio of their root length to that of control seedlings). The growth index among the "clean" species varied between 82 and 94%; among the "forbidden" species, including the horse, 39 to 54%.

Similar experiments were conducted on fresh or frozen flesh from other prohibited (but not specifically named in *Leviticus* 11 or *Deuteronomy* 14) species, including dog, cat, squirrel, rat, ground hog, fox, opossum, hamster, black bear, grizzly bear, and rhinoceros (Table 10.2). Among these species likewise, the growth index was significantly depressed, varying between 43 and 62%.

Concerning fowl, God instructed Moses and Aaron as follows: "And these are they which ye shall have in abomination among the fowls; they shall not be eaten...: the eagle, and the ossifrage [fish hawk, or buzzard], and the ospray, And the vulture, and the kite after his kind; Every raven after his kind; And the owl, and the night hawk, and the cuckow, and the hawk after his kind, and the little owl, and the cormorant, and the great owl, And the swan, and the pelican, and the gier eagle, And the stork, the heron after her kind, and the lapwing, and the bat [mistakenly classified with the fowl]." (*Leviticus* 11:13-19) Thus most of the forbidden avian species were birds of prey, scavengers for carrion, or fish-eating water-fowl.

Table 10.1. Effect of muscle juices of Biblically clean and some forbidden quadrupeds on growth of **Lupinus albus** *(after Macht[14])*

Species of Animal	No. of Experiments	Index of Growth	Species of Animal	No. of Experiments	Index of Growth
Ox	20	91	Swine	20	54
Calf	20	82	Rabbit	20	49
Sheep	20	94	Guinea Pig	20	46
Goat	20	90	Camel	20	41
Deer (Venison)	20	90	Horse	20	39

"But of all clean fowls," Moses explained to his followers, "ye may eat." (*Deuteronomy* 14:20) Thus permitted as food for the Israelites were chicken, duck, goose, turkey, pigeon, and quail. The flesh extracts of these avian species, tested by Macht on his *Lupinus* seedlings, were essentially non-toxic, as evidenced by growth indices of 83 to 93% (Table 10.3). The birds of prey, on the other hand, the owl, hawk, falcon, and crow, all forbidden, inhibited the seedlings, depressing their growth indices to 45 to 63%. Only the swan, among the forbidden species tested, produced a growth index within the range of that of the permitted birds.

Table 10.2. Effect of muscle juices of some other Biblically forbidden quadrupeds on growth of Lupinus albus *(after Macht[14])*

Species of Animal	No. of Experiments	Index of Growth	Species of Animal	No. of Experiments	Index of Growth
Dog	10	62	Fox (silver)	6	50
Cat	10	53	Opposum (*Didelphis virginiana*)	8	53
Squirrel	6	43	Hamster	4	46
Rat (white)	8	55	Black Bear (*Euarctos americanus*)	8	59
Ground Hog (*Arctomys monax*)	6	53	Grizzly Bear	8	55
			Rhinoceros	8	60

Table 10.3. Effect of muscle juices of Biblically clean and forbidden birds on growth of Lupinus albus *(after Macht[14])*

Species of Animal	No. of Experiments	Index of Growth	Species of Animal	No. of Experiments	Index of Growth
Chicken	20	83	Sparrow Hawk (*Falco parverius*)	6	63
Duck (mallard)	10	90	Red Tail Hawk (*Buteo borcalis*)	8	36
Goose (*Anser albifrons*)	6	85	Owl	8	62
Turkey	10	85	Crow	10	46
Pigeon	10	93	Coot	8	88
Quail (*Coturnix communis*)	20	89	Wild Duck (*Aytha americana*)	8	85
Canada Goose (*Branta canadensis*)	7	85	Swan	6	87

The Biblical commands concerning "winged swarming things"[15] are no longer clear, for not all the species can be identified with certainty. "Every creeping thing that flieth is unclean unto you," Moses told the Israelites, "they shall not be eaten." (*Deuteronomy* 14:19) But God had instructed: "Ye may eat of every flying creeping thing that goeth upon all four, which have legs above their feet, to leap withal upon the earth; Even these of them ye may eat; the locust after his kind, and the bald locust after his kind, and the beetle after his kind, and the grasshopper after his kind. But all other flying creeping things, which have four feet shall be an abomination unto you." (*Leviticus* 11:21-22)

Finally, the fishes: In lieu of naming the permitted and the prohibited species, the Bible simply specifies the criteria by which they are so classified. "These ye shall eat," God commanded, "of all that are in the waters: whatever hath fins and scales in the waters, in the seas, and in the rivers, them shall ye eat. And all that have not fins and scales in the seas, and in the rivers, of all that move in the waters, and of any living thing which is in the waters, they shall be an abomination unto you...ye shall not eat of their flesh..." (*Leviticus* 11:9-11) Clams and oysters, we now know, are common vectors of hepatitis virus and Vibrio infections.

As he did with the quadrupeds and birds, Macht made muscle extracts of 54 species of fish and assayed their effect on his *Lupinus* seedlings (Table 10.4). Of the fish with scales and fins, the bonito produced a growth index of 78; all the other 44 species so endowed gave growth indices of 80 or higher, averaging 88.8. Extracts of the fishes without scales and fins, by contrast, including the catfish, eel, moonfish, puffer, skate, shark, stingaree, toadfish, and porcupine fish, proved distinctly toxic to the seedlings, as evidenced by growth indices between 40 and 60, with an average of 51.8. All the fish muscle extracts that inhibited growth of the *Lupinus* seedlings, but none of the others, were likewise toxic to mice, causing depression, convulsions, and death after intraperitoneal injection.[16]

Table 10.4. Effect of fish muscle extracts on growth of **Lupinus albus** *(after Macht[14])*

Common Name	Scientific Name	Growth Index
"Alewife"	*Pomolobus pseudoharengus*	82
Banded drum	*Larimus fasciatus*	80
Black bass	*Micropterus dolomient*	80
Black drum	*Pogonias cromis*	105
Bluefish	*Pomatomus saltatrix*	80
"Bonito"	*Auxis thazard*	78
Bowfin	*Amia calva*	90
Butterfish	*Poronotus triacanthus*	81

Table 10.4. (continued)

Common Name	Scientific Name	Growth Index
Carp	Cyprinus carpio	90
Catfish	Amelurus catus	48
Channel bass	Sciaenops ocellata	80
"Chub"	Chaenobryttus coronarius	91
Cod	Gadus callarias	90
Croaker	Micropogon undulatus	90
Eel	Anguilla rostrata	40
Flounder	Paralichthy dentatus	83
Flying fish	Prionotus carolinus	87
Gambusia		89
Goldfish	Carassius auratus	88
Haddock	Melanogrommus aeglefinus	80
Hake	Urophycis regius	98
Halibut	Phatysomatichthys hippoglossoides	82
Herring	Clupea harengus	100
Kingfish	Tarpon atlanticus	83
Menhaden	Brevoortis tyrannus	90
Moonfish	Vomer setipinnis	51
"Mullet"	Erimyzon sucetta	87
Pike	Esox americanus	98
Pompano	Trachinotus carolinus	110
Porcupine fish	Diodon hystrix	60
Porgy	Stenotomus chrysops	80
Puffer	Spheeroides maculatus	51
Rainbow trout	Salmo gairdneri irideus	81
"Robin"	Lepomis gibbosus	91
Rock	Roccus saxatilis	100
"Salmon trout"	Cynoscion nebulosus	96
Sand flounder	Lophopsetta maculata	85
Sand skate	Pteroplates maclura	59
Smelt	Menidia menidia	90
Sea bass	Centropristes striatus	103
Shad	Alosa sapidissima	100
Shark (dogfish)	Mustelus canis	62
Silver squeteague	Cynoscion nothus	84
Spadefish	Chaetodipterus faber	80
Spanish mackerel	Scomberomorus maculatus	98
Spot	Leinostomos xanthurus	80
Stingaree	Dasyatis say	46
Sturgeon	Acipenser oxyrhynchus	87
Toadfish	Opsanus tau	49
Tuna, bluefin	Thunnus thynnus	88
Weakfish	Cynocion regalis	97
White perch	Pomoxis nigromaculatus	81
Whiting, Carolina	Menticirrhus americanus	84
Yellow perch	Perca flavescens	87

Experiments with blood extracts showed a similar but less pronounced disparity between the two categories of fish. The species without scales and fins caused an average growth index of 49.2 in the seedlings, varying between 31 and 60; while those with scales and fins averaged a growth index of 77.6, varying between 70 and 87.

LAWS OF SLAUGHTER

Kindness to animals has ever been an essential feature of the Jews' holiness code. Moses repeated to the children of Israel the words of God: "Thou shalt not see thy brother's ass or his ox fall down by the way, and hide thyself from them: thou shalt surely help him to lift them up again" (*Deuteronomy* 22:4); and "Thou shalt not muzzle the ox when he treadeth out the corn." (*Deuteronomy* 25:4) Further, "If a bird's nest chance to be before thee in the way in any tree, or on the ground, whether they be young ones, or eggs, and the dam sitting upon the young, or upon the eggs...thou shalt in any wise let the dam go, and take the young to thee..." (*Deuteronomy* 22:6-7)

So in death, the Talmudists decreed, slaughter must be swift and merciful, as Moses presumably intended in his charge to the Israelites: "thou shalt kill of thy herd and of thy flock, which the Lord hath given thee, as I have commanded thee, and thou shalt eat in thy gates whatsoever thy soul lusteth after." (*Deuteronomy* 12:21) Only animals without blemish were acceptable for ritual slaughter. Sick, maimed, or lame animals were excluded. Slaughter of quadrupeds and fowl was to be carried out in a prescribed manner, with a sharp knife free of any nicks or notches; without interruption; by rapid incision through the trachea and esophagus; and exsanguination by transection of the major blood vessels in the neck.[17] Health of the animal was to be confirmed by inspection of its viscera after slaughter.

Pharmacological differences have been demonstrated in the blood and meat of animals according to the method of their slaughter. Using the same assay technique with *Lupinus albus* seedlings, Macht found that fresh arterial blood, or blood serum, from the white mouse, white rat, guinea pig, rabbit, cat, dog, domestic pigeon, and domestic hen was less toxic than blood obtained from the same species killed by asphyxiation or injury to the brain. Most pronounced was the difference in the mouse, in which species decerebration nearly doubled the toxicity (halved the growth index of the seedlings in 24 hours) (Table 10.5). Toxic substances, Macht believed, possibly from the brain itself or from other organs such as the endocrine glands, are liberated into the circulation as a result of asphyxia or brain injury.[18]

Additional experiments were carried out on the frog, goldfish, carp, turtle, domestic hen, domestic duck, pigeon, opossum, white mouse, white rat, guinea pig, rabbit, kitten, cat, dog, sheep, calf, and ox, in which the toxicity of their muscle extracts was assayed after various methods of slaughter, including asphyxiation, injuries to the brain, and

Table 10.5. Effect of method of slaughter on toxicity of blood (after Macht[18])

Animal	Kind of Blood Sera	Growth Index per cent
White mouse	Freshly drawn	63
	After decerebration	33
Rat (mus norvegicus)	Freshly shed	66
	After blow on head	45
Guinea pig	Freshly shed	69
	After blow on head	54
Pigeon	Freshly shed	67
	After breaking neck	58
Hen	Freshly shed	57
	After decerebration	50
Rabbit	Freshly drawn arterial	77
	In extreme asphyxia	66
	Decerebrated	51
Cat	Freshly drawn arterial	70
	Extreme asphyxia	56
	Decerebrated but oxygenated	54
	Decerebrated and asphyxiated	50
Dog	Freshly drawn arterial	68
	Extreme asphyxia	61
	Decerebrated but oxygenated	53
	Decerebrated and asphyxiated	49

electrocution. In every case the toxicity of the muscle extracts obtained after death by arteriotomy (bleeding) was less than after death by decerebration (brain injury) or by asphyxiation. Electrocution, Macht believed, produced greater toxicity of the muscle extracts through the abnormal metabolic products that resulted from the clonic and tonic muscle contractions induced by the current.[19]

In demonstration of biophysical difference attributable to method of slaughter, Macht and associates showed, in nerve-muscle preparations in rats, that nerves lost their viability more quickly after arteriotomy, corresponding to the Judaically required method of slaughter, than after other methods killing. Biochemical differences in the tissues were also demonstrated, in the form of oxidation and reduction reactions, which were inhibited more rapidly after death by arteriotomy.[20]

THE HIND QUARTER

Irrespective of species or method of slaughter, the thighs of quadrupeds are prohibited fare. So generally observed was abstinence from the rear of the animal, some authorities believed,[21] that it was not thought to need specification in the Torah's dietary code, in *Leviticus* 11 and *Deuteronomy* 14. The basis for the prohibition is found in the Biblical narrative of Jacob's encounter, presumably with an angel, or with God Himself. En route to his rapprochement with his brother Esau, Jacob sent his wives, children, and servants ahead, and remained at night by a brook at Peniel: "And Jacob was left alone; and there wrestled a man with him until the breaking of the day. And when he saw that he prevailed not against him, he touched the hollow of his thigh; and the hollow of Jacob's thigh was out of joint, as he wrestled with him... And he said, Thy name shall be called no more Jacob, but Israel: for as a prince hast thou power with God and with men, and hast prevailed... And as he passed over Penuel the sun rose upon him and he halted upon his thigh. Therefore the children of Israel eat not of the sinew which shrank, which is upon the hollow of the thigh, unto this day: because he touched the hollow of Jacob's thigh in the tissue that shrank." (*Genesis* 32:24-32) *Gid hanasheh*, the prohibited part of the hind quarter, is taken to include the sciatic nerve, blood vessels, tendons, joints, and part of the muscle and fascia of the limb. These structures can be removed and the remaining meat thereby rendered kosher, by skilled butchers, through a precise, tedious dissection known as "porging."

MEAT AND MILK

In three places in the Bible, presumably under the separate authorship of the three major sources, E, J, and D,[22] and in the same wording, the prohibition appears: "Thou shalt not seethe a kid in his mother's milk." (*Exodus* 23:19; 34:26; *Deuteronomy* 14:21) Its origins remain unclear. Many explanations have been offered, magical, symbolic, and moral, none convincing. Maimonides, in his *Guide for the Perplexed*, suggested that its intent was to discourage idolatry, in the form of an unspecified pagan rite, not presently known.[23] The prohibition has been compared, by some anthropologists, with magical African customs for preservation of lactation in cattle. Others have seen its motivation as humanitarian. In the Middle East, celebrations were characterized by feasts of meat. Goats were plentiful, their milk abundant. A kid of a fresh litter, cooked in its mother's milk, was standard fare. Such insensitivity to the mother's feelings could not be countenanced: the Torah made it a moral issue.

Rabbinic Judaism made the proscription a fundament of dietary law and extended its meaning to ban the mixing of all meat and milk products. After a meal of meat, according to this tradition, milk or milk products must not be consumed for several hours. The proscription does not apply to fish. Milk, on the other hand, was believed to pass more quickly than meat through an empty stomach. Consumption of meat was therefore permitted after a shorter interval following a meal of dairy foods. Recognizing, perhaps, the hardship that might result from accidental contamination of a milk dish with meat, or vice versa, the Talmud established the principle of *Bateil beshishim* (*B. Hullim* 97 a; *Yoreh Deah* 98:1): that the prohibition would be annulled if the main dish measured at least 60 times the volume of the contaminant. The same principle was to apply to contamination by forbidden foods.[24]

The purpose of the law not being clear, as some allege (if indeed we may demand a "purpose" of the law), some members of the Reform rabbinate see the prohibition of the ingestion of meat and milk products together as "entirely extraneous to the text" of the Biblical injunction.[25] Most Reform Jews have come to disregard it as part of the *halakhah*.

Macht studied the matter experimentally, testing the effects of cow's milk and beef muscle extracts, separately and in combination, on plants and animals.[26] Test objects included *Lupinus albus* seedlings, as in previous experiments; tadpoles and goldfish, which were placed in the solutions; mice, white rats, and guinea pigs, injected intraperitoneally; cats, injected intravenously; and rabbits, to which the solutions were fed by stomach tube. The milk solutions alone were less toxic to both plants and animals than were the meat extracts; but, in all the experiments, a combination of the two solutions produced a synergistic effect, in the form of heightened toxicity. The limit of this synergism was reached when 59 parts of milk were mixed with one part of beef juice. No such potentiation resulted from the combination of milk with fish broth.

Macht continued his experiments on the biochemical level, studying the oxidases of muscle juices with and without milk.[27] Oxidases are enzymes that catalyze oxidation reactions, such as ethanol to acetaldehyde and aldehydes to acids. They are present in various tissues, as liver, kidney, and muscle; and can be measured by the time required for their blanching of the coloration of methylene blue solutions. Milk is poor in oxidases; muscle tissue, relatively rich. Using muscle suspensions or juices from rats and a variety of other animals, Macht and Bryan found that the addition of even a small amount of milk, itself having little effect on the oxidase reaction, produced a pronounced potentiation of the muscle extract's reduction of the indicator solution, diminishing the time for its discoloration. The limit of such potentiation was reached, however, when one part of milk was added to 60 parts of muscle juice. Similar synergism in oxidase activity was observed when small quantities of muscle extract were added to large quantities of milk.

MODERN INTERPRETATION

Although most traditional Judaic scholars emphatically deny any but a religious basis for the Mosaic dietary laws, passages from the Bible attest its authors' nutritional knowledge. "Man doth not live by bread alone," Moses lectured the Israelites. (*Deuteronomy* 8:3) "The Lord shall give you in the evening flesh to eat," he comforted them in the desert, "and in the morning bread to the full." (*Exodus* 16:8) The custom remains with us: grains and cereals for breakfast, meat for dinner.

When Jacob called his sons together before his death he said, of Judah (in Hebrew): "*l'ven schinayim maycholov.*" (*Genesis* 49:12) The *Authorized King James Version* translates the words as "his teeth [shall be] white with milk"; *The New English Bible*, "his teeth whiter than milk." The Union of American Hebrew Congregations' *The Torah* likewise gives the translation "His teeth are whiter than milk," but adds, in a footnote, "or, white from milk.'"[28] The difference in wording is crucial, for the last implies a knowledge of milk's importance in dental structure.

As they prepared for battle against the inhabitants of the land of Canaan, Joshua and Caleb reassured the Israelites: "...neither fear ye the people of the land, for they are bread ["a piece of cake"] for us. (*Numbers* 14:9)

Speaking of God's works and commands, the author or authors of *Deuteronomy*, which contains the Mosaic dietary code, predicted that some of His teachings will amaze "your children that shall rise up after you, and the stranger that shall come from a far land," who may try to interpret them. (*Deuteronomy* 29:22)

SUMMARY

The laws of *kashruth* require that animal slaughter be swift and merciful, by exsanguination following rapid incision of the neck vessels with a sharp knife. The blood and flesh extracts of a large variety of animals slaughtered in this manner, tested similarly on plant seedlings, have been found less toxic than the same fluids obtained after death by asphyxiation, electrocution, or brain injury.

From the Biblical prohibition, "Thou shalt not seethe a kid in his mother's milk," has evolved the rabbinic proscription against the mixing of meat and milk products. In tests on plant seedlings and various species of experimental animals, injections of cow's milk and of beef muscle extracts each had a measurable toxic effect, the meat more than the milk; but a combination of the two solutions produced a synergistic, heightened toxicity. Similar synergism was found in the effect of milk, itself poor in oxidase, on muscle oxidase, a mixture producing marked potentiation of the enzyme's activity.

All of the Earth's creatures, according to the Bible, subsisted on a vegetarian diet during the first ten generations of mankind. Only after the flood did God authorize Noah and his entourage to consume meat.

Many years later Moses instructed the Israelites in detail concerning forbidden foods. Blood and animal fat were to be avoided. Distinction was made between clean and unclean beasts: among the latter, animals without cloven hoofs or that did not chew their cud, such as swine; scavengers or birds of prey; and fish without fins and scales.

Modern medicine recognizes the association between fat consumption and blood cholesterol level and arterial disease; the pig as a vector of trichinosis and the pork tapeworm diseases taeniasis and cysticercosis; rabbits and squirrels, of tularemia; rodents, as carriers of the plague bacillus; and shellfish, as agents for the transmission of the hepatitis virus and vibrio infections. Pharmacologic experiments during the mid-20th century have shown muscle extracts of the forbidden species to have a greater inhibitory effect on the growth of test seedlings than extracts of the "clean" or permitted species.

Notes and References

1. The concept of vegetarianism as a symbol of the ideal world appears again in the vision of Isaiah, who foresaw the carnivores rejoicing the herbivores in their diet of grasses: "And the cow and the bear shall feed: their young ones shall lie down together: and the lion shall eat straw like the ox... The wolf and the lamb shall feed together, and the lion shall eat straw like the bullock." (*Isaiah* 11:7; 65:25)
2. Orthodox Jewish law requires specific preparation of meat, including fowl but not fish, for removal of blood. The meat is soaked in water for one-half hour, salted and left standing for an hour, then washed before cooking (*Shulchan Arukh, Yoreh Deah* 69:1).
3. I Maccabees, 1. *The Apocrypha*. New Hyde Park, N.Y.: University Books 1962:172.
4. II Maccabees, 6. *The Apocrypha*. New Hyde Park, N.Y.: University Books 1962:221.
5. Durant W. *Our Oriental Heritage*. New York: Simon and Schuster 1954:330.
6. Maimonides M. *Guide for the Perplexed*. Translated by M. Friedländer. London: 1881; 370 ff. The main reason for the prohibition of swine flesh, Maimonides believed, was that the animal is dirty in habit and its food therefore loathsome.
7. Yellin D, Abrahams I. *Maimonides*. Philadelphia: Jewish Pub Soc 1903:184.
8. Excepting, of course, the foods proscribed during Passover, a holiday that combined an ancient agricultural festival with the commemoration of the *Exodus* from Egypt. During the 8 days of Passover matzoh is eaten in lieu of bread, and all forms of leavening are prohibited, as are certain grains and legumes, according to regional variations in custom.
9. Encyclopaedia Britannica 1953; 22:468.
10. During the subsequent 3 decades the prevalence of trichinosis in the United States declined to 4.2% (Plorde JJ: Trichinosis. In: Harrison's Principles of Internal Medicine 8th ed. New York: McGraw-Hill 1977; 1100-1102.)

11. Plorde JJ. Cestode (Tapeworm) Infections. In: Harrison's Principles of Internal Medicine, 8th ed. New York: McGraw-Hill 1977:1114.
12. Schantz PM, Moore AC, Munoz JL, Hartman BJ, Schaefer JA, Aron AM, Persand D, Sarti E, Wilson M, Flisser A. Neurocysticercosis in an Orthodox Jewish community in New York City. New Eng J Med 1992; 327:692-727.
13. Soler J. The Dietary Prohibitions of the Hebrews. New York Review of Books 1979; 26:24-30.
14. Macht DI. An experimental pharmacological appreciation of Leviticus XI and Deuteronomy XIV. Bull Hist Med 1953; 27:444-450; Phyto-toxic Properties of Fresh Muscle Juices from Various Animals. Arch Internat Pharmacodyn et de Thérap 1953; 94:23-25.
15. Translation in The Torah. Plaut WG ed. New York: Union of American Hebrew Congregations 1981; 815, 1438, in lieu of "every creeping thing that flieth." Locusts and grasshoppers were part of the dietary of Yemenite Jews as recently as the late-19th century and are still eaten by some peoples in the Middle East.
16. Macht DI, Spencer E. Physiological and toxicological effects of some fish muscle extracts. Proc Soc Exper Biol and Med 1941; 46:228-233.
17. *Shulchan Arukh, Yoreh Deah* 6:1; 18:1 ff.
18. Macht DI. Comparative toxicity of blood after arteriotomy asphyxiation and injuries to the brain. Am J Physiol 1931; 96:662-666.
19. Macht DI, Cook HM. Toxicity of muscle extracts after arteriotomy, asphyxiation, injuries to the brain and electrocution. Am J Physiol 1932; 97:662-667.
20. Macht DI. the Bible as a source of subjects for scientific research. Medical Leaves 1940; 3:174-184.
21. The Torah. WG Plaut, ed. New York: Union of American Hebrew Congregations 1981; 219.
22. The Torah. WG Plaut, ed. New York: Union of American Hebrew Congregations 1981; 593-594.
23. The JPS Torah Commentary: Exodus. NM Sarna, ed. Philadelphia: Jewish Pub Soc 1991; 147.
24. Klein I. A Guide to Jewish Religious Practice. New York: Jewish Theological seminary of America. 1979; 362-368.
25. The Torah. WG Plaut, ed. New York: Union of American Hebrew Congregations 1981; 1439.
26. Macht DI. Synergistic effects of milk and meat solutions. Arch Internat de Pharmacodynamie et de Thérapie 1934; 49:175-188.
27. Macht DI, Bryan HF. Synergistic action of milk and meat oxidases. J Biol Chem 1935; 110:101-105.
28. The Torah. WG Plaut, ed. New York: Union of American Hebrew Congregations 1981; 309.

CHAPTER 11

CONSERVATION: OF EARTH AND PERSON

THE SABBATH

No less than 12 times does the Bible declare the holiness of the Sabbath as a day of rest.

(*Genesis* 2:2-3) Having created the universe, "God ended his work which he had made; and he rested on the seventh day from all his work... And God blessed the seventh day, and sanctified it.

(*Exodus* 20:8-11) "Remember the Sabbath day," God commanded, "to keep it holy. Six days shalt thou labour, and do all thy work: but the seventh day is the Sabbath of the Lord thy God: in it thou shalt not do any work, thou, nor thy son, nor thy daughter, nor thy manservant, nor thy maidservant, nor thy cattle, nor thy stranger that is within thy gates: For in six days the Lord made heaven and earth, the sea, and all that in them is, and rested the seventh day."

(*Exodus* 31:13-16) God to Moses: "Speak thou also unto the children of Israel, saying, Verily my Sabbaths ye shall keep: for it is a sign between me and you throughout your generations...for a perpetual covenant."

(*Exodus* 34:21) But Moses, in his wrath at the Israelites for their worship of the golden calf, shattered the stone tablets on which were recorded God's commandments. On the new tablets that he hewed he again inscribed God's words: "Six days thou shalt work, but on the seventh day thou shalt rest: in earing time and in harvest thou shalt rest."

(*Exodus* 35:2-3) Moses to the congregation of the children of Israel, telling them the words of God: "Six days shall work be done, but on the seventh day there shall be to you an holy day, a Sabbath of rest to the Lord... Ye shall kindle no fire throughout your habitations upon the Sabbath day." Food preparation, he explained, must be done in anticipation of the Sabbath. On Friday he said to them:

(*Exodus* 16:23,29) "Tomorrow is the rest of the holy Sabbath unto the Lord: bake that which ye will bake today, and seethe that ye will seethe; and that which remaineth over lay up for you to be kept until the morning...abide ye every man in his place, let no man go out of his place on the seventh day."

(*Deuteronomy* 5:12) "Keep the Sabbath," repeated Moses, reminding all Israel of the covenant with them and their future generations, "to sanctify it, as the Lord thy God hath commanded thee."[1]

The basis for the Sabbath, as advanced in the Books of *Genesis* and *Exodus,* is essentially cosmological[2]—that God rested on the seventh day; whereas a social motivation for Sabbath observance is provided additionally in *Deuteronomy* 5:15: "And remember that thou wast a servant in the land of Egypt, and that the Lord thy God brought thee out thence... Therefore the Lord thy God commanded thee to keep the Sabbath day." Thus is usually explained the custom of lighting two candles in welcoming the Sabbath.[3]

The Sabbath was hence to serve the physical, social, emotional, and spiritual needs of mankind. It also introduced a new unit of time, the seven-day week, unique because of its independence of the phases of the moon and the positions of the sun and the other heavenly bodies, in contradistinction from the day, month, and year.[4]

Moses had prescribed the work prohibitions of the Sabbath in general terms and mentioned specifically restrictions against fire-making, baking and cooking, harvesting, travel, and wood-gathering, for the last of which a transgressor was stoned to death (*Numbers* 15:32-36). Later rabbis further defined "work", 39 categories of which are detailed in the *Mishnah* (*Shabbat* 7:2): sowing, plowing, reaping, sheaving, threshing, winnowing, cleansing crops, grinding, sifting, kneading, baking, shearing, blanching, carding, dyeing, spinning, weaving, making a minimum of two loops, weaving two threads, separating two threads, tying, untying, sewing a minimum of two stitches, ripping out stitches, hunting a gazelle, slaughtering it, flaying it, salting it, curing, scraping its hide, slicing its hide, writing a minimum of two characters, erasing, building, wrecking, extinguishing, kindling, hammering, and transporting.[5,6]

Lucius Annaeus Seneca, famous Roman statesman and philosopher of the first century, scoffed at the idea of a weekly Sabbath and belittled the Hebrews as an "outrageous people who lose almost a seventh part of their life in inactivity." Major objectives of oppressors of the Jews included, in addition to closure of their institutions of learning and prohibition of circumcision (see chapter 9) and ritual slaughter, their observance of the Sabbath. After the conquest of Judea by the Seleucids in the 2nd century B.C.E. and Antiochus IV Epiphanes' determination to assimilate the Jews, he "wrote to his whole kingdom," the *Apocrypha* relates, "that all should be one people, and every one should leave his laws: so all the heathen agreed according to the commandment of the king. Yea, many also of the Israelites consented to his religion...and profaned the Sabbath. For the king had sent letters by messengers unto Jerusalem and the cities of Judea, that they should...profane the Sabbaths and festival days." (*I Maccabees* 1)

Later, "when Antiochus had carried out of the temple a thousand and eight hundred talents, he departed in all haste unto Antiocha... And he left governors to vex the nation...who coming to Jerusalem, and pretending peace, did forbear till the holy day of the Sabbath, when taking the Jews keeping holy day...slew them all that were gone to the celebration of the sabbath[6]... Not long after this the king sent an old man of Athens to compel the Jews to depart from the laws of their fathers, and not to live after the laws of God... Neither was it lawful for a man to keep Sabbath days or ancient feasts." (*II Maccabees* 5,6)

The *Apocrypha* records the first resistance of the Maccabees under their leader Mattathias and their refusal to fight on the Sabbath: "Then Mattathias answered and spake with a loud voice, Though all the nations that are under the king's dominion obey him, and fall away every one from the religion of their fathers, and give consent to his commandments: yet will I and my sons and my brethren walk in the covenant of our fathers... We will not harken to the king's words, to go from our religion... Now when it was told the king's servants...that certain men, who had broken the king's commandment, were gone down into the secret places in the wilderness, they pursued after them a great number, and having overtaken them...made war against them on the Sabbath day[7]...But they said, We will not come forth...to profane the Sabbath day...they answered them not, neither cast they a stone at them, nor stopped the places where they lay hid... So they rose up against them in battle on the Sabbath, and they slew them, with their wives and children, and their cattle, to the number of a thousand people."

Whereupon Mattathias resolved: "Whosoever shall come to make battle with us on the Sabbath day, we will fight against him; neither will we die all, as our brethren that were murdered in the secret places." (*I Maccabees* 2) Thus was a new principle adopted by the Jews, who had hitherto shunned combat on the Sabbath, even in self-defense. Without this reinterpretation of Sabbath passivity, some scholars believe, the Jews would long since have been annihilated.[8]

Modern commentators have focused on the positive rather than the proscriptive aspects of the Sabbath, emphasizing its use for prayer, study, socialization, and self-assessment. In its observance, Erich Fromm commented, human beings are liberated from "the chain of time," arguing that "the spiritual and moral survival of the Jews during two thousand years of persecution and humiliation would hardly have been possible without the one day in the week when even the poorest and most wretched Jew was transformed into a man of dignity and pride."[9]

Claude Montefiore, who died shortly before the outbreak of World War II, noted: "the gathered experience of humanity that the break in the routine of work one day in seven will heighten the value of the very work itself...the Sabbath is one of the glories of our humanity."[10] Documentation was provided early in the War, when government and industry strove for maximal production. *Science*, the organ of the American Association for the Advancement of Science, editorialized:[11]

"Longer working days may result in decreased output, despite eagerness on the part of both management and worker to rush war production, is indicated by a review of previous experience especially by the British.

"With a tremendous incentive such as the war gives to American workers, men can greatly step up their production and working hours for a short period, without any breakdown resulting. But if this pace is kept up for any length of time production drops off, sickness and accidents increase, and a 'staleness' or lack of morale results. Just how long a man's or a woman's working day should be for maximum production depends on the type of work, on the makeup of the individual and also upon social conditions inside and outside the plant.

"British industrial authorities have found fifty-six working hours a week to be best for their men. This would amount to five 10-hour days with a 6-hour day on Saturday and with Sunday off. After a trial of longer hours at the beginning of the war, hours in England have been cut to 48 a week for women and...54 to 60 for most men. Even in Germany an initial trial of longer hours gave way to a restoration of the eight-hour day. The one rest day in seven recommended in the Bible is still found to be essential for retaining working efficiency in the new World War. Enforced rest periods with an opportunity to take food assist in keeping up the output.

"In the United States where workers may have been geared to higher production rates and more intensive production methods, the optimum hours should very likely be lower than has been found best for British workers... At scientific work the British found that very little more was accomplished in a 66-hour, seven-day week than had been done in the peace time week of 44 hours."

Our skeletal muscles, which comprise 40% of our body mass, require regular exercise for optimal health. They, as well as our psychological apparatus, likewise need periodic rest from tension if we are to minimize deaths from hypertension, coronary heart disease, and stroke.

RETIREMENT

The ages for work prescribed in the Bible provided also for retirement. God instructed Moses concerning the employment of his progeny, the Levites: "From thirty years old and upward until fifty years old shalt thou number them; all that enter in to perform the service, to do the work in the tabernacle of the congregation." (*Numbers* 4:23) A later passage in the Scriptures has the Levites assuming their duties at age 25: "from twenty and five years old and upward they shall go in to wait upon the service of the tabernacle of the congregation:"[12] but retirement remained at 50: "And from the age of fifty years they shall cease waiting upon the service thereof, and shall serve no more." (*Numbers* 8:24-25)

Throughout the industrial world persons with foresight and funds have long been able to provide support for their declining years through annuity insurance. In the United States many business organizations, chiefly among the heavy industries and railroads, created private pension plans for their employees. In Great Britain an act was passed in 1908 providing pensions to the needy, beginning at age 70.

Social security plans are characterized, ideally, by their objective to provide financial protection, through income security, to all citizens or workers against physical contingencies that might affect their livelihood, such programs to be financed, directly or indirectly, by the entire community. By the mid-20th century most European countries and various parts of the British dominions had social security systems, the majority covering the loss or reduction of earnings caused by sickness, maternity, old age, or death.

The U.S. Social Security act of 1935 and its subsequent amendments have developed into one of the most comprehensive programs for social welfare ever undertaken through direct legislation. A major part of the plan was its design to ensure a basic retirement income after age 65 for all workers enrolled under the system. Provided also, through federal grants to the states on a matching basis, was public assistance to families with dependent children and to needy blind persons. By 1949 all the states were cooperating in one or more of the plan's programs, and wage-record accounts had been established for some 80 million persons. Retirement benefits were to be financed by equal taxes on employer and employee, to be paid into a trust fund into which the Congress would make annual appropriations sufficient to provide for the anticipated payments mandated by the old-age insurance plan.

THE LAND

Soon after mankind's creation God made clear its responsibility to the soil: "And the Lord God took the man, and put him into the Garden of Eden to dress it and to keep it." (*Genesis* 2:15) Clear also did God make mankind's status—as tenant, not owner of the land: "for the land is mine," said God, "for ye are strangers and sojourners with me." (*Leviticus* 25:23) A belated move toward this Biblical ideal was made with the creation in 1901 of the Jewish National Fund (*Keren Kayemet L'Yisrael*), to which Jews the world over contributed for the acquisition of land in Palestine, to be the common and permanent property of the Jewish people. Tenants, as individuals and as members of communes, have continued to work the land for use rather than profit, without rights to sale or mortgage. Through the Fund and its program of soil conservation and management much desert and swampland has been reclaimed, fertility of the land has been restored, and sites have been provided for public buildings and industrial development.[13]

Environmentalism was emphasized to mankind from the beginning. A midrash tells of God's warning to Adam:

"In the hour when the Holy One, blessed be he, created the first man, he took him and let him pass before all the trees of the garden of Eden, and said to him: See my works, how fine and excellent they are! Now all that I have created for you have I created. Think upon this, and do not corrupt and desolate my world; for if you corrupt it, there is no one to set it right after you."[14]

Deforestation, common in ancient warfare, was clearly prohibited by the foremost of environmental principles, embodied in the Biblical command of *bal tashchit* (do not destroy): "When thou shalt besiege a city...in making war against it to take it, thou shalt not destroy the trees thereof by forcing an axe against them (for the tree of the field is man's life) to employ them in the siege." (*Deuteronomy* 20:19) Yet tropical rain forests, which help maintain our global climate and provide a home for nearly half of the Earth's species, are being destroyed at a rate of 30 acres per minute; the temperature of our atmosphere continues to rise as a result of its increasing carbon dioxide canopy; the Earth's protective ozone shield is being diminished by refrigerant and propellant chlorofluorocarbons and the chlorinated hydrocarbons in automotive emissions; and one-third of our land mass lies unfit for farming. To mankind's credit, on the other hand, paper, metals, glass, and plastics are being recycled in ever-increasing quantity.

Ezekiel, 2500 years ago, expressed the hope, in the form of a vision, that our polluted environment and the pains of our troubled world would be salved by the healing power of God's holy waters: "Afterward he brought me again unto the door of the house; and, behold, waters issued out from under the threshold of the house eastward: ...and the waters came down from under from the right side of the house, at the south side of the altar. Then brought he me out of the way of the gate northward, and he led me about the way without unto the utter gate by the way that looketh eastward; and, behold, there ran out waters on the right side. ...and he brought me through the waters; the waters were to the ankles. Again he measured a thousand, and brought me through the waters; the waters were to the knees. Again he measured a thousand, and brought me through; the waters were to the loins. Afterward he measured a thousand; and it was a river that I could not pass over: for the waters were risen. ...at the bank of the river were very many trees on the one side and on the other. Then he said unto me, These waters issue out toward the east country, and go down into the desert, and go into the sea: which being brought forth into the sea, the waters shall be healed. And it shall come to pass, that every thing that liveth, which moveth, withersoever the rivers shall come, shall live: and there shall be a very great multitude of fish, because these waters shall come hither: for they shall be healed; and every thing shall live whither the river cometh. And it shall come to pass, the fishers shall stand upon it from En-gedi even unto En-eglaim; they shall be a place to spread forth nets; their fish shall be according to their kinds, as the fish of the great sea, exceeding many. ...And by the river upon the bank thereof, on this side and on that side, shall grow all trees for meat, whose leaf shall not fade, neither shall the fruit thereof be consumed: it shall bring forth new fruit according to his months, because their waters they issued out of the sanctuary: and the fruit thereof shall be for meat, and the leaf thereof for medicine." (*Ezekiel* 47:1-12)

Well into the post-Biblical era the 15th day of the month of *Shevat* (*Tu B'Shevat*) was selected as a special day for the planting of trees in the Holy Land. It is still retained for its symbolism. The Talmud tells that on this quasi-holiday it was customary to plant a cedar for the birth of a boy, a cypress for a girl. At their marriage branches from their trees were woven together for the wedding canopy (*chupah*). An American counterpart of *Tu B'Shevat* is found in Arbor Day, an occasion for tree-planting first observed on April 10, 1872 in Nebraska, made a legal holiday in that state in 1885, and now widely celebrated throughout the country by the public planting of trees, but on different dates in different states.

When speaking to Moses at Mount Sinai God stressed the importance of rest for the land. As the seventh day was to be a Sabbath for mankind, so was the seventh year to be a Sabbath for the soil. "When ye come into the land which I give you," God ordered, "then shall the land keep a Sabbath unto the Lord. Six years thou shalt sow thy field, and six years thou shalt prune thy vineyard, and gather in the fruit thereof; But in the seventh year shall be a sabbath of rest unto the land...thou shalt neither sow thy field, nor prune thy vineyard... That which groweth of its own accord of thy harvest thou shalt not reap, neither gather the grapes of thy vine undressed: for it is a year of rest unto the land." (*Leviticus* 25:2-5)

The reason given here for the land's sabbatical is clearly conservational: "for it is a year of rest unto the land." Some have seen an implication of economic benefit in the command.[15] Worded somewhat differently is the same command in *Exodus* 23:10-11, where the motivation for the land's rest is expressed in social and humanitarian terms: "that the poor of thy people may eat: and what they leave the beasts of the field shall eat."

Anticipating the Israelites' fear of famine, God reassured them: "And if ye shall say, What shall we eat the seventh year? behold, we shall not sow, nor gather in our increase: Then I will command my blessing upon you in the sixth year, and it shall bring forth fruit for three years. And ye shall sow the eighth year, and eat yet of old fruit until the ninth year; until her fruits come in ye shall eat of the old store." (*Leviticus* 25:20-22)

For centuries, according to the *Mishnah* and the Palestinian Talmud, the Israelites faithfully observed the land's Sabbath. The Syrians chose such a year, between 164 and 162 B.C.E., the historian Josephus recorded, for their siege upon the city of Beth-zur, which the Israelites could not withstand because of lack of provisions:

"Then the king's army went up to Jerusalem to meet them, and the king pitched his tent against Judea, and against mount Sion. But with them that were in Bethsura he made peace: for they came out of the city, because they had no victuals there to endure the siege, it being a year of rest to the land. So the king took Bethsura, and set a garrison there to keep it. As for the sanctuary, he besieged it many days. ...Yet at the last, their vessels being without victuals, (for that it was the seventh year, and they in Judea, that were delivered from the Gentiles, had eaten up the residue of the store;) there were but a few left in the sanctuary, because the famine did so prevail against them, that they were fain to disperse themselves, every man to his own place." (I *Maccabees* 6)

Josephus, in his *Antiquities*, tells also of the exemption of the Palestinian Jews from certain taxes by Julius Caesar during sabbatical years. Only in emergencies, as when Roman rulers less tolerant than Julius Caesar refused to relax their exactions, did rabbinic authorities authorize agricultural work during the sabbatical year. Some groups in Israel consider the law of an agricultural Sabbath still operative, not as a matter of land conservation, but as an expression of the divinely ordained Sabbath philosophy.[16]

Plants need rest as does the earth. They undergo seasonal periods of inactivity intrinsically regulated by chemical and physiological factors, in addition to the external stimuli or depressants of light, temperature, and water. In addition they require repeated replenishment of their nutrients, which need is intensified by harvest of their produce.

Plants differ widely in their nutritional requirements. Leafy vegetables, such as lettuce, kale, and cabbage need large amounts of nitrogen. Roots and tubers, as beets, carrots, parsnips, and potatoes, require abundant potash. Seed or fruit crops, as beans, tomatoes, and eggplant demand phosphorus. Rational rotation of crops from year to year, in lieu of consecutive plantings of the same species in the same sites, prevents uneven depletion of the earth's nutrients and reduces the risks from disease-causing organisms in the soil. As a gardener I learned early to alternate my potato patch with that for cucurbits; and not to plant cabbage, broccoli, or cauliflower in the same site in consecutive years.

All food, indeed all life, can be traced back to rock, forerunner of the soil. Twelve and one-half percent of beef by weight, for example, consists of phosphorus, iron, and calcium. A pound of steak thus contains about 2 ounces of rock material, provided by the soil and obtained by plants for the bovine diet. Release of these 2 ounces of elemental nutrients requires long periods of weathering of large quantities of rock. More than 2 tons, corresponding to a 0.007 inch thickness of an acre, must be weathered to yield the elements in 4 tons of alfalfa, an average annual yield per acre. The average rate of rock erosion, estimated at only one inch per 9,000 years, produces only a small fraction of these required nutrients.[17] Rest of the soil is valid in principle; in practice, fertilizers must be added to replace depleted elements.

God's command assured the vigor of fruit trees before the enjoyment of their harvest. "When ye shall come into the land," God ordered, "and shall have planted all manner of trees for food, then ye shall count the fruit thereof as uncircumcised: three years shall it be as uncircumcised unto you: it shall not be eaten of." On the fourth year the fruit was to be given as an offering to the priests for religious celebration: "But in the fourth year all the fruit thereof shall be holy to praise the Lord withal." Only thereafter was the fruit permitted for general consumption: "And in the fifth year shall ye eat of the fruit thereof, that it may yield unto you the increase thereof." (*Leviticus* 19:23-25) *Rosh Hashanah Lailanot* (the New Year of the Trees) became the day to mark their age.

Similarly did I husband the asparagus bed in my garden, according to instructions, during the early years after planting, to ensure the bounty it now produces: "Avoid cutting spears sooner than the third spring after planting; otherwise the plants will suffer and will not yield so well in after years. Do not cut too liberally the first crop-year... Cutting too late in any season reduces the yield of sprouts in the season following."[18]

THE GAIA HYPOTHESIS

For Gaia, the legendary Earth Mother of the ancient Greeks, was named an ecologic concept, originated in the late 1970s by English biochemist James Lovelock and American microbiologist Lynn Margulis. Developed initially as a purely technical explanation for the long-term stability of the Earth's atmosphere, the Gaia hypothesis has been widely embraced by ecologists and philosophers as an expression of the interaction of the biomass itself and the life it supports. Summarized by Margulis: "Gaia, the superorganismic system of all life on earth, hypothetically maintains the composition of the air and the temperature of the planet's surface, regulating conditions for the continuance of life. ...On earth the environment has been made and monitored by life as much as life has been made and influenced by the environment."[19] Herein is restated the challenge of the Scriptures. May mankind meet it!

SUMMARY

Some say that Israel has kept the Sabbath; others, that the Sabbath has kept Israel. It has been termed "one of the glories of our humanity." The Sabbath has preserved the physical, social, emotional, and spiritual needs of mankind; and introduced a new unit of time, the 7-day week, independent of the phases of the moon and the positions of the sun. The experience of World War II, when government and industry strove for maximal production, showed that one rest day in seven was essential for working efficiency.

The Bible lists the general work prohibitions of the Sabbath: fire-making, baking and cooking, harvesting, travel, and wood-gathering. Additional specific restrictions are enumerated in the Talmud.

In their battle of resistance against the Seleucids the Maccabees, under Mattathias, who had hitherto shunned combat on the Sabbath, even in self-defense, took up arms against their persecutors, in the 2nd century B.C.E. Without this reinterpretation of Sabbath passivity, some scholars believe, the Jews would long since have been annihilated.

The Bible prescribed retirement of the Levites from service in the tabernacle at age 50. By mid-20th century most European countries had social security systems covering loss of earnings through sickness or old age. The U.S. Social Security Act of 1935 has developed into one of the most comprehensive programs for social welfare ever undertaken through direct legislation.

The Bible made clear mankind is but a tenant on Earth, not owner of the land: "For the land is mine," said God, "for ye are strangers and sojourners with me." Mankind's responsibility "to dress it and to keep it" was made clear to Adam. Deforestation was prohibited. At Mount Sinai God stressed to Moses the importance of rest for the land. Farmers and gardeners have long recognized the need for crop rotation. The masses of humanity have still to accept their trusteeship of the Earth's resources.

NOTES AND REFERENCES

1. See also *Leviticus* 23:1-3; *Isaiah* 58:13-14; *Isaiah* 66:23; *Jeremiah* 17:24,25,27; Ezekiel 20:10-13, 17-22; and *Nehemiah* 13:15-22.
2. Views of the Biblical World: 1. The Law, B. Mazar, M. Avi-Yonah, A. Malamat, eds. Chicago: Jordan Pub 1959:152.
3. Among other reasons for the lighting of 2 candles: (1) the Bible in one place says "remember the Sabbath," in another, "observe the Sabbath"; (2) to create unity between body and soul, one candle being lit with the body, the other with the soul.
4. The JPS Torah Commentary: Genesis. NM Sarna, ed. Philadelphia: Jewish Pub Soc 1989; 14-15.
5. Fields HJ. A Torah Commentary for Our Times, vol.2, Exodus and Leviticus. New York: UAHC Press 1991; 88-90.

6. Domestic chores such as turning on and off lights may be performed on the Sabbath by trained monkeys or dogs, ruled former Chief Rabbi Ovadia Yosef of Israel, but only by borrowed beasts; for one's own animals must be allowed to rest. (Dateline World Jewry, World Jewish Congress Dec 1991)
7. About 320 B.C.E. Ptolemy invaded Palestine from Egypt and captured Jerusalem on the Sabbath. In the Yom Kippur War of October 1973 the fledgling State of Israel was attacked by its Arab neighbors on the "Sabbath of Sabbaths."
8. Loewe HMJ in Encyclopaedia Britannica 1953; 13:52-53.
9. Fromm E. You Shall Be as Gods. New York: Holt, Rhinehart and Winston 1966:193-197.
10. Fields HJ. The JPS Torah Commentary: Genesis. NM Sarna, ed. Philadelphia: Jewish Pub Soc 1989; 89.
11. Van de Water M. The Eight Hour Day. Science 1942; 95, suppl. 12.
12. Plaut suggests that the first five years may have been a probationary period, or a period for guard service, as it was after age 50. (The Torah WG Plaut, ed. New York: Union of American Hebrew Congregations 1981:1077)
13. The Torah. WG Plaut, ed. 944.
14. Ecclesiastes Rabbah VII, 28; quoted in Hammer on the Rock. NH Glatzer, ed. New York: Schocken Books 1948, 1962; 13.
15. The JPS Torah Commentary: Exodus. NM Sarna, ed. Philadelphia: Jewish Pub Soc 1991:144.
16. The Torah. WG Plaut, ed.,1741.
17. Foster RJ. General Geology. Columbus O: Charles E Merrill 1969:99-100.
18. The New Garden Encyclopedia. E.L.D. Seymour, ed. New York: Wm H Wise 1946:82.
19. Quoted by Roszak T. Beyond the Reality Principle. Sierra:1993; 78:59-62, 80.

CHAPTER 12

SEPARATISM

Back and forth, throughout the colorful tapestry of Jewish tradition, is woven the thread of separatism. "If ye will obey my voice," God told the Israelites, "...and keep my covenant, then ye shall be a peculiar treasure unto me above all people...and an holy nation." (*Exodus* 19:5,6) God commanded Moses: "Speak unto all the congregation of the children of Israel, and say unto them, Ye shall be holy: for I the Lord your God am holy." (*Leviticus* 19:2) Biblical commentators as early as the 3rd century have interpreted the words "ye shall be holy" as "ye shall be separate."[1] The *Oxford English Dictionary* gives as its primary definition of holy: "kept or regarded as inviolate from ordinary use, and appropriated or set apart for religious use or observance."

Moses responded to God: "So shall we be separated, I and thy people, from all the people that are upon the face of the earth." (*Exodus* 33:16) And to the Israelites Moses reported: "For thou art an holy people...the Lord thy God hath chosen thee to be a special people unto himself...thou shalt be blessed above all people." (*Deuteronomy* 7:6, 14) God reiterated: "I am the Lord your God, which have separated you from other people...have severed you from other people, that ye should be mine." (*Leviticus* 20:24,26)

Balaam, Israel's traditional enemy, acknowledged his foe's special status: "How shall I curse, whom God hath not cursed? ...lo, the people shall dwell alone, and shall not be reckoned among the nations." (*Numbers* 23:8-9)

Based on Biblical precepts and post-Biblical customs, the concept of separatism has permeated all the Jew's activities. *Kilayim*, the Hebrew word meaning "of two kinds," is mentioned repeatedly. Forbidden was the planting together of different types of seed: "Thou shalt not sow thy vineyard with divers seeds: lest the fruit of thy seed which thou hast sown, and the fruit of thy vineyard be defiled." (*Deuteronomy* 22:9) Prohibited also was the cross breeding of animals: "Thou shalt not let thy cattle gender with a diverse kind." (*Leviticus* 19:19) Even the harnessing together of different species of draft animals was forbidden:

"Thou shalt not sow with an ox and an ass together." (*Deuteronomy* 22:10) Transvestism was declared an "abomination unto the Lord": "The woman shall not wear that which pertaineth unto a man, neither shall a man put on a woman's garment." (*Deuteronomy* 22:5) Nothing was permitted that interfered with the established order of nature. Sexual contact with animals was sinful: "Neither shalt thou lie with any beast to defile thyself therewith: neither shall any woman stand before a beast to lie down thereto." (*Leviticus* 18:23) Separation of the clean from the unclean animals and of meat from milk, decreed in the Bible, were discussed in chapter 10. A special prayer (*Havdalah*) is recited at the conclusion of the Sabbath and of the holidays, separating the holy from the profane days. In traditional synagogues men and women worshipers are seated in separate sections.

SHAATNEZ

The principle of identity was established and all things, as all species, were to be categorized—and kept separate. First to generalize the concept that it lay beyond the prerogatives of humans to create that which God had not was the 12th-century exegete of northern France, Rabbi Joseph Bekhor Shor. He recognized as a proscription against the creation of hybrids the negative command of *Leviticus* 19:19: "neither shall a garment mingled of linen and woolen come upon thee;" repeated in *Deuteronomy* 22:11: "Thou shalt not wear a garment of diverse sorts, as of woolen and linen together," a mixture known as *shaatnez*. The origin of the term is uncertain, as is the significance of the proscription.

Later codification of Judaic law defined more precisely the prohibition against mixed fibers.[2] Only to a mixture of wool and linen did it apply, and only to its use as clothing.[3] Mixtures of cotton, silk, and other fibers were permissible, as was the use of *shaatnez* for any other purpose. The priestly vestments, however, which were worn only during service in the temple, did indeed contain both wool and linen; and Josephus, himself of priestly descent, suggested in his *Antiquities* (late-1st century C.E.), that *shaatnez* was for this reason prohibited to all others.[4]

Most scholars have classed *shaatnez* among the *chukim*, statutes without rational explanation. The name itself, it has been suggested, is an acronym from the processes of combing, spinning, and weaving.[5] Rashi of Troyes (Rabbi Solomon ben Isaac, 1040-1105) insisted that the proscription of mingling of fibers, as of crossing of species, is as the decree of a king, for which no reason need be given. Maimonides (1135-1204), a century later, associated *shaatnez*, together with shaving of the face and trimming of the beard, with the customs of heathen priests, and viewed the prohibition of these practices as protests against idolatry.[6] Nachmanides (Moses ben Nahman, Barcelona, 1194-ca. 1270), on the other hand, regarded the insistence on these prohibitions and the maintenance of the purity of species as an "apotheosis of alterity," designed to preserve the integrity of creation.[7] As the 20th century draws to a close the possibilities for the modification of species, both plant and animal, through genetic engineering appear without limit. But ringing in my ears are the warning words of Erwin Chargaff, Columbia University's distinguished biochemist: "Posterity will curse us!"

Pious Jewish tailors the world over remain punctilious in their observance of God's command; and special laboratories have been established for the detection of the forbidden mixture of fibers. Clearly, *shaatnez* and its avoidance have had different meanings for different persons. Seeking an objective measure of any biological specificity or uniqueness of wool and linen in combination, beyond Biblical symbolism, David Macht turned again to his *Lupinus* seedlings[8] (see chapter 7). Drugs or chemicals derived from plants, he had found, were relatively non-toxic to these pharmacologic test objects; whereas those of animal origin were, in general, toxic to the plants. Epinephrine, for example, which is derived from the suprarenal glands of animals, proved highly poisonous to the seedlings; while ephedrine, a plant alkaloid with similar pharmacologic action, was relatively innocuous. Macht prepared extracts of undyed cotton, linen, wool, silk, and rayon by boiling the fibers in plant-physiological saline, and used the filtrates as nutrient solution for the *Lupinus albus* seedlings.

The pharmacologic effect of the various extracts was measured by the growth of the seedlings under standard conditions of light and temperature, in comparison with the growth of control plants under identical conditions. The vegetable fiber extracts (cotton, linen, and rayon) had no effect on seedling growth, while those from fibers of animal origin (wool and silk) proved distinctly toxic (Table 12.1). When wool and cotton extracts were combined, the depressive effect on seedling growth diminished as the proportion of wool to cotton decreased (Table 12.2). When wool and linen extracts were combined, by contrast, synergistic enhancement of the wool's toxicity occurred, until its proportion in the nutrient mixture was reduced to 10% (Table 12.3). Combination of linen with wool produced a potentiation of the latter's toxicity.

Table 12.1. Effect of various fiber extracts on seedling growth (after Macht[8])

Fiber	Growth Index
Cotton	100%
Linen	119%
Wool	30%
Silk	56%
Rayon	100%

Table 12.2. Effect of combinations of wool and cotton extracts on seedling growth (after Macht[8])

	Percentage of wool and cotton combined				Growth index	Significance
Wool	100%		cotton	0%	31%	—
Wool	90%	+	cotton	10%	55%	Antagonism
Wool	80%	+	cotton	20%	60%	Antagonism
Wool	70%	+	cotton	30%	64%	Antagonism
Wool	60%	+	cotton	40%	60%	Antagonism
Wool	50%	+	cotton	50%	72%	Antagonism
Wool	40%	+	cotton	60%	84%	Antagonism
Wool	30%	+	cotton	70%	88%	Antagonism
Wool	20%	+	cotton	80%	92%	Antagonism
Wool	10%	+	cotton	90%	98%	Antagonism
Wool	0%	+	cotton	100%	100%	—

Table 12.3. Effect of combinations of wool and linen extracts on seedling growth (after Macht[8])

	Percentage of wool and linen combined				Growth index	Significance
Wool	100%		linen	0%	30%	—
Wool	90%	+	linen	10%	22%	Synergism
Wool	80%	+	linen	20%	24%	Synergism
Wool	70%	+	linen	30%	26%	Synergism
Wool	60%	+	linen	40%	33%	Synergism
Wool	50%	+	linen	50%	52%	Synergism
Wool	40%	+	linen	60%	62%	Synergism
Wool	30%	+	linen	70%	71%	Synergism
Wool	20%	+	linen	80%	71%	Synergism
Wool	10%	+	linen	90%	100%	Synergism
Wool	0%	+	linen	100%	119%	—

DEMOGRAPHICS

Throughout the ages, wherever they have lived, common factors have set the Jews apart. "Their separation came of their piety," noted Will Durant, "...their racial pride was the indispensable prop of their courage through centuries of suffering."[9] Lestchinsky focused on the social determinants. "No matter how different and variable the conditions under which the Jews live," he wrote, "there is one common factor operating on them in the majority of countries, namely, the social structure...almost the same in even the most unlike of countries. There may be considerable differences in the attained social levels, in the class proportions, but with regard to the surrounding population the Jews everywhere stand out as a separate social group... In every Jewish community...are active potent factors of inheritance of a bio-psychic nature...the reason for the linkage or bond that ties the Jews of the various parts of the world together."[10] Shylock's words to Bassanio are echoed in the exclusivity of the social clubs of the 20th century: "I will buy with you, sell with you, talk with you, walk with you, and so following; but I will not eat with you, drink with you, nor pray with you."[11]

From the legendary 70 of Jacob's household, driven out of Canaan to Egypt by famine, the Children of Israel increased to 5 million during the reign of King David. From this, its peak in ancient times, the population of the Jews declined to its nadir during the Middle Ages, depleted by persecution and epidemics of disease. The numbers increased slowly, from about 750,000 in the 12th century to perhaps 1 million in the middle of the 18th. During the next hundred years both increase and dispersion were explosive, leading to diffusion of Jews throughout most habitable lands. Early in the 20th century the world's Jewish population had increased to 12 million; and in 1939, before World War II and the decimation of European Jewry in the Holocaust, had reached more than 18 million, residing in 75 different countries, its highest ever but less than 1% of the earth's total.[12] Raymond Pearl, Johns Hopkins' professor of biometrics, commented: "Would one venture to say that their proportional influence on human affairs is of the order of 1%? Whether 'chosen' or not they are as a people differentiated in a statistical sense from the rest of mankind by the most objective tests—success in life, and influence and power in the control of human affairs on a world-wide scale. And it is equally plain that their differentiation must be constitutional in a biological sense... A differentiated tenth of any herd is never likely to have an easy time. The crowd is against them, and it is a big rough crowd."[13]

WORLD JEWISH POPULATIONS

As the 20th century draws to an end the world's Jewish population is estimated at 13.8 million, about 0.25% of humanity.[14] Despite the Jew's few numbers, Mark Twain wrote, "he is as prominent on the planet as any other people... His contributions to the world's list of great names in literature, science, art, music, finance, medicine, and abstruse learning are also away out of proportion to the weakness of his numbers. He has made a marvelous fight in this world, in all ages; and has done it with his hands tied behind him. All things are mortal but the Jew; all other forces pass, but he remains."[15]

UNITED STATES OF AMERICA

Jewish population 5,835,000,[16] about 3% of the country's population and nearly half of the world's Jewish population, with 1,720,000, the largest concentration of Jews, in the Greater New York area; other major communities in Los Angeles, Chicago, Philadelphia, Miami, Boston, and Baltimore. The first Jewish settlement, in New Amsterdam in 1654, was followed by a second in Newport, Rhode Island in 1677; the first synagogue, in New York, was consecrated in 1730. By 1854 the Jewish population had grown to 100,000; by 1880, had tripled as a result of immigration from Germany and Poland. Eastern Europe added another 2 million Jews to American soil by 1914. Further immigration from Germany and Austria following Hitler's rise in the 1930s made the United States the center of world Jewry. In 1992 approximately half of America's Jewish adults had completed at least 4 years of college. Nearly one-half million are members of 2500 Orthodox congregations, most of which are affiliated with the Union of Orthodox Jewish Congregations of America; one and one-half million, members of 930 Conservative congregations, most affiliated with the United Synagogue; and 1,100,000 are members of about 750 Reform congregations, linked with the Union of American Hebrew Congregations. More than 75 Jewish newspapers are published weekly throughout the country.

ISRAEL

Jewish population 3,755,000 of 4,600,000. The first Jewish state was established, in the same area, following its conquest by Joshua, about 1250-1200 B.C.E., but autonomy was lost to the Romans in the 2nd century C.E. A Jewish community redeveloped after the Ottoman conquest in the 16th century, growing to a population of 85,000 by the beginning of World War I. A nation of 650,000 declared its independence in 1948; since then, has multiplied seven times. In 1991 Israel endured nearly 40 missile attacks from its neighbor Iraq, causing much property damage but claiming only one life. Israel is home to seven institutions of higher education, several theater companies, and the Israeli Philharmonic Orchestra; and has the highest doctor/patient ratio in the world.

RUSSIA AND SATELLITE COUNTRIES

Jewish population 1,450,000. Most of the large Jewish population of Poland, which spawned the movements of Hassidism, Zionism, and Jewish socialism, became subjects of the Russian Empire after the partitioning of the former under Catherine II during the second half of the 18th century. Mass emigrations from Russia, mainly to the United States, followed the pogroms of 1881. Current emigration is largely to Israel. About 62 synagogues and several hundred worship groups still exist in the countries that comprised the U.S.S.R.

FRANCE

Jewish population estimated at 600,000 concentrated mainly in Paris and suburbs, Marseilles, Lyons, Toulouse, and Strasbourg. Jewish settlement in France began soon after the destruction of the second Temple in the year 70 C.E. By the Middle Ages the country had become a center of Jewish scholarship. Much immigration from East Europe, at the turn of the 19th to 20th century, was followed by a heavy influx of German Jews in the 1930s. Some 80,000 were deported during the German occupation of World War II. Nearly a quarter-million immigrants arrived from North Africa after the war, and a smaller number from Egypt. Homes for the Jewish aged and 24 full-time Jewish schools are located in and around Paris; others, in the other major Jewish centers. Three Jewish weeklies, two in Yiddish, are published in France.

UNITED KINGDOM

Jewish population 330,000. Most of Britain's large cities included Jewish communities as early as the mid-12th century. Expelled in 1290 by Edward I, they were permitted to return in 1656 by Oliver Cromwell, Lord Protector of England. Full emancipation of the Jews was achieved in 1858; and large waves of immigration from Russia toward the end of the century were followed by masses of refugees from Germany and Eastern Europe in the 1930s. Most live in London, base of the Orthodox United Synagogue, with smaller communities in Manchester, Leeds, and Glasgow, and are served by four Jewish weekly newspapers. About 85% have a synagogue affiliation. Attached to Oxford University is the Oxford Centre for Postgraduate Hebrew Studies.

CANADA

Jewish population 325,000, its first congregation established in 1768 in Montreal. Mass immigration to Canada followed the Russian pogroms of the late-19th century. Toronto contains about 50 synagogues. Together with Montreal these two cities alone have 12 Jewish schools and five Jewish hospitals. Montreal's Jewish Public Library is the only one of its kind in North America.

ARGENTINA

Jewish population 228,000 beginning with French settlers in the 1860s, followed by immigrants from Eastern Europe toward the end of the century, and subsequently by refugees from Nazi Germany in the 1930s. Buenos Aires is home to some 50 synagogues, 71 Jewish schools, A Jewish hospital, a Jewish museum, and weekly, fortnightly, and thrice-annual Jewish publications.

BRAZIL

Jewish population 150,000. First among the Jewish settlers in the early-16th century were the Marranos, those who had converted to

Christianity. Not until the flood of refugees from Nazi Germany in the 1930s did the Jewish population increase substantially. Major communities are in Sao Paulo, which has two Jewish hospitals, seven schools, and a yeshiva; and Rio de Janeiro, which also has a Jewish hospital, and nine synagogues.

SOUTH AFRICA

Jewish population 120,000. The first settlement, in 1841 in Cape Town, followed by the establishment of a Jewish community in Johannesburg in 1886, was abetted by large-scale immigration from Eastern Europe in the 1880s. Legislation in 1937 banned immigration of Jews from Nazi Germany. Most of the Jews now live in the Johannesburg area, and 65 of the synagogues are affiliated with the mainstream Union of Orthodox Synagogues of South Africa.

AUSTRALIA

Jewish population 90,000. A few were included among British convicts deported after 1788; free immigrants began to arrive in the 1820s, with repeated waves of immigration through the aftermath of World War II. Most live in Melbourne, which has about 20 synagogues and eight Jewish day-schools; and Sydney, with about 15 and 8, respectively. The *Australian Jewish News* and *Australian Jewish Times* are published weekly, the *Australia-Israel Review* fortnightly.

HUNGARY

Jewish population 80,000 estimated, original settlement dating back to Roman times, growing from 400,000 to 725,000 between 1938 and 1940 as a result of incorporation of Slovakia, Carpatho-Ruthenia, Transylvania, and the Southern Territories. After the German occupation about 600,000 died in the Holocaust. With the exception of Russia, Hungary still has the largest Jewish population in Central and Eastern Europe. Most live in Budapest, which houses a Jewish museum and Europe's only rabbinical seminary. Hungary has 26 synagogues, the Dohany Street synagogue being the largest in Europe.

URUGUAY

Jewish population 44,000 beginning in the early-20th century with immigration from Central and East Europe, augmented by refugees from Europe and the Middle East after World War II. Most live in Montevideo, which has about 11 synagogues or prayer rooms. The main newspaper for the Jewish community is the Spanish-language weekly *Semanario Hebrao*.

MEXICO

Jewish population 35,000. Some Marranos accompanied the conquistadors into Mexico in the 16th century, but not until 1885 was the first Jewish community established, by the Sephardi Jews from Aleppo, in northern Syria, who built their first synagogue 2 years later. Many European immigrants arrived after World War I. The majority live in Mexico City, which has 16 synagogues. A small group of 100 Mexican Indians in Pachuca, north of Mexico City, practice Judaism and have their own synagogue.

ITALY

Jewish population 34,500, the oldest Jewish community in Western Europe, dating back to the 2nd century B.C.E. When the Germans occupied Italy in 1943, 8360 Jews were deported to Auschwitz, most of whom were killed. The main centers of Italy's Jewish population are in Milan, Turin, Florence, Leghorn, and especially Rome, which has a Jewish hospital and two-thirds of whose Jewish children attend Jewish schools.

BELGIUM

Jewish population 30,000. The Great Plague of 1348 eradicated most of the Jewish communities, which dated back to Roman times. Marranos from Spain and Portugal re-established Jewish settlements early in the 16th century, Ashkenazis from Central Europe in the 18th century. About 100,000 Jews were living in Belgium in 1940. Many fled before the German invasion. Some 25,000 were hidden by Christian Belgians. Of 25,631 Jews deported only 1244 survived. The Jews of Belgium now reside mainly in Brussels and Antwerp, each of which has several synagogues and Jewish schools and its own Jewish weekly.

GERMANY

Jewish population 28,400, most of which lives in what was West Germany. Records of Jewish settlement date back to the 4th century. More than one-half million Jews were living in Germany when the Nazis came into power. Between 1933 and 1938 half of them fled the country. An estimated 160,000 to 180,000 were murdered by the Nazis or died from persecution. Many synagogues remain in both parts of Germany, and Jewish weekly publications are produced in Düsseldorf and Munich.

IRAN

Jewish population 25,000, dating back to the 6th century B.C.E. as Persians, one of the oldest Jewish communities of the Diaspora. A period of prosperity for the Iranian Jews ended with the revolution and overthrow of the Shah in 1979, following which more than half fled the country, the majority to Israel, Most of those who remain live in Tehran, where they have three synagogues but are banned from working in governmental agencies or teaching in non-Jewish schools.

The Netherlands

Jewish population 25,000. Marranos from Spain, Portugal, and Turkey began to settle in Holland in numbers during the 16th century, where they were granted freedom of worship; and by the 17th century and for the next hundred years the country was the main center of world Jewry. Of the 140,000 Jews that were living there when the Nazis invaded in 1940 some 100,00 had perished by war's end. About half of the present Jewish community lives in Amsterdam, which has 12 synagogues and three Jewish day-schools; with smaller communities in Rotterdam and the Hague. The weekly *Nieuw Israelitisch Weekblad*, 120 years old, enjoys a circulation of 5500.

Romania

Jewish population 23,000, dating back to Roman times. The country became a haven for Jewish refugees from Hungary in the 14th century, from Spain in the 16th, and from Poland and the Ukraine in the 17th; but restrictions on the Jews were imposed during the 19th century, and some 17,000 departed the country early in the 20th. The Jewish population stood at 800,000 before World War II; about 385,000 perished in the Holocaust. Of the present residents about half live in Bucharest, which still has 41 functional synagogues, 25 Hebrew schools, and a Jewish journal, published fortnightly in Romanian, English, Hebrew, and Yiddish.

Turkey

Jewish population 23,000. Expelled from Spain in 1492, many took refuge in the Ottoman Empire, augmenting the community that had been established at Bursa in 1326 with settlements in Istanbul, Edirne, and Izmir. About 37,000 Jews departed for Israel after World War II, and internal violence in the late 1970s led to further mass emigration. The larger cities of Turkey have synagogues, but Turkish law prohibits ethnically or religiously based associations. *Shalom*, the only Jewish newspaper, is mostly in Ladino.

Venezuela

Jewish population 20,000. Settlement began in the early-19th century with immigrants from the Middle East and North Africa, and is concentrated mainly at present in Caracas, which has nine synagogues and a weekly Jewish newspaper. Nearly all the country's Jewish children are educated in Jewish schools. Venezuela's is South America's sole Jewish community that is currently expanding.

Switzerland

Jewish population 18,300. Although Jews began to settle in Switzerland as early as the 13th century, they did not gain full civil rights until 1866. The country sheltered 23,000 Jews during the Holocaust.

The largest of about 25 current Jewish communities are in Zurich, which has four synagogues; Geneva, three; and Basel, two.

CHILE

Jewish population 17,000. Settlement began with the immigration of some Marranos in the 17th century, followed by an influx of Jews after Chile's liberation from Spain in 1810. Large numbers came from Germany in the late 1930s. Most live in Santiago, which now has 12 synagogues. Nearly half of the Jewish children attend Jewish day-schools.

SWEDEN

Jewish population 16,000. A Jewish community was established in the 18th century, achieved civil rights near the end of the 19th, when refugees began to arrive from Poland and Russia. During World War II and in its aftermath Sweden offered asylum to more than 200,000 refugees, including Norwegian, Danish, Hungarian, and Polish Jews. More than half of Sweden's present Jewish population consists of refugees from Central and Eastern Europe. Stockholm has three synagogues, Gothenburg two, and Malmö one.

ETHIOPIA

Jewish population 15,000. The Falashas, dating back to the 2nd or 3rd century, remained isolated from world Jewry and had not known of white Jews until 1868, when the Alliance Israélite Universelle established contact with the community and initiated its education. These North African Jews began leaving their homes in Gondar and Tigre provinces in 1974 in response to oppression by the governing Marxist regime, and within 10 years 5,000 had reached Israel. Rescue missions by the Israeli government have continued.

MOROCCO

Jewish population 13,000, dating back to Roman times. Fez and Sigilmasa were established as centers of Jewish scholarship in the 11th century; the Maimonides family settled in the former in 1160. After a long period of suppression under Muslim rule the status of the Jews improved when Morocco was made a French protectorate in 1912; and in 1956, when Morocco gained independence, its 285,000 Jews were granted full rights of citizenship. During the 2 decades after World War II 226,000 Moroccan Jews emigrated to Israel. The country's remaining Jewish population is concentrated mainly in Casablanca.

AUSTRIA

Jewish population 12,000. Jews lived in Austria at least as early as 906. In the 13th and 14th centuries Vienna was prominent among the world's Jewish communities. Viennese Jews were important figures in culture and science during the 19th and early-20th centuries. About

120,000 of Austria's 183,000 Jews managed emigration after Germany's 1938 *Anschluss*. Almost all who remained were murdered in the Holocaust. Most of the Jews now in Austria, more than half over age 60, live in Vienna, which has a synagogue, several prayer rooms for the ultra-Orthodox, and two kosher restaurants.

Czechoslovakia

Jewish population 12,000 (before division into the Czech Republic and Slovakia in 1992). Jews lived in Moravia in the 9th century, in Bohemia at least as early as the 10th, and comprised an important part of the Prague community by the end of the 16th. More than 350,000 lived there in 1935. By the end of World War II only 42,000 Jews remained in Czechoslovakia. The country had 13 synagogues in 1991, including the 11th-century Altneuschul, one of the oldest in Europe, but no rabbi.

Spain

Jewish population 12,000. Jews lived in Spain from the Roman era until their expulsion in 1492, when some 50,000 fled the country. They began to return after 1869, when rights of residence and religious practice were granted to non-Catholics. In the 1930s and during World War II several thousand Central European Jews took refuge in Spain. Separation of church and state was established by the Constitution of 1978. Spain's Jewish population is concentrated mainly in Madrid, Barcelona, and Malaga, which have modern synagogues, resident rabbis, and Jewish day-schools.

Colombia

Jewish population 7000. Significant Jewish immigration began after World War I with the arrival of European refugees, but was banned during the period of Hitlerian oppression, 1934-1945. Most Colombian Jews live in Bogota.

Poland

Jewish population 6000. Some settlement having begun in the 9th century, the country became renowned for its Jewish culture and scholarship during the 16th and 17th centuries. With the partitioning of Poland in the late-18th century, most of the country's Jews came under Russian rule. Persecution in the late-19th century led to mass emigration. At the end of World War I Jews still comprised one-third of the population of newly-independent Poland, and about 3.5 million at the onset of World War II. Three million were killed in the Holocaust. The Jews remaining in Poland, mostly elderly, are concentrated mainly in Warsaw, Wroclaw, Cracow, and Lodz.

INDIA

Jewish population 5600. According to legend, Jews lived in India in King Solomon's time; but the earliest documentation of their residence, in Cochin, dates to 1000 C.E. Present Jewry in India, concentrated in Greater Bombay, consists of two groups: the larger, Bene Israel, claiming descent from refugees from ancient Israel in the 2nd century B.C.E., who have adopted some local Muslim and Hindu customs; and a smaller community of Baghdadi Jews, descendants of Middle Eastern immigrants. Eighteen of a larger number of synagogues and prayer halls remain open, but India lacked the services of a rabbi in 1991. Most Indian Jews now live in Israel.

YUGOSLAVIA

Jewish population 5500, among the several political entities into which the country was divided in 1991. Early Jewish settlement, dating back to Roman times, was augmented by refugees from Spain in 1492 and by immigrants from Austro-Hungary after World War I, when Yugoslavia was founded. Eighty percent of its Jewish population, some 60,000 souls, were killed in the Holocaust. Most of the survivors emigrated to Israel after that State was established. The remaining, elderly population resides mainly in Belgrade, Zagreb, and Sarajevo, which have 12 synagogues.

PERU

Jewish population 5000, nearly all in Lima, which has four synagogues and two Jewish newspapers. Peru's earliest Jews, who practiced their religion secretly, were put to death in the Inquisition, between 1581 and 1776. Jewry became established in Peru at the end of the 19th century through immigrants from North Africa, with additional arrivals between the two World Wars from the Middle East and Nazi Germany.

GREECE

Jewish population 4800, living mainly in Athens, with a smaller community in Salonica; together they have eight synagogues. Europe's oldest Jewish communities were established on mainland Greece in the 3rd century B.C.E. and in Chalcis, on Euboea Island, about 20 B.C.E. At the outbreak of World War II Greece was home to 77,000 Jews, most of whom were killed during the Holocaust. By 1945 only 11,000 remained.

NEW ZEALAND

Jewish population 4800. Jews began to settle in New Zealand in 1829; and after British annexation of the country in 1840, established communities in Auckland and Wellington, where most of the present Jewish population, augmented by European immigrants in 1882 and after 1933, live. Synagogues are maintained in these and three other cities.

BULGARIA

Jewish population 4000. Jews lived in Bulgaria, in small but increasing numbers, since the Roman era. Of their population of 50,000 at the end of World War II some 44,000 emigrated to Israel. Most that remain live in Sofia, whose synagogue is one of the largest and most beautiful in the Balkans. Plovdiv also has a synagogue.

SYRIA

Jewish population 4000. The region served as home for Jews before the Greek conquest of the 4th century B.C.E. Their numbers were increased by refugees from Spain in the 15th and 16th centuries. Many were killed in anti-Zionist attacks in the 1940s. Some 30,000 Jews still lived in Syria in 1943, most of whom have since emigrated, mainly to Israel. Of those who remain, most live in segregated communities in Damascus, which has a synagogue.

PANAMA

Jewish population 3800, the largest and most vigorous Jewish community in Central America. Settlement began in the mid-19th century and continued into the 20th, with the arrival of Jews from the Middle East and Eastern Europe, followed by refugees from Germany and Austria in the 1930s. Most live in Panama City, which has three synagogues—Sephardi, Conservative, and Reform.

TUNISIA

Jewish population 3500. Jews lived in Tunisia, under Muslim rule, at least 1800 years ago. Kairouan became a center of Jewish scholarship. The position of the Jews began to deteriorate in the mid-11th century as a result of Muslim repression and subsequent Spanish persecution, and worsened after Tunisia attained independence, the Jewish population declining steadily from a peak of 105,000 in 1949. During the Nazi occupation of 1942-43 the Jews of Tunisia were subjected to confiscation of property, deportation, and execution. The remaining Jewish population is concentrated in Tunis and on the island of Djerba, which has several synagogues.

COSTA RICA

Jewish population 2500. Turkish and Polish Jews began to arrive soon after World War I, followed by refugees from Germany and Austria in the 1930s. Most live in San Jose, which has a synagogue and a Jewish school, and where the Spanish language *Hayom* is published monthly.

IRELAND

Jewish population 2000. Immigration from Central and Eastern Europe, England, and Holland began in the 17th century, the Jewish population reaching 3800 by the beginning of the 20th century. Most of the Jewish community is concentrated in Dublin, which has six synagogues and four Jewish day-schools.

PUERTO RICO

Jewish population 2000. The first Jewish community began to form during World War II with the influx of U.S. troops. Many American Jews subsequently settled there, and were joined by co-religionists who left Cuba after its revolution in 1959. The Jewish community center with its attached synagogue is the focal point of Jewish life in Puerto Rico.

FINLAND

Jewish population 1200. Previously under Russian rule, Jews acquired full civil rights in Finland only after the country's attainment of independence in 1918. The Jewish population peaked at 2000 between the two World Wars. Most of the present Jewish community lives in Helsinki, which has a synagogue, a Jewish day-school, and a Jewish hospital, and where *Ha-Kehila* is published four to six times a year. Turku also has a synagogue.

LUXEMBOURG

Jewish population 1200. The country's small Jewish community, massacred in 1349, was reincarnated in 1791, when Luxembourg was joined with France under Napoleon I. Refugees flowing into Luxembourg in the 1930s brought its Jewish population to 3500 before its decimation by the Nazis. Many perished in the Holocaust. Their synagogue, destroyed by the invaders, has been replaced by a new building, financed by the state.

ZIMBABWE

Jewish population 1200, its first congregations established by immigrants from Lithuania in the early-20th century. Jewish immigrants also arrived from Rhodes during the years between the two World Wars, the population peaking in the 1960s but subsequently declining. The Jewish community is now divided between Harare, which has Ashkenazi, Sephardi, and Progressive congregations; and Bulawaya, which has an Orthodox Ashkenazi synagogue.

CUBA

Jewish population 1000. Cuban independence at the beginning of the 20th century was followed by an influx of nearly 6000 Jews from Syria and Turkey. By 1948 some 12,000 had settled on the island, but most departed after the revolution in 1959. Most of the present small population lives in Havana, where four rarely used synagogues remain.

Ecuador

Jewish population 1000, stemming mainly from immigration from Germany during the years between the World Wars. Quito, where most live, has a synagogue and a rabbi.

Monaco

Jewish population 1000, its beginnings in 1948, mostly retired and nearly half of British origin. In the early 1960s Jews from North Africa joined the community, which in 1972 acquired premises to serve as a synagogue and community center.

Yemen

Jewish population 1000, virtually all in what was formerly North Yemen, which records Jewish settlements as early as the third century and where Jews have probably lived since Biblical times. Nearly 49,000 were airlifted to Israel in 1949-50 in "Operation Magic Carpet". The remaining Jews, mostly artisans and small traders, are banned from public service and land ownership. Their community is scattered and has little contact with world Jewry.

Norway

Jewish population 950. Not until 1851 were Jews legally admitted. A large influx from Eastern Europe took place toward the end of the century, and congregations were founded in Oslo in 1892 and in Trondheim in 1905. The Quisling government during the Nazi occupation permitted the deportation of nearly half of the country's 1800 Jews to Auschwitz; about half escaped to Sweden; a few remained in hiding. Jewish survivors of the war, about 800, were invited back by the Norwegian government. Most of the present community live in Oslo, a smaller number in Trondheim. Each has a synagogue.

Paraguay

Jewish population 900, its main organization the Unión Hebraica del Paraguay having its roots in the immigrants from Greece and Turkey about 1917 and those from Russia and Poland a few years later. Most live in Asunción, where nearly all Jewish children attend the Jewish school. More than 10,000 Jewish immigrants from Central Europe passed through Paraguay between 1933 and 1947 en route to Argentina.

Guatemala

Jewish population 800. Immigration, mostly from Germany, began in the late-19th century, intensifying during the years immediately preceding World War II. Many have since left the country. Most of the remaining Jews live in Guatemala City. Guatemala has three synagogues and a Jewish school, but no rabbi.

JAMAICA

Jewish population 800. Some Marranos, it is believed, had settled in Jamaica long before the British occupation of the island in 1665. Jews subsequently came from the Mediterranean countries and from England, forming a unified community in 1921. Many left after Jamaica achieved independence in 1962, apprehensive of future governmental stability, a fear based on the Marxist revolution in Cuba.

HONG KONG

Jewish population 700. Jews first settled in Hong Kong in the mid-19th century and were followed a century later by refugees form Europe; but their communal life ceased with the Japanese occupation of the colony in 1941. Of those still there after the war many emigrated, but were soon replaced by Jews fleeing communist China. Most of the present Jewish community are expatriate British business people, their religious center the Ohel Leah Synagogue.

JAPAN

Jewish population 700. Jews from Poland and Russia settled in Japan in 1861, Jewish merchants from Iraq soon thereafter. In the 1930s refugees came from Germany, Russia, and China. Like other foreigners, Jews are ineligible for Japanese citizenship. Currently they comprise a small religious community, with a synagogue in Tokyo and another in Kobe.

BOLIVIA

Jewish population 600, the majority living in La Paz, which has two synagogues. The first Jewish settlers arrived in 1905. Others followed, from the Soviet Union, Germany, and Austria, until immigration was stopped in 1940, when the Jewish population peaked at about 10,000. The country's Jewish community near the end of the 20th century appears threatened by emigration of its younger members.

CURAÇAO

Jewish population 600. Settlement of Jews in Curaçao was encouraged by a charter and tract of land granted by the Dutch West India Company in 1652. Jews fleeing from persecution on South America's mainland later took refuge there. Most of the present residents are 20th-century Ashkenazi immigrants who, together with a minority of 17th-century Sephardi settlers, maintain three synagogues and a Reform temple.

GIBRALTAR

Jewish population, static at 600 for the past 40 years, is entirely Sephardic, dating back to the British occupation in 1704. The Jewish community numbered 2000 in the mid-19th century, but most left the country during World War II and did not return. Of its four synagogues the Shaar Hashamayim, constructed in 1768, is Gibraltar's most historic building.

U.S. VIRGIN ISLANDS

Jewish population 500. Most live in St. Thomas, whose Sephardi synagogue is the oldest in the United States and its Territories. Jews have lived in the Virgin Islands since the mid-17th century, but most of the present population are immigrants from mainland U.S. or their descendants, who settled on the Islands after World War II.

SURINAM

Jewish population 350, comprising the oldest permanent Jewish settlement in the Americas, to which Marranos fled from Portuguese persecution in Brazil in 1639. Many Jews have left in recent years. Those that remain, nearly all of whom live in the capital, Paramaribo, maintain two synagogues.

KENYA

Jewish population 330. The first Jewish community, established in 1904, was augmented by an influx of immigrants from Europe in 1945. The Nairobi Hebrew Congregation serves as the center for Jewish communal and religious life.

PORTUGAL

Jewish population 300, dating back to the 13th century. From the end of the 15th century many were forcibly converted to Christianity, as in Spain. During World War II about 70,000 Central European Jews passed through Portugal, but some remained. Most of the present small Jewish community lives in Lisbon, which has two synagogues: a Sephardi and an Ashkenazi.

SINGAPORE

Jewish population 300. Founded in 1841 by Baghdadi traders, the Jewish community was decimated in the Japanese invasion during World War II. The rebuilt community maintains two synagogues but is declining as a result of steady emigration, mainly to Australia and the United States.

ALGERIA

Jewish population 250, dating back to Roman times, possibly earlier. With the influx of Sephardim from Spain in the late-14th and

15th centuries Algeria became the spiritual center of Jewry of Northwest Africa. Almost all of the country's 140,000 Jews departed after Algeria gained independence from France in 1962—some 125,000 to France, 10,000 to Israel; but a synagogue is still maintained in Algiers.

EGYPT

Jewish population 240. Land of four centuries of enslavement of the Children of Israel, until the Exodus, about 1250 B.C.E., Egypt has remained a major factor in Jewish history. In the late-4th century B.C.E. the Jews established a community in Alexandria, then under Greek rule, and another in Cairo in the 10th century C.E. It was here that Maimonides wrote most of his works, in the late-12th century. Anti-Zionist riots after World War II led to a rapid decline in the Jewish population of Egypt, from 75,000 in 1948 to 2500 by 1967. Jewish rights in Egypt were restored after the Camp David peace accord with Israel in 1979. Despite the present small population, four synagogues are maintained in Cairo and one in Alexandria.

BAHAMAS

Jewish population 200. The first Jew to land in the Bahamas was Columbus' interpreter, Luis de Torres, for whom is named the synagogue in Freeport. A few Jews came to the islands from Poland, Russia, and the United Kingdom after World War I. About 40 Jewish families were living in Nassau and Freeport in the 1980s.

IRAQ

Jewish population 200. Here was born the patriarch Abraham, about 2000 B.C.E., in Ur of the Chaldees; here was established the first Jewish community of the Diaspora, when Babylonia conquered Judea, in 586 B.C.E.; and here was recorded the Jewish law of the Babylonian Talmud, about 200 C.E. About 150,000 Jews were living in Iraq in 1947. After a pro-German revolt and anti-Jewish pogroms in 1941 many had already left when, in 1950-51 the Jewish Agency and the Israeli government salvaged 113,545 by airlift. By 1958 the Jewish community of Iraq was virtually obliterated. A few old people remain and one synagogue is still maintained, in Baghdad.

THAILAND

Jewish population 200, its community established in the 1960s by a mixture of foreign nationals, who maintain a modern synagogue. A small group of Orthodox Sephardim conduct separate services in a converted private home.

ZAIRE

Jewish population 200, settled initially by Jews from South Africa in the early-20th century, followed by Sephardim from Rhodes. The

Jewish population numbered as high as 2500 in 1959, concentrated in Elizabethville (now Lubumbashi), which still has a synagogue, and Leopoldville (Kinshasa).

Taiwan

Jewish population 180, its community and synagogue founded jointly by Israelis and Americans working in Taipei.

Dominican Republic

Jewish population 150, mainly German and Austrian, divided between Santa Domingo and Sosua, each of which has a synagogue. The Dominican Republic was alone of the 32 countries at the Evian Conference in 1938 in agreeing to accept a substantial number of Jewish refugees from Europe. Only about 600 arrived on Dominican shores, but some 5000 more survived because of their Dominican visas.

Haiti

Jewish population 150, consisting of 20th-century immigrants from Syria, Egypt, and Germany, without communal organization. A settlement of Marranos in the 17th century was killed or expelled during a revolution in the 19th.

Honduras

Jewish population 150, concentrated largely in Tegucigalpa, consisting of the families of immigrants from Central and East Europe between the two World Wars. San Pedro Sula has a synagogue but no rabbi.

Philippines

Jewish population 150. The first Jewish community, stemming from traders from Alsace-Lorraine who settled in the late-19th century, built a synagogue in 1924. Jews began to flee here from Europe and Shanghai in the 1930s. Some 2000 arrived between 1939 and 1940. All were interned during the Japanese occupation in 1943. The present small community, re-established in 1945, is augmented by about the same number of temporary residents from Israel.

Channel Islands

Jewish population 140; most live on Jersey. Jews began to settle in the Channel Islands in the mid-18th century, built a synagogue in the mid-19th century. Most had escaped by the time of the German invasion in 1940; a few returned after the war.

El Salvador

Jewish population 100, originating with 19th-century settlers from France. Additional immigrants arrived, from Eastern Europe and the

Orient, between the two World Wars, and from Germany after World War II. One hundred-twenty Jewish families were living in El Salvador in 1976, but the country's civil war caused many to leave and the synagogue to close.

LEBANON

Jewish population 100, dating from ancient times. Numbering 10,000 in 1952, many left after the Six-Day War in 1967; others after the civil war of 1976. Prominent Lebanese Jews were kidnapped and murdered. The country's Shiite Muslims are hostile to neighboring Israel.

ZAMBIA (FORMERLY NORTHERN RHODESIA)

Jewish population 85, mostly in Lusaka, linked with the larger Jewish population of neighboring Zimbabwe. Jewish settlement, which began in Zambia early in the 19th century, was increased by German refugees arriving in the 1930s, reaching 1200 in the 1950s but declining sharply after Zambian independence in 1964.

AFGHANISTAN

Jewish population less than 50. The country's modern Jewish community began in 1839 as an offshoot of Persian Jewry, grew to 40,000 in the second half of the 19th century. Emigration to Palestine began after World War I. Few Jews remained by the early 1950s, but Kabul still has a synagogue.

ALBANIA

Jewish population less than 50. Some Sephardim took refuge in Albania after their 1492 expulsion from Spain, and were joined by Jews from Southern Italy soon thereafter. Most of Albania's small Jewish population was annihilated by the Germans in 1944. Practically all of the survivors emigrated to Israel or the United States in 1991.

ARUBA

Jewish population less than 50. The small settlement, dating to 1924, maintains the Beth Israel Congregation but has no rabbi.

BARBADOS

Jewish population less than 50, originating with refugees from northeast Brazil when that country was re-conquered by Portugal in the mid-17th century. The small Jewish community, in Bridgetown, is represented by the Jewish Community Council.

BERMUDA

Jewish population 50. A few Jewish merchants have lived on the island since the 18th century, but without an organized Jewish community.

Burma

Jewish population 20. Iraqi Jews founded a congregation in Rangoon in 1857. Most of Burma's 3000 Jews had fled the country by the time of the Japanese invasion during World War II.

China

Jewish population less than 50. Some one thousand Jews from India and Persia are believed to have settled in Kaifeng, Hunan Province, during the 9th and 10th centuries, but were subsequently assimilated into the Chinese community. Jewish merchants settled in China in the 1840s, after Hong Kong became a British colony; later, immigrants came from Russia, after its 1917 Revolution, and from Nazi Germany. Almost all of the 30,000 Jews living in China in the 1940s left after the communist takeover in 1949. A few Jews were still living in Kaifeng in 1988.

Cyprus

Jewish population less than 50. The island had a substantial Jewish population as early as the first century C.E. Many were interned by the British during World War II while trying to enter Palestine. A few Jews still live there, without synagogue or rabbi.

Indonesia

Jewish population less than 50. The families of Dutch and Iraqi Jews who settled there in the 19th century were joined in the 20th by immigrants from Eastern Europe and Germany. Most of the Jewish population of 3000 left after Indonesia gained independence from the Netherlands in 1949.

Libya

Jewish population less than 50, first settlement dating back to the 3rd century B.C.E. After a long absence from the country Jews settled there again following their expulsion from Spain in 1492. They suffered repeated persecution during the ensuing years; and after the Six-Day War in 1967 virtually all of those still living in Libya fled to Israel.

Maylasia

Jewish population less than 50. With no formal community, practically all the Jews who lived there, mostly Russian refugees, have left.

Malta

Jewish population less than 50. The original settlement, dating back to Roman times, was eliminated by the expulsion of Jews in 1492. Jewish immigrants arrived from North Africa in the late-18th century. A new synagogue was inaugurated in 1984.

Nicaragua

Jewish population less than 50. Immigrants began to arrive from France, Germany, and Holland in 1848, followed by an influx from Eastern Europe after World War I. An earthquake devastated Managua in 1972. By 1976 only 150 Jews remained there, and virtually all of them fled the country after the assumption of power by the Sandinistas in 1979.

Pakistan

Jewish population less than 50. A small settlement began in the 19th century in what is now Pakistan and built a synagogue, which still remains, in Karachi; but only one Jewish family is believed to remain in the country.

South Korea

Jewish population less than 50, consisting of U.S. military personnel who arrived after World War II and a small number of Russian refugees, who settled there during the Japanese occupation.

Trinidad and Tobago

Jewish population less than 50, mostly elderly, with no synagogue, the remainder of a once vigorous community of some 800 who had come from Central Europe before and during World War II.

Diaspora

The history of the Jew in the Diaspora was summarized by Will Durant: "The story of the Jews since the Dispersion is one of the epics of European history. Driven from their natural home...scattered by flight...persecuted and decimated...shut up within congested ghettos...mobbed by the people and robbed by the kings...outcast and excommunicated, insulted and injured...this wonderful people has maintained itself in body and soul, has preserved its racial and cultural integrity, has guarded with jealous love its oldest rituals and traditions...has emerged in greater number than ever before, renowned in every field for the contributions of its geniuses, and triumphantly restored, after 2000 years of wandering, to its ancient and unforgotten home. What drama could rival the grandeur of these sufferings, the variety of these scenes, and the glory and justice of this fulfillment?"[17]

WHO IS A JEW?

As Moses wed the Midianite Zipporah; as Boaz took to wife the Moabite Ruth; and as Shakespeare's Jessica ran off with the Venetian Lorenzo,[18] intermarriage has ever been a fact of life among the Jews. Its startling increase in the late-20th century has required a re-examination of the question: "Who is a Jew?" Before 1965 about 6% of Jews from Conservative families "married out." According to the Council of Jewish Federation's 1990 National Population Study, 52% of Jews married in recent years have chosen spouses who were not born Jewish.

For the Orthodox and most Conservatives the issue is clear, and relatively simple. The *halakhah* of the Talmud decrees that a Jew is any person born of a Jewish mother or who has been converted to Judaism by proper rabbinic authority and according to rigorous, established procedure. Thus the child of a Jewish father and non-Jewish mother, according to traditional law, is a Gentile, and would have to be formally converted in order to qualify as a Jew.[19]

The Reform movement has adopted a more liberal stand on the issue of parentage as a determinant of status. In both Biblical and rabbinical tradition the paternal line has been decisive in tracing descent. Accordingly, the Central Conference of American Rabbis on March 15, 1983 adopted the Report of its Committee on Patrilineal Descent on the Status of Children of Mixed Marriages, declaring "that the child of one Jewish parent [whether it be mother or father] is under the presumption of Jewish descent. The presumption of the Jewish status of the offspring of any mixed marriage is to be established through appropriate and timely public and formal acts of identification with the Jewish faith and people." Such a child is accepted as Jewish by Reform Judaism, without a formal conversion, if he or she attends a Jewish school and follows a course of studies leading to Confirmation.

THE CHOSEN PEOPLE

Some Jews began to bridle at the concept of their "chosenness" over a century ago. *Jewish Tidings*, a Reform weekly published in Rochester, New York during the late-19th century, editorialized: "The Jews of the world have a proper appreciation of what they have done for mankind, but they do not glory in the fact that they are a distinctive people."[20] The fundamentals of Judaism, the editors insisted, were good government, liberty, and freedom of conscience; the achievement of these goals required the elimination of Jewish social separatism. They coupled social progress of Jews with the destruction of any trace of Jewish distinctiveness. *Jewish Tidings* foresaw even the abandonment of Jewish ritual in its vision of a proper relation of the American Jew with his Christian neighbor: "Old customs and ceremonies that hinder Jewish progress," the editors predicted, "are dying out and will, before the century closes, be pleasant memories of bygone days. Disagreeable habits and customs that prevent the Jew from occupying the social station he deserves will drop away with his increasing merit, and the American Jew of the future will be a polished and cultured cosmopolitan."[21]

More modest was the view of Mordecai Kaplan (1881-1983), founder of the Reconstructionist movement in the first half of the 20th century. While emphasizing the primacy of Zion and the Jewish people and the identification of Judaism with moral value and cosmic purpose, he rejected the traditional notion of the Jews as a chosen people and insisted on its elimination from Jewish theology and its liturgy. Such a view, he held, could not be dissociated from the objectionable implication that some nations are superior to others. "The idea of Israel as the Chosen People," Kaplan wrote, "must...be understood as belonging to a thought-world which we no longer inhabit... Nowadays for any people to call itself 'chosen' is to be guilty of self-infatuation." The earlier accent in the doctrine of election, he believed, "was not on national self-awareness as such, but on being the most privileged of all peoples, by virtue of possessing God's Torah." Kaplan insisted that *"Judaism can certainly not afford to harbor any doctrine which is in conflict with the ethical basis of democracy.* That basis is the intrinsic worth of the individual human soul, a worth which is independent of the people, race or church to which one belongs."[22]

Prominent figures in Reform Jewry concur. Referring to special election or chosenness, W. Gunther Plaut wrote: "In times of stress it was a source of hope and reassurance, and Jewish survival might not have been possible without the conviction that Israel was indeed God's beloved... From this, some have drawn the conclusion that in fact the concept of the Chosen People was essentially a survival mechanism...in an age which decries inequality of every kind, the doctrine of special election has no further place and should forthwith be disavowed... it was productive, but has become counterproductive."[23] Alexander M. Schindler, President of the Union of American Hebrew Congregations, added: "Separation is bad for Jews... Our survival is for a far higher purpose: to heal a fractured world."[24]

Kaplan and others articulated what many had long recognized: that fulfillment of the Jew's legitimate spiritual and intellectual wants required replacement of the doctrine of election by the doctrine of vocation in his Jewish consciousness; that in viewing his life as a divine calling he must be engaged in needful work in which his best powers are called into use and through which he can contribute to the welfare of mankind. The doctrine of election had long been a pillar in the barrier of anti-Semitism that excluded Jews from a number of professions in America. Perhaps most egregious were the obstacles encountered by Jews in the medical profession, denying them admission to medical school, hindering their opportunities in residency training, and closing to them the doors to academic appointments, especially departmental chairmanships. Two astute observers of the American scene commented, in 1931: "The question of discrimination against Jews in medicine is the most delicate and difficult chapter in the whole history of prejudice in America. There is less frankness here, more cross currents and divisions of opinion, greater danger that an intrusion of comment may bring down the wrath alike of those who discriminate and those discriminated against... It would be going too far to ascribe belligerent hatred to the medical colleges. They are honestly disturbed by what they consider menacing conditions."[25]

For more than a thousand years Jews have sought to become physicians in greater proportion than have other segments of the population in which they lived. In pre-Nazi Germany, for example, in which Jews made up but 1% of the population, Jewish doctors constituted an estimated 30% of their profession. In ten major American cities surveyed over 5-year periods, the number of Jewish medical students graduated as physicians increased from seven in 1875-1880 to 2313 in 1931-1935.[26] During the latter period more than 60% of the 33,000 applications to medical schools on file at any one time were from Jews.

New York City, with its large Jewish citizenry and its several medical schools, presented the problem in microcosm. At Columbia University, President Nicholas Murray Butler in 1918 enunciated a policy of "selective admissions" specifically designed to limit the enrollment of the city's growing Jewish population in favor of what was termed its "natural constituency." First of the professional schools to implement this policy was the University's medical school, the College of Physicians and Surgeons, in which, according to one study, Jewish admissions fell from 14% in 1920 to less than 4% by 1948. Quota systems kept the proportion of Jewish students similarly low at Harvard, Yale, and Cornell medical schools during these years. Analogous restrictions, imposed throughout the country, resulted in bitterness and disillusionment among students facing rejection, causing many to go abroad for a medical education or to turn to related professions such as dentistry, optometry, and pharmacy. More than 90% of the more than two thousand Americans studying medicine in Europe between 1932 and 1933 were Jewish.[28]

Jewish graduates from New York's City College encountered particular discrimination in their efforts to gain admission to medical schools before mid-century. Discouraged by Columbia's College of Physicians and Surgeons' exclusionary policy, none even applied for an endowed scholarship there for a City College graduate during a period of 9 years, the scholarship going begging. Despite such obstacles, no less than four of City College's graduates of that era were subsequently awarded the Nobel Prize in Physiology or Medicine.[27]

By the end of World War II the mood of the country, and especially of the Jewish community, had changed. Returning veterans were not to be denied; and concerted efforts by a number of Jewish organizations led to confrontation with private institutions and ultimately to legislation prohibiting discriminatory admissions policies. In 1948 the New York State legislature declared that "the American ideal of opportunity requires that students, otherwise qualified, be admitted to educational institutions without regard to race, color, religion, creed or national origin."[29] Sensitivity to discriminatory quotas was a major factor in the creation of the State University of New York, which took over three medical schools, previously private and in financial straits: the Syracuse College of Medicine and the Long Island College of Medicine, both in 1950; and the Buffalo Medical School, in 1962. Two new medical schools, under Jewish sponsorship but nonsectarian, were created in New York City around the same time, "to alleviate the shortage of health personnel, to insure young men and women with necessary talent the opportunity for medical education, to advance the medical sciences, to carry on a great tradition of the Jew in medicine, and to make a collective Jewish contribution to American life that would earn the gratitude of all humanity":[27] the Albert Einstein College of Medicine of Yeshiva University, chartered in 1951; and the Mount Sinai School of Medicine, which came into being in 1965.

Admissions policies of medical schools, as of other professional schools, are now, happily, quite open. The discrimination fostered by separatism has been superseded by preferential admission for minority candidates. In 1950, of the approximately 100,000 physicians in the United States, an estimated 12 to 15% were Jewish; although Jews constituted less than 4% of the population.

SUMMARY

Passé is the concept of the Jews as "the Chosen People"; but the thread of separatism is woven throughout their history, traditions, and rituals. *Kilayim*, meaning "of two kinds," is mentioned repeatedly in the Bible; the holy is clearly distinguished from the profane. Forbidden was the planting together of different types of seed, the crossbreeding of animals, or even the harnessing together of different species of draft animals. Nothing was permitted that interfered with the established order of nature. Transvestism was decreed an abomination. Men and women are still seated separately at Orthodox religious services.

Shaatnez, a curious Biblical proscription against the wearing of a garment of mixed linen and wool, has been interpreted by some as symbolizing the prohibition of the creation of hybrids. An objective measure of the biological specificity of mixtures of wool and linen extracts has been provided by plant seedlings. Wool extracts proved toxic, inhibiting growth; linen extracts, innocuous. Combined with wool, however, linen, unlike other vegetable fiber extracts, as those of cotton and rayon, produced a potentiation of wool's toxicity.

Wherever they have lived, Jews have been set apart. At the close of the 20th century they inhabit virtually every country, although comprising only 0.25% of the world's population. The Talmudic definition of a Jew, as any person born of a Jewish mother or who has been converted to Judaism by proper rabbinic authority, has been amended by the Reform movement, which declares that the child of one Jewish parent, whether mother of father, is under the presumption of Jewish descent.

Notes and References

1. Fields HJ. A Torah Commentary for Our Times, vol. 2. Exodus and Leviticus. New York: UAHC Press 1991; 132.
2. Shulchan Arukh: Yoreh Deah 295:1.
3. Shaatnez is permitted in a shroud for a corpse (Niddah 61).
4. The Torah. WG Plaut, ed. New York: Union of American Hebrew Congregations 1981; 901.
5. Lehmann J. A Guide to Shaatnez. Spring Valley New York: Feldheim Pub 1988.
6. Maimonides, Moses. The Guide for the Perplexed. Translated from the Arabic by M. Friedländer. New York: Dover Pub 2nd ed. (1904), 1956:335,338.
7. Wieseltier L. "Leviticus," in Congregation, David Rosenberg, ed. San Diego: Harcourt, Brace, Jovanovich 1987:36.
8. Macht DI. Phytopharmacological reactions of extracts from textile fibers. Protoplasma 1939; 33:341-344.
9. Durant W. Our Oriental Heritage. New York: Simon and Schuster 1954:335.
10. Lestchinsky J. The natural increase of Jewish people during the last century. Medical Leaves 1940; 3:130-140.
11. Shakespeare W. The Merchant of Venice. I, iii, 36-39.
12. Morrison H. A biologic interpretation of Jewish survival. Medical Leaves 1940; 3:97-103.
13. Quoted by H Morrison. A biologic interpretation of Jewish survival. Medical Leaves 1940; 3:97-103.
14. Estimate of Sergio della Pergola of the Hebrew University of Jerusalem (Dateline World Jewry March 1992).
15. Quoted by Alan M Dershowitz in Chutzpah. Boston: Little, Brown 1991:128.
16. Population figures and other data from The Jewish Communities Handbook. New York and London: Institute of Jewish Affairs and World Jewish Congress 1991.
17. Durant W. The Story of Philosophy. Garden City, New York: Garden City Pub Co 1926: 161-162.
18. The Merchant of Venice.
19. Such qualification would be required, according to traditional law, for marriage to a Jew or for synagogue membership.
20. Jewish Tidings. November 30, 1888; quoted by Stuart E. Rosenberg: Some Attitudes of Nineteenth Century Reform Laymen, in Essays of Jewish Life and Thought, JL Blau et al. eds. New York: Columbia University Press 1959:412.
21. Jewish Tidings, September 24, 1887; quoted by Stuart E. Rosenberg. Some Attitudes of Nineteenth Century Reform Laymen, in Essays of Jewish Life and Thought, JL Blau et al. eds. New York: Columbia University Press 1959:412.

22. Kaplan MM. The Future of the American Jew. New York: Macmillan 1948:211-230.
23. The Torah. WG Plaut, ed. New York: Union of American Hebrew Congregations 1981; 526.
24. Reform Judaism, 20, no. 2, Winter 1991.
25. Broun H, Britt G. Christians Only. A Study in Prejudice. New York: Vanguard 1931:137-145.
26. Goldberg JA. Jews in the medical profession: a national survey. Jew Soc Stud 1939; 1:327-336.
27. Sokoloff L. The rise and decline of the Jewish quota in medical school admissions. Bull NY Acad Med 1992; 68:497-518.
28. Collins KJ. Go and Learn: The International Story of Jews and Medicine in Scotland. Aberdeen: Aberdeen Un Press 1988.
29. Report of the Temporary Commission on the Need for a State University. Albany, New York: Legislative Document no. 30; Feb 10,1948.

CHAPTER 13

MEDICAL-ETHICAL ISSUES

THE ROLE OF THE PHYSICIAN

During most of early recorded history the professions of medicine and religion were undifferentiated, with common origin and common purpose. The first centers of healing were the temples; the healers, the priests. Monotheism among the Hebrews replaced the thaumaturgy of the Egyptians and surrounding peoples and their reliance on magic and worship of idols and animals for healing. The Torah taught that both disease and cure emanate from God: "I kill, and I make alive; I wound, and I heal." (*Deuteronomy* 32:39) Man was but God's agent. Jesus ben Sira extolled him, about 200 B.C.E.: "Honour a physician with the honour due unto him for the uses which ye may have of him: for the Lord hath created him. For of the most High cometh healing, and he shall receive honour of the king. The skill of the physician shall lift up his head: and in the sight of great men he shall be in admiration. The Lord hath created medicines out of the earth; and he that is wise will not abhor them." (*Ecclesiasticus* 38:1-4)

Medical discussions in early rabbinic literature were usually subordinate to other matters, hence incidental and not organized; but from them emerged three main principles, all endorsed by modern medicine: (1) the importance of a weekly day of rest; (2) the concept of personal and communal hygiene: cleanliness, prophylaxis, and quarantine; and (3) recognition of organic changes resulting from disease.

A commitment to medical ethics, similar in many respects to the Hippocratic Oath, familiar to all modern medical graduates, was required of the disciples of Assaph the Physician, the earliest Hebrew medical author whose writings are extant, and his colleague Yohanan, 6th-century residents of Northern Palestine:

"Ye shall not harden your hearts against the poor and needy but shall heal them.

"Ye shall not call good evil or evil good.

"Ye shall not walk in the ways of sorcerers to cast spells, to enchant, and to bewitch...

"Ye shall not make use of any manner of idolatry to heal thereby...

"Let not a spirit of haughtiness cause you to lift up your eyes and your hearts in pride.

"Wreak not vengeance upon a sick man and alter not your prescriptions for them that do hate the Lord our God."

Three centuries later, in his book *On Medical Ethics*, Isaac ben Solomon Israeli (Isaac Judaeus) included the precepts:

"Never rely in treatment upon wonder-working cures, for these depend mostly upon ignorance and superstition...

"Make it thy special concern to visit and treat poor and needy patients, for in no other way canst thou find more meritorious service...

"Too large a practice confuses the judgment of the physician and causes him to give mistaken directions."

The reverent appreciation accorded physicians by the Talmud and the rabbinic literature of the Middle Ages attracted to medical practice many religious scholars and philosophers, notably Judah Halevi (11th century), Moses Maimonides (12th century), Moses Nachmanides (13th century), and Levi Gersonides (14th century). Perhaps best known is Maimonides, who placed health care first among the communal services that a city needed to provide for its residents.

Maimonides, known also as Rabbi Moses ben Maimon, was born in Cordova, Spain, in 1135. The Jewish populace, subjugated by the Almohades in 1148, had to embrace Mohammedanism or be killed. Maimonides' family fled to southern Spain, migrated to Fez in North Africa in 1160, and in 1165 to Palestine, where they stayed but a short time before settling in Egypt. After the death of his father and brother Maimonides, now a rabbi, turned to the practice of medicine in order to support his mother and sister. He soon became physician to the Sultan Salah-Al-Din (Saladin). In Egypt Maimonides wrote his codification of Jewish law, the *Mishneh Torah*, and his *Guide for the Perplexed*, and supervised the preparation of the pharmacopoeia of Cairo, which contained drugs for the treatment of snake bites, scorpion bites and other poisonings. Toward the end of the century he wrote, in Arabic, philosophy, astronomy, mathematics, a number of medical treatises, and translated into Hebrew the *Canon of Avicenna*. He died in Cairo, December 18, 1204, at age 69. The "*Morning Prayer of a Physician*," often attributed to Maimonides, was probably penned by the 17th-century rabbi-physician Jacob Zaholon:

"Inspire me with love for my art and for Thy creatures. Do not allow thirst for profit, ambition for renown and admiration to interfere with my profession, for these are the enemies of truth and love for mankind and they can lead astray in the great task of attending to the welfare of Thy creatures. Preserve the strength of my body and of my soul that they may ever be ready cheerfully to help and support rich and poor, good and bad, enemy as well as friend... Let me be contented in everything except in my quest for knowledge of the great science of my profession..."

Jewish physicians helped found the first European universities, at Salerno and Montpellier, but were soon barred from them; and during the 15th and 16th centuries they were swept up by the hysteria of the Inquisition. An anecdote of the 16th century tells that Francis I of France, suffering from a lingering illness (probably syphilis), requested the Holy Roman Emperor's Jewish physician. Upon his arrival the king taunted the doctor about his Judaism; whereupon the latter hastened to inform the king that he was no longer a Jew, having converted to the true faith. Indignant, the king promptly dismissed him, demanding a real Jewish physician. During the 20th century more than 20% of the recipients of the Nobel Prize in Physiology or Medicine have been Jews.

DOCTOR-PATIENT RELATIONSHIP

For centuries medical ethics remained a distinct category of immutable moral precepts, the domain solely of the profession.[1] Revulsion over the atrocities of Nazi physicians and their medical experiments during World War II led to a complete re-examination of the principles of medical ethics and the widespread adoption of the doctrine of informed consent in all doctor-patient relations. At the close of the 20th century medical ethics is a subject of broad debate and public concern. Four general principles, enunciated by Beauchamp and Childress,[2] have been generally accepted: nonmaleficence, beneficence, autonomy, and justice. The first two characterize the Hippocratic obligation, always to act in the patient's best interests and to do no harm. Autonomy, on the other hand, rejects the authoritarianism of the Hippocratic ethic in favor of the principle of self-determination, central to the temper of American life. The concept of justice in medical ethics has become increasingly prominent as disparities in health care have become more glaring, and the development of new and expensive technology has required triage of patients and rationing of available medical resources.

Not always do the values of the patient coincide with those of the physician in medical decision making, the Emanuels[3] point out, a conflict between autonomy and health sometimes resulting. Their four models of the physician-patient interaction illustrate the different understandings of the goals of the doctor-patient relationship, the physician's obligations, the role of the patient's values, and the concept of patient autonomy. Different models may be appropriate in different circumstances.

In the paternalistic model the physician serves as the patient's guardian, implementing what he or she believes best for the patient and soliciting consultation when necessary. The paternalistic model is clearly proper in emergencies; few believe it suitable for most other doctor-patient interactions.

In the informative model the physician provides the patient with all relevant information concerning the nature of the illness, diagnostic and therapeutic options, and probability of risks and benefits. The physician serves as a purveyor of technical expertise; the patient makes the decisions. In this model the caring approach that the patient expects of a physician is lacking. Moreover the patient may not possess the fixed values that the informative model presupposes.

In the interpretive model the physician strives to ascertain the patient's values and to help the patient make the proper choice to realize them. The physician serves as a counselor, providing the services as in the informative model but also attempting to arrive with the patient at a joint understanding. Technical specialization has grown so diverse, however, that the physician may lack the skills necessary to this model. Further, with limited time and interpretive talent, the physician may fail to ascertain the patient's values. The interpretive model merges easily into the paternalistic.

In the deliberative model the physician, knowing the patient and acting as teacher and friend, indicates not only what the patient can do but also what the patient should do, helping to elucidate and choose the best health-related options. Is it proper, some ask, for the physician to judge the patient's values? The physician's values may conflict with the values of other physicians and with those of the patient. The physician's function, many insist, is to render health care, not moral guidance or value revision. The Emanuels, to the contrary, view the deliberative model as the embodiment of the ideal physician-patient relationship. "The essence of doctoring," they write, "is a fabric of knowledge, understanding, teaching, and action, in which the caring physician integrates the patient's medical condition and health-related values, makes a recommendation on the appropriate course of action, and tries to persuade the patient of the worthiness of this approach and the values it realizes. The physician with a caring attitude is the ideal embodied in the deliberative model, the ideal that should inform laws and policies that regulate the physician-patient interaction."

AIDS

Some physicians have refused to treat patients with acquired immunodeficiency syndrome (AIDS), in accordance with American common law that a physician is under no obligation to treat any patient in the absence of a consensual physician-patient relationship.[4] The Jewish physician, on the other hand, has a clear responsibility to do so. The Talmud decrees that every life is worth saving, and makes no distinction as to person, whether criminal, sinner, or model citizen. The degree of obligation on the physician relates to the magnitude of the risk involved. Rabbinic authorities are in general agreement that when life is imperiled and the danger to the rescuer is great, he is under no obligation to attempt rescue. When the risk to the rescuer is small, he is encouraged but not required to attempt rescue. If the risk to the rescuer is remote, on the other hand, he is required to save the endangered person if possible. The risk to physicians in caring for patients with AIDS is considered extremely small. The physician's compassion in treating such patients implies no condonation of aberrant homosexual behavior or abusive drug practices:[5] "...neither shalt thou stand against the blood of thy neighbor... Thou shalt not hate thy brother in thine heart: thou shalt in any wise rebuke thy neighbour, and not suffer sin upon him." (*Leviticus* 19:16-17)

Israel's Sephardic Chief Rabbi Mordecai Eliahu in 1991 issued an order, non-binding, that Jewish couples living outside Israel be tested before marriage for the virus associated with AIDS.

ALZHEIMER'S DISEASE

Named for Alois Alzheimer (1864-1915), German neuro-psychiatrist who described its manifestations in 1907, Alzheimer's disease is a common, progressive disorder of aging characterized by mental deterioration, loss of memory, depression, and diminishing motor coordination. In its late stages its victims are often reduced to a mere vegetative level. Associated with Alzheimer's disease and probably responsible for its manifestations is atrophy of the cerebral cortex; but the cause remains unknown and treatment ineffective. The disease presents the Jewish physician with a number of ethical problems.[6] As with AIDS the physician is required to treat Alzheimer patients, as others, as best he can. In the absence of curative treatment he is limited to symptomatic and supportive care, and possibly experimental therapy. Britain's Chief Rabbi Lord Immanuel Jakobovits, considering the principles of Jewish law covering experiments on humans, concluded that hazardous experiments may be performed only if potentially helpful to the patient, if no effective safe treatment is available, if carried out by the most expert medical team, and after prior experimentation on animals or other nonhuman models.[7]

In terminal stages of the disease euthanasia is prohibited, but no measures may be taken to artificially delay the patient's imminent demise (see later paragraphs on life-support). No treatment need be given that prolongs suffering without possibility of cure. Artificial resuscitation and life-support systems are inappropriate for patients terminally ill with Alzheimer's disease and with hopeless prognosis. Supportive care, however, is mandated by Jewish law until the patient's death, indicated by cessation of brain function and spontaneous cardiorespiratory activity.

Autopsy, normally permissible in Jewish law only to save the life of another patient immediately at hand (see later paragraphs on autopsies), has been sanctioned by some scholars for victims of Alzheimer's disease. The disease has become so common and widespread, and communication within the world medical community so rapid, that the "here and now" requirement for autopsies is satisfied, they conclude, when the information sought relates to the cause, treatment, and possible cure.[6]

ORGAN TRANSPLANTATION

God promised, through Ezekiel: "And a new heart also will I give you, and a new spirit will I put within you: and I will take away the strong heart out of your flesh, and I will give you an heart of flesh." (*Ezekiel* 36:26)

At the close of the 20th century organ transplantation has become a growth industry. Between the late 1950s and the early 1980s only kidneys were transplanted, in small numbers and in few hospitals.[8] Since 1963 the majority of Americans have been insured for this procedure through the Medicare or Medicaid programs. Between 1981 and 1990 the number of kidney transplants performed annually in the United States increased by 50%. During the same period the number of heart transplants increased 12 times; the number of liver transplants, over 16 times. Referring to the last, the *Wall Street Journal* commented, April 1, 1993, on "what had become a $500 million market that was growing so fast that hospitals were offering million-dollar signing bonuses to lure coveted transplant surgeons: Since 1988 the number of liver transplant programs in the U.S. has nearly doubled to 105 as hospitals have sought to build their technical reputations, boost billings, fill beds, generate media attention, keep local patients in town for treatment and even lift staff morale."[9]

Transplantation of kidneys, hearts, and livers has become accepted treatment for a number of end-stage organ diseases. More than 16,000 such operations are performed annually in the United States, with one-year survival rates over 90% and 5-year survival rates over 50%. Transplants of bone marrow, corneas, and other tissues have become routine. The success rate of solid organ transplantation was greatly enhanced by cyclosporin, an immunosuppressive agent that came into common clinical use in 1983, and by monoclonal antibody technology, which made possible the production of an anti-T cell agent, highly effective in allaying tissue rejection.

The National Transplant Act of 1984 made organ transplantation the only medical discipline guided by a federal health policy, its governing body the Organ Procurement and Transplant Network, which is operated, under contract with the federal government, by a not-for-profit foundation, the United Network for Organ Sharing. Through it a system has been constructed, albeit controversial, that exercises quality control of organ transplantation; determines where, how, and by whom the transplants are performed; and mandates how the organs are obtained, preserved, distributed, and transported.

Despite the Network's efforts organ transplantation remains encumbered by major practical and ethical problems. The procedure is expensive, requiring an allocation of scarce medical resources. Selection of recipients is difficult in the face of a chronic scarcity of organs. The threat of graft rejection is ever-present, despite immunosuppressive drugs, which themselves increase the risk of infection. Especially troublesome to some is the removal of still-beating hearts from brain-dead patients, for transplant.

In a thoughtful recent book Fox and Swazey[10] have criticized transplant surgeons and researchers for their zeal to keep patients alive at all costs, and institutions for bypassing the protections of formal review processes in their pursuit of wealth and glory. They express the fear that in viewing organs as spare parts we have adopted a therapy that "has become an overly zealous medical and societal commitment to the endless perpetuation of life," with resultant "social, cultural, and spiritual harm."

A sharp dichotomy has developed among rabbinic scholars as to the permissibility of organ transplantation. The majority view, summarized by Rosner[11] in 1986, concerning transplantation of kidney, heart, liver, lung, pancreas, colon, or other organs, has undergone recent modification. Rosner had stated that, with consent of donor or next of kin, organ transplantation is permissible to save the life of the recipient. Only if death of the recipient was a certainty without transplantation and the risk to the donor was small might a live donor be used. Otherwise, where danger to the donor was great or death certain, only might a donor be used that is dead according to Jewish legal criteria; that is, with no cerebral or spontaneous cardiorespiratory activity. In such a case, if a life might be saved, the Biblical proscriptions against desecration of the dead were waived.

A major change in transplantation policy resulted from the landmark decision of the 1000 member Orthodox Rabbinical Council of America in 1991 approving organ donation from brain-dead patients who satisfied only the death criterion of loss of cerebral activity.[12] A proxy, to be provided to patients urging their designation of an agent to make health-care decisions in case of incapacitation, read in part concerning organ donation:

"The saving of a life takes precedence over all but three halakhic imperatives—murder, idolatry, and adultery.

"Therefore, no halakhic barriers exist to the donation of the organs of the deceased if they are harvested in accord with the highest standards of dignity and propriety.

"Vital organs such as heart and liver may be donated after the patient has been declared dead by a competent neurologist based upon the clinical and/or radiological evidence... Since organs that can be life-saving may be donated, the family is urged to do so. When human life can be saved, it must be saved. Cornea transplants that can restore sight to the blind are treated in halakha as life-saving surgery.

"The halakha therefore looks with great favor on those who facilitate the procurement of life-saving donations."

Prompt and sharp disagreement was expressed by other Orthodox authorities, notably the Union of Orthodox Rabbis of the United States and Canada, known as the *Agudas Harabonim*, which issued a statement of refutation: "Let it be known clearly and emphatically that according to Jewish law ruled by the greatest *poskim* [judges], scholars and halakhic decisors both in America and in Israel, it is absolutely prohibited to perform such an operation."

Early resolution of the conflict between the differing Orthodox groups concerning organ transplantation appears unlikely.

END-OF-LIFE DECISIONS

"To every thing there is a season... A time to be born, and a time to die..." (*Ecclesiastes* 3:1-2) Medical techniques developed during the second half of the 20th century have made possible the artificial maintenance of ventilation and circulation and the elimination of metabolic waste products in bodies with irreversibly functionless brains. "A dead brain in a body whose heart is still beating," Pallis lamented, "is one of the more macabre products of modern technology."[13] "Ventilating corpses," as he referred to attempts to resuscitate bodies beyond salvage, produces needless grief to surviving families and friends and problems of morale among those responsible for the care of dying patients. Brain death, distinguished from irreversible loss of consciousness, is physiologically equivalent to decapitation. Its victim is not terminally ill but dead. A Uniform Determination of Death Act, approved in 1981 by the President's Commission, the American Medical Association, the American Bar Association, the National Conference of Commissioners on Uniform State Laws, the American Academy of Neurology, and the American Electroencephalographic Society, states: "An individual who has sustained either (1) irreversible cessation of all circulatory and respiratory function, or (2) irreversible cessation of all functions of the entire brain, including the brain stem, is dead."[14] Few informed persons, regardless of religious orientation, would disagree that attempts to maintain semblances of life in such cases are inappropriate.

More difficult is determination of the physician's responsibility for life support in cases of damage to the cerebral hemispheres resulting in a chronic state of unconsciousness, a condition commonly termed "persistent vegetative state."[15] In such a state, which may follow any of a variety of insults including stroke, poisoning, infection, trauma, or degenerative disease, the body sleeps and awakes cyclically but gives no evidence of cognitive function or of ability to respond in a meaningful manner to external events. Provided with fluid, nutrition, other supportive measure, and nursing care, some persons may survive in this condition for months or even years. Nearly all maintain near-normal body temperature but remain incontinent of bladder and bowel.

Cardiorespiratory activity, swallowing, and digestive and other non-neurological vital functions are usually preserved. With the neural apparatus for suffering impaired or destroyed, pain cannot be experienced. Few if any who become vegetative as a result of asphyxia, as after cardiac arrest, recover after 1 month, and virtually none regain cognitive function after 3 months of impairment. Based on the handful of reported cognitive recoveries in relation to the estimated number of cases of persistent vegetative state in the United States, the odds of recovery are calculated as less than one in one thousand.[15]

Withdrawal of supportive measures, known as "passive euthanasia" (from the Greek *eu*, meaning "good" or "pleasant;" and *thanatos*, "death") has become increasingly popular in recent years, with the growing resort to "living wills," which eschew unusual or heroic measures in the face of a hopeless prognosis. The American Hospital Association estimates that fully 70% of the 6000 deaths that occur daily in the United States are in some way timed or arranged by physicians in concert with patients and their families.[16]

Widely debated for several decades have been the ethical questions involved, and the role of the physician, in the withdrawing or withholding of life support measures from patients judged permanently unconscious. The Council on Ethical and Judicial Affairs of the American Medical Association in 1989, while affirming the social commitment of the physician to sustain life and relieve suffering, stated that a physician, with informed consent, may "cease or omit treatment to permit a terminally ill patient to die when death is imminent. ...Even if death is not imminent but a patient is beyond doubt permanently unconscious, and there are adequate safeguards to confirm the accuracy of the diagnosis, it is not unethical to discontinue all means of life-prolonging medical treatment [including] artificially or technically supplied respiration, nutrition or hydration."[15]

In such cases the physician cannot play a purely passive role in his interactions with the patient and his or her family—nor may the physician violate their wishes because of differences in ethical values. If the physician cannot in conscience comply with their directives, the family must be so informed and the patient transferred to the care of another physician whose ethics are more compatible with those of the patient and family.

A large segment of today's rabbinate interpret Jewish law as not requiring heroic measures for the prolongation of life in the hopelessly ill, but as forbidding their withdrawal once initiated.[11] In such cases Jewish law makes no distinction between "natural" measures, such as food and fluids, and "artificial," such as drugs and mechanical support of respiration and circulation. The traditional rabbinate therefore refuses to sanction "living wills" or Natural Death Acts as enacted by a number of state legislatures, which bind the physician to the patient's wishes in withholding or withdrawing life-sustaining measures.[17]

Traditional Judaism, ever proclaiming the sanctity of human life, insists that the physician's divine license is only to heal, not to hasten death. When unable to heal, the physician, together with all close to the patient—family, friends, nurses, and social workers—are obligated to provide supportive care to the end, including fluids and nutrition. At no time may such care be abandoned to hasten the patient's demise.[18] Only in the case of a *gosses*, one in a dying condition, whose expected survival is less than 3 days, may factors be withdrawn that might artificially delay death. In keeping with Judeo-Christian teaching, a Catholic group under the sponsorship of the Pontifical Academy of Sciences in 1965, distinguishing between treatment that may be withdrawn and care which may not, from permanently comatose patients, likewise placed feeding and hydration in the latter category.[19]

ACTIVE EUTHANASIA

"Better death than a life of misery, eternal rest than a long illness." (*Ecclesiasticus* 30:17)[20] The deliberate termination of a patient's life has been controversial throughout the history of medicine. The Hippocratic Oath (4th century B.C.E.), keystone of medical ethics, clearly condemns it: "I will give no deadly drug to any, though it be asked of me, nor will I counsel such." Classical philosophers, on the other hand, considered death an honorable alternative to hopeless illness. In the view of Seneca, 1st-century Roman Stoic, "death is a punishment to some, to some a gift, and to many a favor." Sir Thomas More advocated voluntary euthanasia in his *Utopia* (1516).

Whether the death of King Saul, in the year 1013 B.C.E. was by suicide or euthanasia is still debated by Scriptural scholars. In his battle with the Philistines three of his sons had already been killed, when Saul himself was mortally wounded. "Then said Saul unto his armourbearer, Draw thy sword, and thrust me through therewith; lest these uncircumcised come and thrust me through, and abuse me. But his armourbearer would not; for he was sore afraid. Therefore Saul took a sword, and fell upon it... So Saul died." (*I. Samuel* 31:4, 6) Some rabbinic scholars believe that Saul, who had been anointed by Samuel (*I. Samuel* 10:1), was permitted to shorten his life to prevent a desecration of the divine name (*Sefer Hasidim*, chapter 723).[21]

Different, however, is the account of Saul's death conveyed by the Amalekite to David: "And David said unto the young man that told him, How knowest thou that Saul and Jonathan his son be dead? And the young man that told him said...He said unto me...Stand, I pray thee, upon me, and slay me: for anguish is come upon me, because my life is yet whole in me. So I stood upon him, and slew him, because I was sure that he could not live after that he was fallen." (*II. Samuel* 1:5-10)

In the Netherlands, near the end of the 20th century, active euthanasia, although technically illegal, is resorted to in perhaps as many as 20,000 cases annually. Public policy has established three requisite conditions: (1) voluntariness: a persistent, conscious, and free request by the patient; (2) a state of illness with intolerable suffering, judged beyond recovery; and (3) consultation with a medical colleague.[22] In the United States public support for voluntary euthanasia and assisted suicide appears to be growing.[23] Membership in the Hemlock Society, an organization dedicated to their legalization, has doubled within the last few years to approximately 33,000. In nation-wide surveys between 1950 and 1991, the year when the voters in Washington State defeated an initiative to legalize physician aid-in-dying by a narrow margin, 63% of those polled felt that euthanasia should be legalized, responding affirmatively to the question: Should doctors be allowed to end the life of a patient with incurable disease if the patient or his or her family requests it? Nearly three-fourths, however, stated that they would not personally assist relatives or friends to end their lives. In most cases the burden to act rests ultimately with the physician.[23] At the same time the American Medical Association's Council on Ethical and Judicial Affairs took the position that "what is termed 'active euthanasia' is a euphemism for the intentional killing of a person; this is not part of the practice of medicine, with or without the consent of the patient... The intentional termination of the life of one human being by another—mercy killing—is contrary to public policy, medical tradition, and the most fundamental measure of human value and worth."[24]

The case was well stated by Howard W. Haggard, Yale University's medical philosopher: "The judge may in dignity, with self and public respect, condemn a man to death, but he may not then in the same dignity and respect step down from the bench and execute the man. Similarly a physician may in dignity and respect give as his opinion that the sufferer is entitled to the benefits of euthanasia but he will not, I believe, retain his dignity and respect if he practices public euthanasia. The physician cannot serve two masters—life and death."

Question has been raised, also, as to the validity of informed consent given by the patient long in advance. "Will we not sweep up, in the process," Kamisar asks, "some who are not really tired of life, but think others are tired of them; some who do not really want to die, but who feel that they should not live on, because to do so when there looms the legal alternative of euthanasia is to do a selfish or cowardly act? Will not some feel an obligation to have themselves 'eliminated' in order that funds allocated for their terminal care might be better used by their families or, financial worries aside, in order to relieve their families of the emotional strain involved?"[25] More than one-fourth of Medicare program expenditures go for patients in the last 6 months of life. Approximately 5% of the American population now accounts for half of the nation's total expenditures for medical care.[26] The physician, however, Kass insists, "serves only the sick. He does not serve the relatives or the hospital or the national debt inflated due to Medicare costs."[27]

The fabric of human relations, or what has been termed the social ecology, is damaged, Bellah pointed out, "not only by war, genocide, and political repression. It is also damaged by the destruction of the subtle ties that bind human beings to one another, leaving them frightened and alone."[28] Never must "medical reform" permit this to happen to the relation between the physician and his dying patient, visualized by Lord Horter.[29] "The two extremes of dying in pain and being killed," he wrote, "do not exhaust the possibilities of the stricken patient, because there is a middle course created by a kindly and skillful doctor who gives assistance in an equally kindly nature, and that is what is implicit in the patient's question: 'You will stand by me, won't you?' and the doctor's assurance: 'Yes, I will.'"

AUTOPSY

In tribute to Giovanni Battista Morgagni, famed 18th-century professor of anatomy at the University of Padua and author of the monumental *The Seats and Causes of Disease...*,[30] which, through detailed autopsy records, correlated clinical features of disease with postmortem findings, Henry Sigerist, my professor of the history of medicine, wrote: "From every physician we expect tact and moral earnestness, but we expect them from a pathologist in a supreme degree. It is the dead who are brought to the latter, persons whom medical practitioners have been powerless to save. All too often an autopsy demonstrates the insufficiency of human knowledge. In such cases the pathologist must not play the part of judge, but must be a helper and an exhorter."[31]

Very little advance in human anatomic knowledge had been made until the 16th century, for corpses for dissection were hard to obtain and the conditions for anatomic study and demonstration were rigidly prescribed by the civil authorities. On the rare occasions when dissections were carried out in conjunction with courses in anatomy at the universities, the professor read aloud from Galen, whose authority remained beyond question, while assistants performed the dissections. For 1500 years the grossest errors were thus perpetuated, until the anatomic renaissance of the 16th century, ushered in by Sylvius, Vesalius, Fabricius, Eustachius, and Falloppio, when the autopsy opened the portals of scientific medicine. From a means of anatomic study the autopsy rapidly became an instrument of instruction, a mechanism for correction, a pathway to discovery, a storehouse of valuable supplies, and a handmaiden of the law.[32]

Virtually everyone's body harbors one or more diseases, in early or intermediate stages, either unrecognized or ignored, in addition to that which ultimately causes death. Only through postmortem examination can they be discovered. The autopsy permits the final critical analysis of life's end point. Through it many new diseases have been discovered. The autopsy provides tissues, often life-saving, for transplantation to the living: kidney, bone marrow, cornea, major blood vessels, fascial strips, bone, liver, and heart; makes possible the evaluation of new and potent drugs, and the evaluation of radiation therapy; and the establishment of valid mortality statistics. New and intricate surgical procedures, after development on experimental animals, may require final rehearsal on the dead before being attempted on the living.

Perhaps most important, the autopsy fosters accuracy in clinical diagnosis and resultant improvement in medical care. The medical literature is replete with examples of discrepancies between diagnoses made before and after death,[33,34] differences in diagnosis between that reported on the death certificate and that made at autopsy ranging from 25 to 56%. Among several hundred randomly selected autopsies from one university hospital during the late-20th century about 10% revealed a major undiagnosed condition, detection of which might have led to a change in therapy and prolongation of life.

Despite its emphasis on the preservation of life, traditional Jewish law permits autopsy only when of immediate value to the living: where a specific person exists in the same locality suffering from the same disease as the dead, and whose life might be saved as a result of the postmortem examination.[35] This dictum governing autopsies, which stems from an 18th-century responsum of Rabbi Ezekiel Landau (*Yoreh Deah*, 210), has served as the basis of all subsequent traditional rabbinic opinion on the subject. Modern communication, however, having in effect converted the world into "one great parish," has led to a liberal interpretation of this requirement. Routine autopsy and postmortem examination solely for medical research are still banned. They are named in the Talmud and Jewish legal codes as *nivul hameth* (dishonor of the dead). In cases when sanctioned by *halakhah*, autopsy is not only permitted but required, in accordance with the physician's obligation to do all within his power to effect cure.[36]

The Chief Rabbinate of Israel and the administration of the Hadassah University Hospital in Jerusalem, in a mid-20th-century formal concordat, agreed that autopsy may be performed (1) in accordance with requirements of the law (e.g., in cases of suspected foul play); (2) in cases in which the physician cannot ascribe the death to a specific cause; in which circumstance permission for autopsy is granted after consultation and certification by the physician in charge, the director of the hospital, and the director of the pathology department; (3) to save the life of a living patient; and (4) in cases of hereditary disease, for guidance of the surviving family. At the conclusion of the investigation the remains of the deceased are to be transferred to the Chevra Kadisha (Ritual Burial Society) for burial according to Jewish law.

A consent form for limited autopsy, issued by the Sub-Committee on Medical Ethics of the Committee on Religious Affairs of the Federation of Jewish Philanthropies of New York, requires that the physician state in precise clinical terms the information sought, the site to be incised, and the organs to be examined for this purpose. The authorization, signed by the next of kin, thus limits the procedure to that necessary to obtain pertinent and potentially life-saving information of immediate applicability, and specifies that all organs, tissues, and body fluids be returned for burial as specified by Jewish law. Incision extending over the entire length of the abdomen and chest, with examination of all internal organs; and opening of the cranium, for examination of the brain, routine in the usual autopsy, are not permitted by Jewish law if the needed information can be obtained by more limited investigation.[37] Cremation, regarded by traditional law as desecration of a human being, is not allowed.

SUMMARY

Judaic doctrine has ever stressed the ethical basis of medical practice. Modern ethicists continue to debate the proper role of the physician and the nature of the doctor-patient relationship in the light of 20th-century technology. The Talmud teaches that every life is worth saving and makes no distinction as to person. The degree of the physician's obligation to treat a patient relates to the magnitude of the risk involved. Although some physicians refuse to treat patients with AIDS, the Jewish physician has a clear responsibility to do so. In the current absence of curative treatment for Alzheimer's disease, as for a number of other diseases, his efforts are limited to symptomatic and supportive care; and after appropriate consultation and with informed consent, to experimental therapy. The permissibility of organ transplantation remains a matter of debate among rabbinic scholars.

Traditional Judaism insists that the physician's divine license is only to heal, not to hasten death. When unable to heal, he is obligated to provide supportive care to the end. A large segment of the rabbinate, however, interpret Jewish law as not requiring heroic measures for the prolongation of life in the hopelessly ill. Routine autopsy is banned, but postmortem examination is permitted when it offers the prospect of benefit to the living.

REFERENCES

1. Pellegrino ED. The metamorphosis of medical ethics. JAMA 1993; 269:1158-1162.
2. Beauchamp TL, Childress JF. Principles of Biomedical Ethics 3rd ed. New York: Oxford Univ Press 1989.
3. Emanuel EJ, Emanuel LL. Four models of the physician-patient relationship. JAMA 1992; 267:2221-2226.
4. Annas GJ. Legal risks and responsibilities of physicians in the AIDS epidemic. Hastings Center Reports 1988; 18 April/May suppl.:26-32.
5. Rosner F. The physician's obligation to heal AIDS patients in Jewish law. JAMA 1988; 260:2837-2838.
6. Rosner F. Alzheimer's disease and Jewish law. Bull New York Acad Med

1990; 66:181-192.
7. Jacobovits I. Medical Experimentation on Humans in Jewish Law. In: Jewish Bioethics. Rosner F, Bleich JD, eds. New York: Sanhedrin Press 1979:377-383.
8. McDonald JC. The politics of transplantation. Bull Am Coll Surgeons 1993; 78:10.
9. Scott McCartney. Wall Street Journal, April 1, 1993; 128:1.
10. Fox RC, Swazey JP. Spare Parts. Organ Replacement in American Society. New York: Oxford Univ Press 1992.
11. Rosner F. Modern Medicine and Jewish Ethics. Hoboken, New Jersey: Ktav and Yeshiva Univ Press 1986: 271.
12. The Jewish Week. June 28-July 4, 1991:32.
13. Pallis C. ABC of brain stem death: reappraising death. Brit Med J 1982; 285:1409-1486.
14. President's Commission for the Study of Ethical Problems in Medicine and Biomedical and Behavioral Research: Defining Death, A Report on the Medical, Legal and Ethical Issues in the Determination of Death. Washington, D.C. Govt. Printing Off 1981.
15. Council on Scientific Affairs and Council on Ethical and Judicial Affairs, American Medical Association: Persistent Vegetative State and the Decision to Withdraw or Withhold Life Support. JAMA 1990; 263:426-430.
16. New York Times. June 9, 1990.
17. Bleich JD. Judaism and Healing. Hoboken, New Jersey: Ktav Pub 1981:138-139.
18. Rosner F. Withdrawing fluids and nutrition: an alternate way. Bull New York Acad Med 1988; 64: 363-375.
19. Meeting of the Pontifical Academy of Sciences: Ethical, Medical, and Legal Questions on the Artificial Prolongation of Life, Declaration Adopted by Scientists. O'Osservatore Romano 1965:10.
20. The New English Bible. Oxford Univ Press and Cambridge Univ Press 1970:159.
21. Herring BF. Jewish Ethics and Halakhah for Our Time. New York: Ktav Pub 1984:72.
22. de Wachter MAM. Active euthanasia in the Netherlands. JAMA 1989; 262:3316-3320.
23. Council on Ethical and Judicial Affairs, American Medical Association: Decisions Near the End of Life. JAMA 1992; 267:2229-2233.
24. Blendon RJ, Szalay US, Knox RA. Should physicians aid their patients in dying? JAMA 1992; 267:2658-2662.
25. Kamisar Y. Some nonreligious views against proposed "mercy killing" legislation. Minn Law Rev 1958; 42:969-1042.
26. Knaus WA, Wagner DP, Lynn J. Short-term mortality predictions for critically ill hospitalized adults: science and ethics. Science 1991; 254:389-394.
27. Kass LR. "I will give no deadly drug": why doctors must not kill. Am Coll Surgeons Bull 1992; 77:6-17.

28. Bellah RN. Habits of the Heart: Individualism and Commitment in America Life. New York: Harper and Row 1986:284.
29. Thomas Jeeves Horter (1871-1955), First Baron, Physician to King George VI, Queen Elizabeth II, and King Edward VIII.
30. De Sedibus, et Causis Morborum per Anatmen Indagatis, Libri Quinque. Venice, 1761.
31. Sigerist HE. The Great Doctors. New York: WW Norton 1933:229-236.
32. Gall EA. The necropsy as a tool in medical progress. Bull New York Acad Med 1968; 44:808-829.
33. Prutting JM. Symposium on medical progress and the postmortem. Introduction. Bull New York Acad Med 1968; 44:793-798.
34. Kircher LT. Autopsy and mortality statistics: making a difference. JAMA 1992; 267:1264.
35. Kottler A. The Jewish attitude on autopsy. New York State J Med, May 1, 1957: 1649-1656.
36. Bleich JD. Authorization for limited autopsies. Intercom 1977; 16:3-5.
37. Bleich JD. Autopsy consent, issued by Federation of Jewish Philanthropies. Intercom 1977; 16:5-6.

CHAPTER 14

SCRIPTURAL MISCELLANY

PHYSICAL EXERCISE[1]
"I have two doctors—my left leg and my right."—Anonymous

The popular belief that physical exercise helps preserve life and its desirable qualities into old age dates back to antiquity. A number of Biblical heroes, probably products of "the sovereign invigorator of the body," as Thomas Jefferson characterized exercise, are noted for their valor, strength, and athletic prowess. Saul and David, we are told, "were swifter than eagles, they were stronger than lions." (*II. Samuel* 1:23) The Talmud (*Avot* 5:23) and the Midrash (*Numbers Rabbah* 20:24) accordingly urged that a man be fierce as a leopard, swift as an eagle, fleet as a hart, and strong as a lion in the performance of God's will. David demonstrated his skill with the sling in his contest with Goliath. Runners were essential as guards, for communication, and for military protection. The Bible tells of a courier who ran from Aphek to Shiloh, a distance of some 60 miles, to notify the High Priest that the ark of the covenant had been taken by the Philistines: "And there ran a man of Benjamin out of the army, and came to Shiloh the same day with his clothes rent, and with earth upon his head." (*I. Samuel* 4:12) Renowned also for his long distance running was Ahimaaz, who volunteered to carry word to King David "that the Lord hath avenged him of his enemies... Then Ahimaaz ran by the way of the plain, and overran Cushi [another runner]." (*II. Samuel* 18:19, 23) The "stone of Zoheleth," where David's son Adonijah "slew sheep and fat cattle," (*I. Kings* 1:9) served as a test of strength of those who sought to move it, according to 11th-century Rashi.

None could compare with Samson, foremost of Biblical strong men: "Then went Samson down...and came to the vineyards of Timnath: and, behold, a young lion roared against him. And the Spirit of the Lord came mightily upon him, and he rent him as he would have rent a kid, and he had nothing in his hand." (*Judges* 14:5-6) After the Philistines had "bound him with two new cords...the Spirit of the Lord came mightily upon him, and the cords that were upon his arms became as flax that was burnt with fire, and his bands loosed from off his hands. And he found a new jawbone of an ass, and put forth his hand, and took it, and slew a thousand men therewith." (*Judges* 15:13-15) Having lain with a harlot in Gaza, Samson "arose at midnight, and took the doors of the gate of the city, and the two posts, and went away with them bar and all, and put them upon his shoulders, and carried them up to the top of an hill..." (*Judges* 16:1-3) To subdue him for the Philistines, Delilah bound him with "seven green withs [partitions between flues in a chimney stack] which had not been dried... And he brake the withs, as a thread of tow is broken when it toucheth the fire... Delilah therefore took new ropes, and bound him therewith... And he brake them from off his arms like a thread." (*Judges* 16:8-9, 12) When the hair of Samson, now blinded by the Philistines, had regrown and his strength had returned, he called unto God, "that I may be at once avenged of the Philistines for my two eyes. And Samson took hold of the two middle pillars upon which the house stood, and on which it was borne up, of the one with his right hand, and of the other with his left... And he bowed himself with all his might; and the house fell upon the lords, and upon all the people that were therein." (*Judges* 16:28-30)

Physical effort was held meritorious by the sages; its reward, repose: "the sleep of a labouring man is sweet." (*Ecclesiastes* 5:12) Rabbi Yochanan recommended that one-third of one's waking hours be spent in walking (*Ketubot* 111 a). Rabbi Chananel, 11th-century commentator, advised calisthenics, as extending the arms alternately forward and backward while doing deep knee-bends. Swimming too was highly valued; according to the Talmud a father was obligated to teach this skill, as well as a craft, to his sons (*Kiddushin* 29a, b). Jonathan, in his battle with Bacchides, the *Apocrypha* related, owed his life and that of his men to their swimming prowess: "Bacchides...came to the banks of the Jordan on the Sabbath with a powerful force. Jonathan said to his men: '...we are today in worse plight than ever: the enemy in front, the water of Jordan behind, to right and left marsh and thicket; there is no escape. Cry to Heaven to save you from the hands of the enemy.' ...Then Jonathan and his men leapt into the Jordan and swam over to the other side; but the enemy did not cross the river in pursuit." (*I. Maccabees* 9:43-49)

Streets were playgrounds for the children: "And the streets of the city shall be full of boys and girls playing in the streets thereof." (*Zechariah* 8:5) Isaiah's warning to the Persians suggests the prevalence of ballplaying: "He [God] will surely violently turn and toss thee like a ball into a large country." (*Isaiah* 22:18)

Dancing, described in both the Palestinian and Babylonian Talmuds, served as a medium of celebration and worship as well as physical exercise. The Midrash cites 80 different dances performed by Pharaoh's daughter in one night (*Leviticus Rabbah* 12:5) and predicted that the righteous would one day dance before God with zest (*Song of Songs Rabbah* 1:3). The dancing of the Israelites around the golden calf, however, enraged Moses as he approached them with the tablets of the law: "And it came to pass, as soon as he came nigh unto the camp, that he saw the calf, and the dancing: and Moses' anger waxed hot, and he cast the tablets out of his hands, and brake them beneath the mount." (*Exodus* 32:19) David invoked dance in God's praise: "Let Israel rejoice in him that made him... Let them praise his name in the dance." (*Psalms* 149:2-3) Dance continues to figure prominently in Hasidic prayer ritual.

Maimonides, both in his *Mishneh Torah* and his *Medical Aphorisms*, recommended that exercise be continued throughout life. "No elderly person should rest and repose," he wrote, "without having done some exercise." In his treatises on the *Regimen of Health* he concurred with Hippocrates, that "the maintenance of health lies in forsaking the disinclination to exertion. Nothing is to be found," he insisted, "that can substitute for exercise in any way, because in exercise the natural heat flames up and all the superfluities are expelled...exercise will expel the harm done by most of the bad regimens that most men follow... What is termed exercise is powerful or rapid motion or a combination of both, that is, vigorous motion with which the respiration alters, and one begins to have sighs... Although not everyone can endure exertion, or needs it, it is nonetheless better in the conservation of health than the omission of exercise." Maimonides specifically recommended (1) a warm-up before exercise, held important by most athletes; and (2) coordination of exercise with physiologic conditions. "It is proper," he urged, "to precede physical exercise by running and massaging the body. One should then begin exercise slowly, speeding up until an optimum level is reached... It is not advisable to exercise except upon an empty stomach and after expulsion of the superfluities, that is, the urine and the feces. Nor should one exercise in the intense heat or in the intense cold... If one washes with warm water after the exercise, so much the better. After this, one should wait a little and then eat."

Authorities have differed as to the propriety of exercise on the Sabbath. Walking, because it was held as beneficial to digestion and other functions, was not only permitted but recommended on the Sabbath (*Tosefta Peah* 4:10; *Tosefta Shabbat* 16:7). Running, by contrast, was prohibited for exercise, but permitted only for the delivery of important messages. Joseph Caro, in his *Shulchan Arukh*, ruled in one place that "one is not allowed to exercise on the Sabbath, that is to say, to forcibly exercise the body to tire oneself and to perspire" (*Orach Chayim* 328:42); but in another, opined that running and jumping, if enjoyable, are permitted on the Sabbath (*Orach Chayim* 301:2). Some regarded ballplaying as a proper recreational activity for the Sabbath and holidays (*Tosafot, Betzah* 12a); but according to others, ballplaying was a desecration of the Sabbath (*Yerushalmi Taanit* 4:5; *Shulchan Aruch, Orach Chayim* 309:45).

MEDICAL STUDIES

Medical literature has long attested the benefits of physical exercise. One hundred years ago a physiologist noted: "It has been known for fully a century that systematic exercise may markedly increase both height and weight."[2] Warren P. Lombard, Professor of Physiology in the University of Michigan, added, in the field's leading text of that era: "Exercise is the most effective method of increasing not only the strength but the endurance of muscle...a lack of exercise soon results in a loss of strength."[3] Physicians of the late-20th century teach: "There would be many fewer back problems if adults kept their trunk muscles in optimal condition by regular exercise such as swimming, walking briskly, running, and calisthenic programs."[4]

HEART DISEASE

In 1980 a group of British medical scientists reported a long-term study of the cardiac health of 17,944 middle-aged office workers in relation to their physical activity. Those who engaged in vigorous sports during leisure time experienced less than half the incidence of clinical episodes of coronary heart disease, even less of fatal attacks, than did their colleagues who recorded no vigorous exercise. The disparity in coronary heart disease between the two groups was found among all sub-groups examined, including men with a family history of the disease, the obese, those short of stature, the cigarette smokers, and men with severe hypertension. The generality of the differential pointed clearly to the protective effect of exercise for the aging heart.[5] Several subsequent studies have shown that the level of high-density lipoproteins, protective against coronary disease, increases with vigorous exercise.

A few years later a physician and epidemiologists from Stanford and Harvard Universities calculated the mortality rates and longevity of 16,936 Harvard alumni, aged 35 to 74, who entered college in the period 1916 to 1950, and were subjected to 12 to 16 years of follow-up. Mortality was significantly lower among the physically active, relating inversely to amount of exercise, as in walking and sports. A small gradient effect of walking, as distance was increased from less than 3 miles to 9 miles or more per week, was reflected in a 21% reduction in death risk. Death rates were one-fourth to one-third lower among alumni expending 2000 or more kilocalories per week in exercise than among the less active, declining steadily as energy expended in such activity increased from less than 500 to 3500 kilocalories per week. By age 80, 1 to more than 2 years of additional life was attributable to adequate exercise, as compared with sedentariness.[6]

The evidence that exercise is beneficial has often been termed "only circumstantial;" but modern clinical and laboratory studies, supplementing statistical reports, continue to demonstrate mechanisms through which exercise influences body systems essential to cardiovascular and skeletal health, as by altering serum lipoprotein patterns and metabolic processes. Reliance on diet alone, Paffenbarger and colleagues point out, is no longer considered adequate for the control of obesity, but should be accompanied by regular vigorous exercise. Similarly, the prescription of medication for the control of hypertension and stress may be inadequate without a hygienic program that includes regular exercise.[7] Maintenance of cardiovascular health may require constancy of habit, with regular exercise during 9 or more months of the year.[8]

Osteoporosis

Osteoporosis, an abnormal porosity of bone that occurs with aging, rendering it increasingly susceptible to fracture, afflicts an estimated 24 million Americans.[9] About 1.3 million osteoporosis-related fractures occur in the elderly each year, including 538,000 new cases of spinal fracture and more than 250,000 hip fractures, approximately 40% of the latter proving fatal within 6 months and half of the survivors requiring nursing home care.[10] Osteoporosis is more common in women than in men, especially after the menopause. By age 90 about one-third of all American women sustain a hip fracture, about 17% of men. The cause of osteoporosis remains unknown. Increased dietary intake of calcium and estrogen replacement therapy in women are believed by some authorities to be helpful preventive measures; virtually all agree that regular physical exercise is a valuable prophylactic.[11-13]

Other Benefits

Exercise may also help prevent or ameliorate other diseases. A recent study of male physicians showed an association of regular, vigorous exercise with a diminished risk of development of diabetes.[14] Stroke, similarly, was prevented in men by exercise, occurring in only one-sixth as many of those who exercised vigorously as among a control inactive group.[15] Patients of both sexes with chronic, painful osteoarthritis of one or both knees experienced benefit from a supervised walking program, as evidenced by the increase in distance they were able to walk and by their lessened pain and need for medication.[16]

GOURD POISONING

After the Prophet Elisha's resuscitation of the Shunammite woman's child (see chapter 4), "Elisha came again to Gilgal: and there was a dearth in the land; and the sons of the prophets were sitting before him: and he said unto his servant, Set on the great pot, and seethe pottage for the sons of the prophets. And one went out into the field to gather herbs, and found a wild vine, and gathered thereof wild gourds his lap full, and came and shred them into the pot of pottage: for they knew them not. So they poured out for the men to eat. And it came to pass, as they were eating of the pottage, that they cried out, and said, O thou man of God, there is death in the pot. And they could not eat thereof. But he said, Then bring meal. And he cast it into the pot; and he said, Pour out for the people, that they may eat. And there was no harm in the pot." (*II. Kings* 4:38-41)

Biblical scholars and philologists agree that the Hebrew *paqqu'ot*, translated in the King James Version as "wild gourds," means the fruit of either the colocynth or elaterium. The root *paqa*, meaning to burst or break open, may refer to the character of the ripe fruit; also to the drastic effects of the drugs derived from them, violent purgatives and emetics. Botanical evidence suggests colocynth as the correct translation here, for *Ecballium elaterium*, although common in Mediterranean countries, has no tendrils and is not a vine. *Citrullus colocynthis*, on the other hand, is a true vine, which climbs over shrubs and herbs by means of its powerful tendrils. It grows widely in the Jordan valley, where the Biblical gatherers could easily have mistaken it for another plant of the same family, the *Cucumis prophetarum*, or globe cucumber, also common in Samaria.[17]

The colocynth fruit, or bitter apple, is globular in shape, 2 to 4 inches in diameter, and has a smooth, marble-green surface. Its white, spongy pulp separates readily into 3 carpels, each containing ovoid, white or light-brown seeds (Fig. 14.1). Two of the fruit's constituents, colocynthin and colocynthitin, are powerful purgatives. Even small doses may produce severe intestinal irritation; larger doses, dangerous enteritis, with vomiting, bloody stools, anuria, collapse, and convulsions. Four grams of colocynth pulp are fatal to humans.

The plant has been described from antiquity, in the writings of Pliny, Dioscorides, Theophrastus, and others; and its poisonous nature was well known in the Middle East. In his *Travels in Arabia Deserta* (1888) C.M. Doughty said of *Citrullus colocynthis*: "To human nature it is of so mortal bitterness that little indeed, and even the leaf, is a most vehement purgative. They say it will leave a man half-dead, and he may only recover his strength by eating flesh meat."[18]

To further study the symptoms of colocynth poisoning Macht made extracts of the apples, for administration to dogs by stomach-tube. Intense salivation, attributed to the infusion's contact with the buccal mucous membrane, occurred immediately after the tube's withdrawal. This primary symptom, Macht believed, corresponded with the exclamation of the Biblical victims of the poisoning: "there is death in the pot." In the dogs, vomiting and violent purging ensued within 2 hours, with bloody stools, collapse, and after large doses, death the following day.

Elisha had added flour meal to the pot of gourds as an antidote, for the relief of the symptoms of the suffering sons of the prophets. To a second group of dogs Macht administered the colocynth extract in the same or larger dose, but with the admixture of corn and wheat

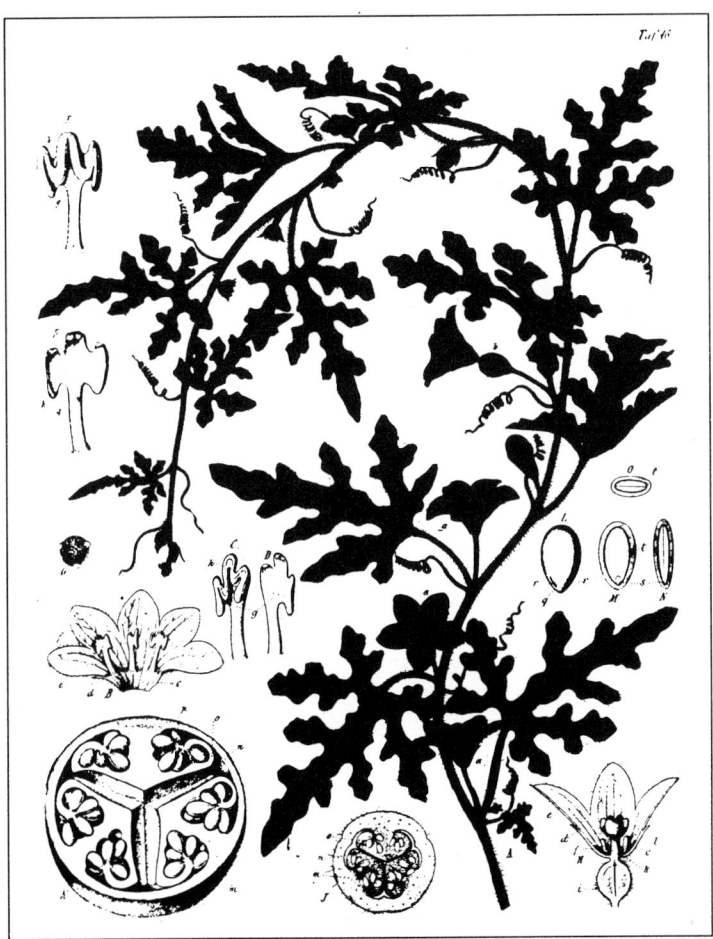

Fig. 14.1. Citrullus colocynthis

flour. Salivation was minimal, vomiting and bowel irritation failed to occur, and the animals remained in normal health. Flour has long been popular, and has a rational basis, in first-aid after ingestion of some types of poisons. Modern pharmacology has abundantly confirmed the effect of colloidal and other materials, themselves inert, in delaying both the absorption of foods and the action of some toxins.

PI

Perhaps most famous of all mathematical relationships is *pi*, the ratio between the circumference of a circle and its diameter. The concept of *pi* dates back at least to the mid-17th century B.C.E., when the scribe Ahmes wrote of it in a Middle Kingdom papyrus. After centuries of study it is now known to be an irrational number; that is, one incapable of expression as a ratio of two integers. It was named for the Greek letter **p** by William Jones, an English mathematician, in his book *A New Introduction to the Mathematics*, published in 1706. Archimedes of Syracuse (ca. 287-212 B.C.E.) had calculated its value as something greater than $3^{10}/_{71}$ and less than $3^{1}/_{7}$. The latter figure (or 3.14) has been universally accepted as the correct, practical approximation of its true value.

Could the Bible have erred, in expressing *pi* as 3? In the building of the temple "King Solomon sent and fetched Hiram out of Tyre. He was a widow's son of the tribe of Naphtali, and his father was a man of Tyre, a worker in brass: and he was filled with wisdom, and understanding, and cunning to work all works in brass. And he came to King Solomon, and wrought all his work... And he made a molten sea, 10 cubits [a cubit being about 21.8 inches] from one brim to the other: it was round all about, and his height was five cubits: and a line of thirty cubits did compass it round about." (*I. Kings* 7:13-14, 23) The same description of the cistern, or "molten sea," is repeated in *II. Chronicles* 4:2. Thus the Bible apparently assigns to *pi*, the ratio of the circumference to the diameter, the number 3 (30 cubits/10cubits). The Talmud also states: "That which in circumference is three hands is one hand broad."

Rabbi Nehemiah, who lived in Palestine in the mid-2nd century C.E., author of the *Mishnat ha-Middot*, the earliest known Hebrew geometry, sought to reconcile the biblical *pi* with the approximate Archimedean value of $3^{1}/_{7}$. Focusing on the verses in *I. Kings* 7 and *II. Chronicles* 4, Nehemiah wrote: "The circle has three aspects: the circumference, the thread, and the roof. Which is the circumference? That is the rope surrounding the circle; for it is written: 'And a line of thirty cubits did compass it round about.' And the thread? That is the straight line from brim to brim; for it is written: 'from the one brim to the other.' And the roof itself is the area... And if you want to know the circumference all around, multiply the thread into three and one-seventh..." To account for the discrepancy between the two values for *pi*, Nehemiah explained: "Now it is written: 'And he made a molten sea, ten cubits from one brim to the other: it was round all about' and yet its circumference is thirty cubits, for it is written: 'and a line of thirty cubits did compass it round about.' What is the meaning of the verse 'and a line of thirty cubits' and so forth? Nehemiah says: Since the people of the world say that the circumference of a circle contains three times and one-seventh of the thread, take off that one-seventh for the thickness of the walls of the sea on the two brims, then there remains 'thirty cubits did compass it round about."

Nehemiah had noted, three verses later, in *I. Kings* 7:26, the description of the cistern's wall: "And it was an hand breadth thick [about 4 inches], and the brim thereof was wrought like the brim of a cup, with flowers and lilies: it contained two thousand baths." He thus explained the Biblical *pi* of 3, by assuming the inner measurement of the vessel as its circumference, while its diameter was measured from outer rim to outer rim. The thickness of the wall accounted, in his interpretation, for the difference of one-seventh between Biblical and secular *pi*.[19] The internal circumference, according to Nehemiah, would have been 30 x 21.8 inches (a cubit), or 654 inches; the internal diameter, 10 x 21.8 inches minus 48 inches, or 210 inches; and their ratio, 3.114, in acceptable agreement with the Archimedean approximation for *pi*.

Pi remains elusive, forming an apparently random sequence of decimals. With the aid of powerful computers Gregory and David Chudnovsky, research mathematicians at Columbia University, have probed the ratio to two billion two hundred and sixty million three hundred and twenty-one thousand three hundred and thirty-six digits, which, if printed in ordinary type on a tape, would stretch from New York to Southern California. The fact that *pi* can be expressed by a simple formula, they insist, means that it is orderly, albeit incomparably complex. Although they have been unable to detect any pattern in its long sequence of digits, they wonder whether, among them, lies a hidden rule, "close to the mind of God."[20]

REFERENCES

1. Exercise in Judaism has been discussed in essays by Sussman Muntner (Leibesübungen bei den Juden von den ältesten Zeit bis auf die Gegenwart, Vienna, 1926) and by Fred Rosner and Ira L. Weg (Exercise in Judaism, Bull New York Acad Med 1989; 65:842-850), to whom I am indebted for numerous citations.
2. Beyer HG. The influence of exercise on growth. J Exper Med 1896; 1:546.
3. Lombard WP. In: An American Text-Book of Physiology. WH Howell ed. 2nd edition. Philadelphia: WB Saunders 1901; 2:76-77.
4. Mankin HJ, Adams RD. In: Harrison's Principles of Internal Medicine. 8th edition. New York: McGraw-Hill 1977:47.
5. Morris JN, Everitt MG, Pollard R, Chave SPW, Semmence AM. Vigorous exercise in leisure-time: protection against coronary heart disease. Lancet ii 1980:1207-1210.
6. Paffenbarger Jr, RS, Syde RT, Wing AL, Hsieh C. Physical activity, all-cause mortality, and longevity of college alumni. New Eng J Med 1986; 314:605-613.
7. Paffenbarger RS, Hyde RT, Wing AL, Steinmetz DH. A natural history of athleticism and cardiovascular health. JAMA 1984; 252:491-495.
8. Magnus K, Matroos A, Strackee J. Walking, cycling, or gardening with or without seasonal interruption in relation to acute coronary events. Am J Epidemiol 1979; 110:724-733.
9. Consensus developmental panel: osteoporosis. JAMA 1984; 252:799-802.
10. Evans JG, Prudham D, Wandless I. A prospective study of fractured proximal femur: incidence and outcome. Pub Health 1979; 93:235-241.

11. Dalen N, Olsson KE. Bone mineral content and physical activity. Acta Orthop Scand 1974; 45:170-174.
12. Smith EL, Reddan W. Physical activity—a modality for bone accretion in the aged. Am J Roentgenol 1976; 126:1297.
13. Aloia JF, Cohn, SH, Ostuni JA et al. Prevention of involutional bone loss by exercise. Ann Int Med 1978; 89:356-358.
14. Manson JE, Nathan DM, Krolewski AS et al. A prospective study of exercise and incidence of diabetes among U.S. male physicians. JAMA 1992; 268:63-67.
15. Wannamethee G, Shaper AG. Physical activity and stroke in British middle aged men. Brit Med J 1992; 304:587-601.
16. Kovar PA, Allegrante JP, MacKenzie R et al. Supervised fitness walking in patients with osteoarthritis of the knee. Ann Int Med 1992; 116:529-534.
17. Macht DI. A pharmacological appreciation of a Biblical reference to mass poisoning, II Kings IV, 38-41. Johns Hopkins Hosp Bull 1919; 30:38-42.
18. Quoted by Macht. A pharmacological appreciation of a Biblical reference to mass poisoning, II Kings IV, 38-41. Johns Hopkins Hosp Bull 1919; 30:38-42.
19. After Beckmann P. A History of p (PI). New York: St Martin's Press 1971:74-76.
20. Preston R. The mountains of Pi. The New Yorker, March 2, 1992; 68:36-67.

INDEX

A

Aaron, 24, 26, 31, 38, 45, 46, 50, 51, 53, 98, 156, 157, 160, 161
Abba bar Aivu, Rabbi, 113
Abed-nego, 61
Abel, 84
Abigail, 96
Abihu, 27
Abimelech, King, 63, 73
Abiram, 26, 53
Abishag, 69
Abortion, 80, 123-125
Abrabanel, Isaac, 11
Abraham, 62, 63, 73, 96-97, 113, 140
Abrahams, Abraham Isaac, 143
Abram, 62, 63. See also Abraham
Absolom, 61
Abulafia, Meir, 123
Adam, 113, 155, 176
Adler, Ludwig, 106
Adrenogenital syndrome, 74
Agudas Harabonim, 220
Ahimaaz, 229
Ahithophel, 61
Ahmes, 235
AIDS, 216-217
Alcohol
    in pregnancy, 79-80
    use and abuse, 56-58
Alfvén, Hannes, 10
Algae, 25
Alligators, 20
Alvarez, Luis, 16
Alzheimer's disease, 217-218
American Gynecological Society, 12
Amnesic shellfish poisoning, 25
Amniotic fluid embolism, 86
Amoraim, 3
Anaphylaxis, 92
Annals of Cuauhtitlan, 13
Antenatal care, 78-80
Anthrax, 35
Antiochus Epiphanes, 142, 157, 172, 173
Anti-Semitism, 207-208
Anxiety syndrome, 58
Aphasia, 69
Aphrodisiacs, 75-76, 122

Apollo moon landings, 12, 16
Archimedes, 236
Aristeas, 2
Aristotle, 8, 99
Artificial insemination, 80, 107, 127-128
Asher, Jacob ben, 4
Ashtaroth, 74, 75
Assaph the Physician, 213-214
Asteroids, 14-20
Astruc, Jean, 1
Autopsy, 217-218, 224-226

B

Baal, 74
Baal-peor, 80
Bacchides, 230
Bacillus anthracis, 34
Balaam, 48, 59, 183
Ballplaying, 230, 231-232
Barad, 17, 25
Baraita, 114, 116
Barbour, Ian, 10, 11
Barzillai, 69
Bateil beshishim, 167
Bathsheba, 96
Beard, John, 115
Beauchamp, T. L., 215-216
Bellah, R. N., 224
Bemisia tabaci, 29
Benjamin, 86
Ben-oni, 86
Big Bang, 9, 10
Bilhah, 73, 97, 126
Birds, 160-161
Birth-stools, 83
Bischoff, T. L. W., 105
Bitter apple, 234-235
Bleich, David, 129
Blood, 24-25
Boaz, 57-58
Briffault, R., 142
Brith Milah Board, 143-144
Brown, Louise, 128
Bubonic plague, 52-53
Butler, Nicholas Murray, 208

C

Caleb, 40, 168
Canaan, 57
Caro, Joseph, 4, 114, 116, 231
Catastrophists, 15
Celsus, 142
Cervical cancer, 148
Cesarean section, 83, 118
Chargaff, Erwin, 185
Chevta Dor Yeshorim program, 123
Chevra Kadisha, 225
Childress, J. F., 215-216
Cholesterol, 156
Chosen people, 206-207
Chudnofsky, David and Gregory, 237
Chukim, 186
Circumcision, 139-154
    anesthesia for, 147
    Biblical background, 140-142
    bleeding from, 145-146
    physiologic sidelights, 145-146
    pros and cons, 146-151
    timing, 144-145
    and urinary tract infections, 150
Citrullus colocynthis, 234-235
Clarke, Edward C., 100
Clusters, 11, 14-15
Cocaine in pregnancy, 125
Coccus manniparus, 38
Codex Chimalpopoca, 13
Coitus interruptus, 116, 128
Colet, John, 8
Colitis, 54
Colocynth, 234-235
Comets, 14-20, 27, 28
Conception, 76, 105-108
Concubinage, 96-97
Condom, 116
Conduplicato corpore, 85
Coniine, 39
Conservation, 171-181
Contraception, 88, 93, 113-119
    oral, 115
Copernicus, Nicholaus, 8
Cosmic Background Explorer, 9
Cosmic events, 11-20
Cosmic plasma, 10
Craters, 14-20
Creation, 7-11
Cremation, 226
Cretaceous/Tertiary boundary, 16, 19
Crocodiles, 20
Cup of roots, 115
Cushi, 229
Cuvier, Georges, 159-160

Cysticercosis, 158-159
Cytomegalovirus, 124

D

D source, 2
Dabney, Herbert, 3
Dancing, 230-231
Daniel, 26, 61-62
Darkness, 27-28, 36, 37
Dathan, 26, 53
David, 60-61, 66, 69, 74, 96, 229, 231
Davis, Edward P., 118
Dead Sea Scrolls, 1
Death, 31, 37
    maternal, 85-86
Delilah, 230
Delivery, position for, 82-83
Demographics, 186-206
Deuteronomy, 1
Dew, J. H., 67
Diabetes, 233
Diaphragm, 116
Diaspora, 205
Dick-Read, G., 82
Dietary laws, 157-170
Dinah, 73, 126, 129
Dinosaurs, 17
Dioscorides, 75
Doctor-patient relationship, 215-216
Doctrinal sources, 1-5
Documentary hypothesis, 1
Doubleday Co., 12
Doughty, C. M., 234
Dreams, 62-66
Drinking during pregnancy, 79-80
Drugs in pregnancy, 125
Durant, Will, 186, 205

E

E source, 2
Earth's variable rotation, 13-14
Eclampsia, 91-94
Ectopic pregnancy, 99
Edwards, Robert, 128
Eichhorn, J. G., 1
Eleazar, 47
Eli, 81
Eliahu, Mordecai, 217
Elijah, 54, 67
Elisha, 67, 233-234
Elkanah, 74
Emanuel, E. J. and L. L., 215-216
Embryology, 76
Empedocles, 78
End-of-life decisions, 220-224

Environmentalism, 176-179
Esau, 56, 84, 166
Essenes, 2
Euglena sanguinea, 34
Euthanasia
    active, 222-224
    passive, 221
Eve, 84, 113, 155
Execution in pregnancy, 125
Exercise, 229-233
Exodus, 1
Exodus, the, 32-41
Extinctions, 14-20
Ezekiel, 59, 96, 139, 176, 218
Ezra, 2

F

Fallopio, Gabriele, 116
Feinstein, Moses, 123
Fertility, 73-76, 113-137
Fetocide, 123
Fire, 26-27
Fish, 162-164
Fletcher, J., 129
Forbidden foods, 155-164
47 Tucanae, 14
Fowl, 160-161
Fox, R. C., 219
Freud, Sigmund, 62
Frogs, 34-35
Frozen embryos, 131-132

G

Gabriel, 18
Gaia hypothesis, 179
Galen, 86-87, 142, 224
Galileo, 8
Ganapathy, R., 16
Gaucher's disease, 122
Gemara, 3, 119
Genesis, 1
Genetics, applied, 120-123
German measles, 124-125
Gershom ben Judah, Rabbi, 97
Gersonides, 8, 214
Gigantism, 65-66
Gilbert, G. K., 15
Gill, Dan, 49
Global warming, 20
Golden calf, 231
Goliath, 66, 229
Gomer, 88
Goren, Shlomo, 129
Gosses, 221
Gourd poisoning, 233-235
Gräfenberg, Ernst, 116

Gräfenberg ring, 117
Grasshoppers, 29-31
Greenblatt, Robert, 56
Guide for the Perplexed, 214

H

Hadrian, Emperor, 142
Haematococcus pluvialis, 34
Hagar, 74, 97
Haggadah, 23
Haggard, Howard W., 223
Hail, 17, 25, 36
Halakhah, 4, 127, 167, 206, 219, 220, 225
Ham, 57
Hammurabi, laws of, 96
Hannah, 73, 74
Hansen's disease, 50-53
Harris, Seale, 55
Hartman, Carl G., 105
Harvey, William, 81
Hash-hatat-zera, 114, 116, 128
Havdalah, 184
Hawking, Stephen, 10, 11
Heart disease, 232
Heat stress, 55
Hell Creek Formation, 20
Hellebore, 39
Hemiplegia, 59
Hemlock, 39
Hemlock Society, 223
Hemorrhoids, 52
Herodotus, 139
Hertig, Arthur, 107
Hezekiah, King, 17, 48, 49, 82
Hezekiah's tunnel, 48-50
Hillel, 98
Hind quarter, 166
Hippocrates, 77, 231
Hippocratic Oath, 213, 222
Hiram, 236
Hitschmann, Fritz, 106
Hobbes, Thomas, 1
Holocaust, 187
Homosexual marriage, 97-98
Hort, Greta, 33
Horter, Thomas Jeeves, 224
Hosea, 58, 80, 88, 96
Hoyle, Fred, 9
Hubble, Edwin P., 9
Hunter, John, 127
Hushai, 61
Hutton, James, 15
Huxley, Aldous, 132
Hydatidiform mole, 99
Hypoglycemia, 55-56
Hypo-ovarianism, 74

I

In vitro fertilization, 128-129
Infant, care at birth, 86-87
Infertility, 73-76
Inflationary hypothesis, 10
Insects, 28-29
Insemination, artificial, 80, 127-128
Intermarriage, 205-206
Intrauterine device, 116
Isaac, 69, 84, 87
Isaiah, 18, 37, 58, 96
Ishmael, 140

J

J source, 1-2
Jacob, 56, 64, 74, 75, 78, 84, 113, 120-122, 126, 166
Jacobi, Mary Putnam, 101
Jacobovits, Immanuel, 131, 217
Jarvis, C. S., 39
Jastrow, Robert, 8
Jehoram, 54
Jehovah, 1
Jereboam, King, 59
Jericho, 40-42
Jethro, 141
Jeremiah, 58, 82
Jew, criteria of, 205-206
Job, 76, 80, 95
Job's Disease, 53
Jonah, 55
Jonathan, 60-61, 230
Jones, William, 236
Jordan, 40, 41
Joseph, 23, 64-65, 76, 84, 129
Josephus Flavius, 2, 178, 184
Joshua, 13, 17, 40, 41, 74, 142, 168
Josiah, King, 2
Judah, 75, 85, 114
Judah Halevi, 214
Judah ha-Nasi, 3
Jung, Leo, 143
Jupiter, 18

K

K/T period, 19
Kamisar, Y., 223
Kansan pioneers, 29-31
Kaplan, Mordecai, 206-207
Kashruth, 157-170
Kass, L. R., 223
Kattina, Rabbi, 126
Khamsin, 36
Knaus, Hermann, 117

Kodashim, 3
Korah, 26, 53

L

Laban, 75, 78, 120-122
Labor, 81-82, 85-86
Lactation, 88
Lamaze, 82
Lamm, Norman, 108-109
Landau, Ezekiel, 225
Larson, Roger, 27
Leah, 73, 75, 76, 121, 126, 129-130
Leidy, Joseph, 158
Lemaitre, Georges, 9
Lemuel, King, 57
Leprosy, 50-53
Lesbianism, 98
Lestchinsky, J., 186-187
Levi, 75
Levirate marriage, 96
Leviticus, 1
Lewis, Joseph, 147
Lex regia, 83
Lo-ammi, 88
Locusts, 29-31
Lot, 57
Lovelock, James, 179
Lungren, S. S., 118
Lyell, Charles, 15

M

Maacah, 96
Maccabees, 173
Macht, David I., 92, 160-165, 185-186, 234-235
Macmillan Company, 12
Maimonides, Moses, 4, 8, 124, 143, 158, 166, 184, 214, 231
Malformations, congenital, 78-80
Mandrakes, 75-76, 129
Manna, 38, 156
Manoah, 79
Margulis, Lynn, 179
Mars, 12, 18
Marvin, Ursula, 16
Masturbation, 128
Maternal impressions, 78-79
Mattathias, 173
Mauriceau, François, 14
Mayer, 92
McCoy, G. W., 158
Meat and milk, 166-167
Medical-ethical issues, 213-228
Medical schools, 208-209
Mendel, Gregor, 120

Menotoxin, 99-105
Menstruation
  coitus during, 84, 98-99
  mythology, 99-100
  work during, 100-101
Meshach, 61
Meteorites, 14-20, 24
Mezizah, 143
Michael, 18
Michal, 74, 96
Midrash, 4, 7, 18, 26, 32, 40, 96, 115, 229, 230
Midwives, 23, 76-78
Mikveh, 98-99
Milah, 143
Milcah, 73
Milcom, 75
Miriam, 50, 80
Miscarriage, 80
Mishnah, 3, 97, 124, 125, 145, 172, 178
Mishneh Torah, 4, 143, 214
Moed, 3
Mohel, 143, 144, 149
Mokh, 116
Monogamy, 95
Monsters, 84
Montefiore, Claude, 173-174
Montgomery, William F., 80
Morgagni, Giovanni Battista, 224
Morning Prayer of a Physician, 214-215
Moses, 1-3, 23, 24, 26, 27, 29, 37, 38, 40, 41, 45, 50, 51, 80, 86, 97, 98, 141-142, 155-157, 159, 160, 161, 164, 171-172, 175, 177, 183
Mosquitoes, 35
Mount Pelée, 32
Mount Sinai theophany, 13
Multiple birth, 84-85. See also Twins
Mycobacterium leprae, 50

N
Nachmanides, Moses, 184, 214
Nadad, 26
Naegele, Franz Carl, 81
Naegele's rule, 81
Nahor, 73
Nashim, 3
Natural Death Acts, 221
Nebuchadnezzar, 61-62
Nehemiah, Rabbi, 236-237
Neuro-psychiatric disorders, 58-62
New Testament, 4
Newborn, 86-87
Nezikim, 3
Niddah, laws of, 105-109, 128
Niemann-Pick disease, 122

Nile, 33-37
Nivul hameth, 225
Noah, 56, 57, 73, 113, 155
Nof, Doron, 33
Noga, 18
Nuclear force, strong, 10
Numa Pompilius, 83
Numbers, 1

O
Obnayim, 83
Obstetrics, Biblical, 73-90
Og, King of Bashan, 66
Ogino, Kayusaka, 117
Old Testament, 4
Onan, 114
Oral Torah, 2
Organ transplantation, 218-220
Osteoporosis, 233
Ovum transplantation, 129-130
Owen, Richard, 158

P
Paget, James, 158
Paldor, Nathan, 33
Paré, Ambroise, 84
Passover, 23, 31, 36
Pearl, Raymond, 187
Penile cancer, 147-149
Peninnah, 74
Penrose, Roger, 10
Pentateuch, 1
Permitted animals, 159-162
Persistent vegetative state, 220-221
Petit mal, 59
Petroleum, 27
Peyrère, Isaac La, 1
Pharaoh, 23, 28, 31, 33, 37, 64-65, 77, 87, 139
Pharez, 85
Pharisees, 2
Philocrates, 2
Phinehas' wife, 81-82, 85, 92
Phocomelia, 79
Physical exercise, 229-233
Physician, role of, 213-215
Physicians, Jewish, 208, 215
Pi, 235-237
Plague, 52-53, 159
Plagues of Egypt, 23-37
Plato, 8
Plaut, W. Gunther, 207
Pleasure principle, 113-114
Pliny the Elder, 99-100
Poinsettia strain, 29

Polarity, Earth's, 14
Polyandry, 95-96
Polydactyly, 66
Polygamy, 96-97
Pope Paul V, 8
Population, Jewish, 187-205
   Afghanistan, 203
   Albania, 203
   Algeria, 200-201
   Argentina, 189
   Aruba, 203
   Australia, 190
   Austria, 193-194
   Bahamas, 201
   Barbados, 203
   Belgium, 191
   Bermuda, 203
   Bolivia, 199
   Brazil, 189-190
   Bulgaria, 196
   Burma, 204
   Canada, 189
   Channel Islands, 202
   Chile, 193
   China, 204
   Colombia, 194
   Costa Rica, 196
   Cuba, 197-198
   Curacao, 199
   Cyprus, 204
   Czechoslovakia, 194
   Dominican Republic, 202
   Ecuador, 198
   Egypt, 201
   El Salvador, 202-203
   Ethiopia, 193
   Finland, 197
   France, 189
   Germany, 191
   Gibraltar, 200
   Greece, 195
   Guatemala, 198-199
   Haiti, 202
   Honduras, 202
   Hong Kong, 199
   Hungary, 190
   India, 195
   Indonesia, 204
   Iran, 191
   Iraq, 201
   Ireland, 197
   Israel, 188
   Italy, 191
   Jamaica, 199
   Japan, 199
   Kenya, 200
   Lebanon, 203
   Libya, 204
   Luxembourg, 197
   Malaysia, 204
   Malta, 204
   Mexico, 190-191
   Monaco, 198
   Morocco, 193
   Netherlands, 192
   New Zealand, 195-196
   Nicaragua, 205
   Norway, 198
   Pakistan, 205
   Panama, 196
   Paraguay, 198
   Peru, 195
   Philippines, 202
   Poland, 194
   Portugal, 200
   Puerto Rico, 197
   Romania, 192
   Russia and satellite countries, 188
   Singapore, 200
   South Africa, 190
   South Korea, 205
   Spain, 194
   Surinam, 200
   Sweden, 193
   Switzerland, 192-193
   Syria, 196
   Taiwan, 202
   Thailand, 201
   Trinidad and Tobago, 205
   Tunisia, 196
   Turkey, 192
   United Kingdom, 189
   United States of America, 187-188
   Uruguay, 190
   U. S. Virgin Islands, 200
   Venezuela, 192
   Yemen, 198
   Yugoslavia, 195
   Zaire, 201-202
   Zambia, 203
   Zimbabwe, 197
Porging, 166
Pork, 157-159
Position for delivery, 82-83
Potiphar, 64
Preeclampsia, 92-93

Index

Pregnancy
  duration, 80-81
  execution in, 125
  intervention in, 125-126
  postterm, 81
Priah, 143
Promised land, 41, 53
P'ru ur'vu, 115
Pschoses, 59-62
Puerperium, 86
Pythagoras, 99

Q
Quails, 38-39

R
Rachel, 73-77, 85, 121, 129-130
Rahab, 18
Rashi, 145, 184, 229
Raup, David, 19
Rebekah, 56, 74, 84, 85
Red Sea, 25, 32, 33, 37
Rehoboam, 73
Responsa, 4-5, 117, 118, 119, 124, 225
Resuscitation, 66-68
Retirement, 174-175
Reuben, 75
Richter, Richard, 116
Robinson, William J., 100
Rock, John, 107
Rosengarten, 77
Rosh Hashanah Lailanot, 179
Rosner, Fred, 219
Rösslin, Eucharius, 77
Rubella, 124-125
Running, 231
Ruth, 57-58, 205

S
Sabbath, 171-174, 231-232
Sachs, Bernard, 121
Sadducees, 2
Safe period, 117-118
Sahagun, 13
Sammangelof, 79
Samson, 79, 229-230
Samuel, 96, 222
Sanitary code of Israelites, 45-47
San-Senori, 79
Sarah, 62, 63, 96-97, 140
Saul, King, 59-61, 66, 222
Schick, Béla, 101-103

Schindler, Alexander M., 207
Schultze, Bernhard S., 67
Sea of Passage, 32
Seixas, Moses, 143
Seneca, Lucius Annaeus, 172, 222
Senility, 68-69
Sennacherib, 17, 49
Senoi, 79
Separatism, 183-211
Sepkoski, Jack, 19
Septuagint, 2
Sewell, H., 92
Sex ratio, 108
Sex selection, 126-127
Sexually transmitted disease, 47-48
Shaatnez, 184-186
Shadrach, 61
Shammai, 98
Shettles, Landrum B., 108, 127
Shor, Joseph Bekhor, 184
Shulchan Arukh, 4, 231
Siamese twins, 84
Sigerist, Henry E., 224
Silvester, Henry R., 67
Simeon, 75
Singer, Isaac Bashevis, 11
Skin ailments, 50
Slaughter, laws of, 164-166
Smallpox, 54
Smith, George Van S. and Olive, 104
Smoking in pregnancy, 125
Social Security, 175
Solomon, 48, 58, 73, 74, 87, 95, 97, 235
Soranus, 77, 78
Spallanzani, Lazaro, 127
Spinoza, Baruch, 1
Spontaneous evolution, 85
Sputnik I, 16
Steady state, 8
Steptoe, Patrick, 128
Sterilization, 118-119
Stern, William, 130
Stomoxys calcitrans, 35
Stone of Zoheleth, 229
Stroganov, Vasili, 91
Stroke, 233
Strong nuclear force, 10
Sudden infant death syndrome (SIDS), 87
Sulfanilamide, 79
Superclusters, 11
Surrogate motherhood, 130-131
Swaddling, 86-87
Swazey, J. P., 219

T

Taeniasis, 158
Takkanah, 97
Tamar, 85
Tamarisk, 38
Tanach, 4
Tay, Warren, 122
Tay-Sachs disease, 122-123
Teharot, 3
Teitelbaum, Yekutiel, 124
Teratogens, 78-80
Thalidomide, 79, 124
"The Test of Time", 13
Theophany at Mount Sinai, 39-40
Trance, 59
Transvestism, 184
Treponema pertenue, 53
Trichinosis, 158
Tropical Roterde, 34
Tsunami, 17
Tu B'Shevat, 177
Tucanae, 47, 14
Tularemia, 158
Twins, 56, 85
　　Siamese, 84
Typhus, 159

U

Uniform Determination of Death Act, 220
Uniformitarianism, 15
Uterine rupture, 86

V

Van Allen Belt, 12
Vaucouleurs, Gérard de, 11, 12
Vegetarianism, 155
Velikovsky, Immanuel, 11-14, 18, 19, 24, 25, 27, 28, 31, 33, 37, 40, 41
Venereal disease, 47-48
Venus, 12, 13, 18, 26
Viruses, 124-125
Vitamin K, 145-146

W

Waldenberg, Eliezer, 123, 127
Walking, 231
Water, 37
Water for Jerusalem, 48-50
Weaning, 87-88
Wellhausen, Julius, 1
Whitehead, Mary Beth, 130
Williams, John Whitridge, 91, 118
Wine, 56-58
"Worlds in Collision," 12

Y

Yaweh, 1
Yersinia pestis, 52
Yohanan, 213-214
Yosef, Ovadiah, 129
Yotze dofen, 83

Z

Zadok, Rabbi, 126
Zaholon, Jacob, 214
Zalman, Shneur, 124
Zarah, 85
Zechariah, 59
Zenker, Friedrich von, 158
Zeraim, 3
Zilpah, 73, 126
Zimri, 53
Zipporah, 50, 141, 205
Zoheleth, stone of, 229
Zophar, 48

In this scientific commentary on the Scriptures, Harold Speert brings Judaic doctrine, based on the Torah, the Talmud, the Midrash, and rabbinic Responsa, together with the discoveries and enlightenment of the twentieth century. Creation of the universe and other cosmic events are considered in the light of the Big Bang theory and species extinctions. Scientific explanations of the plagues of Egypt and the parting of the waters are offered; medicine in the Bible is discussed; and modern interpretations are given for the dietary laws, circumcision, and the Sabbath. From his vantage as an obstetrician-gynecologist and medical historian Dr. Speert provides special insight into Biblical obstetrics, the conjugal relationship, and fertility and its control, and analyzes current medical-ethical issues, including the doctor-patient relationship, surrogate motherhood, organ transplantation, and end-of-life decisions.

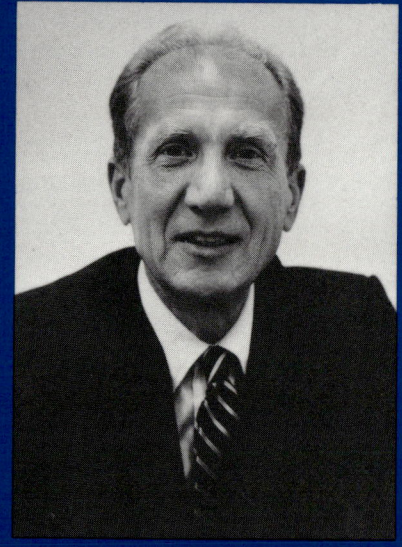

ISBN 1-57059-256-X